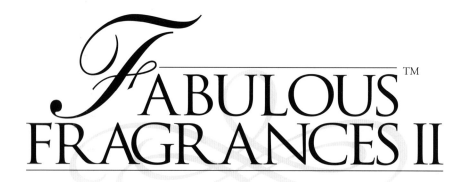

Fabulous™ Fragrances II

❧ A GUIDE TO PRESTIGE PERFUMES ❧
for Women and Men

Countess JAN MORAN

CRESCENT HOUSE PUBLISHING
BEVERLY HILLS

For Inquiries Contact:
CRESCENT HOUSE PUBLISHING
P.O. Box 718
La Quinta, CA 92253
(310) 364-0551
www.fabulousfragrances.com
Orders: (888) CLUB-FAB

Fabulous Fragrances is available for special promotions,
premiums, and content licensing. For details, contact
Crescent House Publishing, as listed above.

Library of Congress Card Number: 00-106051

ISBN 0-9639065-4-2 (hardcover)

Disclaimer: In *Fabulous Fragrances* we (Crescent House
Publishing and Jan Moran) have relied on information
provided by third parties and have performed reasonable
verification of facts. While we believe that these sources
are reliable, we assume no responsibility or liability for
the accuracy of information contained in this book. No
representations or warranties, expressed or implied, as to
the accuracy or completeness of this book or its contents
are made. The information in this book is intended for
entertainment purposes only.

Every effort has been made to locate the copyright holders
of materials used in this book. Should there be any errors
or omissions, we apologize and shall be pleased to make
acknowledgements in future editions.

Note: Some components in perfumes may cause allergic
reactions, so reasonable care should be taken in use.
If symptoms arise, consult a physician.

Printed in Hong Kong, China.

For my mother, Jeanne, whose love of perfume inspired me.

For the men in my life—
my son, Eric, and my husband, Jim.

And for all who enjoy fabulous fragrances.

FOREWORD

It is with great pleasure that I write the foreword to *Fabulous Fragrances II*. It is a privilege to have been selected for such an honor, when, as this book illustrates, there are countless designers marketing a broad spectrum of fragrances. I had the distinct pleasure of introducing the Countess Jan Moran's first foray into the subject, *Fabulous Fragrances*, at my Bijan showrooms in New York and Los Angeles. Her book was compelling and useful in explaining the complexities of the vast world of fragrance. This edition upholds and builds upon that foundation.

I am a fragrance designer, not merely a manufacturer. A designer pours his sensitivity, his expertise, his passion, and his very soul into the creation of a fragrance. Any fragrance designer will tell you that the process of arriving at the perfect scent is a lengthy one. For me, as the process begins, I strive to embrace the power of fragrance. The formula should create a magic that stirs the heart and soul. In creating a women's perfume, I believe it must captivate the senses, evoke an aura of bliss, and embody femininity. For men, I believe the scent should evoke style and presence; a fine scent is a hallmark of the well-dressed man.

Quality, elegance, and simplicity are the tenets of great style; they are also the tenets of a great fragrance.

Designing fragrance is a natural extension of my clothing design business. I enjoy helping people look and feel great by providing the finest in clothing, jewelry, and fragrance. My first fragrance, Bijan Perfume for Women, was created to reflect a sensual state of mind. The woman who wears my perfume is certainly not afraid to be noticed. She is definitive about her personal style, and is as sophisticated as she is alluring. She is a woman who makes a statement.

Fragrance is the most intimate expression of style. Scent, like fashion, conveys a message. Correspondingly, fragrance designers, like fashion designers, have their own vision. Yet, due to each individual's unique chemistry, fragrance is further personalized on the wearer, rendering the designer's interpretation a little different on each person.

My passion for fragrance design does not end with the formula. The best designers understand the aesthetics of creating a flacon that embodies the character of their fragrance. To design a fragrance is to design the total package: A complete impression.

Recently I returned to the drawing board for my latest creations—Bijan With a Twist, one version for men, and one for women. When they are unveiled, the pair will further enhance my fragrance family, which includes DNA and Bijan Light—as well as the scents of my good friend and partner, Michael Jordan Cologne and Jordan by Michael. I hope you enjoy them, and I wish you happiness and delight in your fragrant explorations!

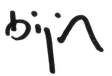

Beverly Hills

ACKNOWLEDGMENTS

It is a pleasure to express my gratitude to those without whom this book would not have been possible. As always, my loving appreciation goes to my husband, Jim Halper. To my son, Eric Moran, and my nephew, Mitch Hollenbeck, for working alongside me in so many phases of the business– that's "Entrepreneurship 101."

To my editor, Eileen Heyes, once again, for her marvelous expertise. Kudos again to Howard Yang, Sherri Yu, and Angela Chu of Wonder Studio, for the book and web site design, and all other design wonders. To Linda Rothstein, office *Übermanager*, for her unfailing assistance. To my legal eagles, Ken Artis and Ron Ostrin, for protecting my copyright and life's work—you're the tops. To Richard Panzarasa, Michel Mane, and Marvel Fields of V. Mane Fils and Mane, U.S.A., for an incredible fragrant journey. To my research and editorial assistant, Pamela Patrick, for her persistence and dedication. To Carolyn Youssef, of Carolyn's Colognes in Torrance, California, for her knowledge and wit. And to my stylist, Harriet Root, and photographer, Marc Glassman. What a team!

For their gracious words of praise, my heartfelt appreciation to Bijan, Mr. Blackwell, Elizabeth Taylor, Gale Hayman, Annette Green, Oleg Cassini, Dr. Linda Hill, and William Owen. A special debt of gratitude goes to Brett Neubig, super publicist and friend. My appreciation to the fragrance houses that contributed information and photography. To the retailers, the buyers, and their staffs, who helped elevate the first *Fabulous Fragrances* to the bestseller list. Thank you for believing in us.

And to my dear friends, for their love and laughter: Aly Spencer, Vana Margolese, and the Marquise Josette Banzet Roe de Bruyenne. Thank you for your generous hospitality. I am indebted to so many lovely people who have graciously given of their time, information, assistance, and enthusiasm. May your kindness be returned in abundance.

And above all, thanks to God.

JM

Contents

LIST OF FRAGRANCE PROFILES

WOMEN'S AND UNISEX FRAGRANCES

HONORABLE MENTIONS

WOMEN'S AND UNISEX FRAGRANCES

Following are a few more fragrances worthy of mention. Some are new, some are old, some are in limited edition.

FRAGRANCE	HOUSE/DISTRUBUTOR	SCENT TYPE
Adrienne Vittadini	Adrienne Vittadini	Semi - Oriental
Andiamo*	Borghese	Floral - Green
Animale (1)	Suzanne de Lyon	Chypre - Floral
Anne Klein (1)	Anne Klein	Floral
Anne Klein II* (1)	Anne Klein	Oriental - Ambery
Antilope (1)	Weil	Floral - Aldehyde
April Fields	Coty	Floral - Fresh
Arôme 3 (♀♂)	D'Orsay	Floral
Asja (1)	Fendi	Floral - Oriental
AV	Adrienne Vittadini	Floral - Fresh
Azzaro (1)	Loris Azzaro	Chypre - Fruity
Baby Doll	Yves Saint Laurent	Floral
Balahé (1)	Léonard	Floral - Ambery
Basic Black (1)	Bill Blass	Floral - Fruity
Believe	Nu Skin	Floral
Bill Blass (1)	Bill Blass	Floral
Black Tie	Oleg Cassini	Floral
Bulgari Black (♀♂)	Bulgari	Chypre
By Woman	Dolce & Gabbana	Oriental
Cachet	Prince Matchabelli	Chypre - Floral Animalic
Capricci (1)	Nina Ricci	Floral
Carita	Carita	Marine
Carrière	Gendarme	Citrus
Caylx (1)	Prescriptives	Floral - Fruity
C'est La Vie!* (1)	Christian Lacroix	Floral - Ambery
Charles of the Ritz (1)	Charles of the Ritz	Floral - Oriental
Charlie	Revlon	Floral
Cherry Blossom*	Guerlain	Floral - Fruity
Cielo Napa Valley	Susan Costner-Kenward	Chypre
Coeur-Joie (1)	Nina Ricci	Floral
Colors (1)	Benetton	Semi - Oriental
Commes des Garçons (♀♂)	Commes des Garçons	Chypre
Courrèges in Blue (1)	André Courrèges	Floral
D & G	Dolce & Gabbana	Floral - Aldehyde
Demi-Jour* (1)	Houbigant	Floral
Désirade (1)	Parfums Aubusson	Floral Semi - Oriental
Di Borghese* (1)	Borghese	Floral - Oriental
Diamonds and Emeralds* (1)	Elizabeth Taylor	Floral
Diamonds and Rubies* (1)	Elizabeth Taylor	Floral - Oriental
Diamonds and Sapphires* (1)	Elizabeth Taylor	Floral - Fruity
Dilys* (1)	Laura Ashley	Floral
E.N.C.O.R.E. (1)	Alfred Sung	Floral - Oriental
Eau de Fleurs de Cédrat (♀♂)	Guerlain	Citrus
Eau du Fier	Annick Goutal	Marine
Eau Fraîche (♀♂) (1)	Léonard	Citrus
Ecco* (1)	Borghese	Floral
Elige	Mary Kay	Semi - Oriental
Elysium (1)	Clarins	Floral - Fruity
Émeraude	Coty	Oriental
Empreinte (1)	André Courrèges	Chypre - Floral Animalic
Energizing Fragrance	Shiseido	Floral - Green
Enjoli	Revlon	Floral
Etiquette Bleue (♀♂)	D'Orsay	Citrus
Exclamation	Coty	Floral - Fruity

Fantasia	Fendi	Floral
Farouche (1)	Nina Ricci	Floral - Aldehyde
Feminité du Bois (1)	Shiseido	Chypre
Fiamma* (1)	Borghese	Floral - Oriental
Fire & Ice	Revlon	Oriental
Fleur de Fleurs (1)	Nina Ricci	Floral - Aldehyde
Fleurage	Parfums Arslanian	Floral - Aldehyde
Fleurs d'Elle (1)	Nettie Rosenstein	Floral - Green
Forever Spring	Connie Stevens	Floral - Fresh
Forever	Alfred Sung	Floral
Fred Hayman's Touch* (1)	Fred Hayman/Parlux	Floral
Gabriela Sabatini (1)	Muelhens	Floral
Gai Mattiolo	Gai Mattiolo/ICR	Floral - Oriental
Galanos (1)	James Galanos	Floral - Oriental
Galore (1)	Germaine Monteil	Floral - Oriental
Gènèration*	André Courrèges	Floral - Fruity
Gianfranco Ferré 20	Gianfranco Ferré	Floral - Oriental
Gieffeffe	Gianfranco Ferré	Floral - Fruity
Giò (1)	Giorgio Armani	Floral - Fruity
Givenchy III (1)	Givenchy	Chypre - Floral Animalic
Gucci No. 1 (1)	Gucci	Floral - Aldehyde
Gucci No. 3 (1)	Gucci	Chypre - Floral
Guess? (1)	Guess	Oriental - Ambery
Guet-Apens*	Guerlain	Oriental
Helmut Lang	Helmut Lang	TBA
Histoire D'Amour (1)	Parfums Aubusson	Chypre - Floral
Hot (1)	Bill Blass	Oriental
Ice Water (1)	Pino Silvestre	Floral
Ici	Coty	Floral - Oriental
In Love Again*	Yves Saint Laurent	Floral
Interlude	Frances Denney	Oriental
Intoxication	D'Orsay	Floral - Oriental
Intuition	Estée Lauder	Oriental
IO	La Perla	Chypre - Green
Isadora	Parfums Isadora Paris	Oriental - Fruity
Ivana	Ivana Trump	Floral
Jean Nate	Revlon	Citrus
Jolie Madame (1)	Pierre Balmain	Chypre - Floral Animalic
Josie	Josie Natori/Avon	Floral - Fruity
K de Krizia (1)	Krizia	Floral
Kenzo (1)	Kenzo	Floral
KL (1)	Karl Lagerfeld	Oriental - Spicy
L'Effleur	Coty	Floral
La Coupe d'Or	Rosine Paris	Floral - Oriental
La Prairie (1)	La Prairie	Floral - Fruity
Lady Stetson	Coty	Floral - Aldehyde
Laura Ashley No. 1 (1)	Laura Ashley	Floral - Fruity
Le Muguet de Rosine	Rosine Paris	Floral - Fresh
Le Temps d'une Fête	Patricia de Nicolaï	Citrus
L'Eau de Monteil	Germaine Monteil	Floral
Léonard de Léonard (1)	Léonard	Floral - Green
Les Copains	Les Copains	Floral - Oriental
Lily Chic*	Escada	Floral - Fruity
Listen* (1)	Herb Alpert	Floral - Fruity
Longing	Coty	Floral - Oriental
Loving Bouquet*	Escada	Floral - Fresh
Lucé (♀♂)	Beth Terry	TBA (lavender/ginger)
Lumière	Rochas	Floral
Lutèce (1)	Parquet/Houbigant	Floral - Aldehyde
Mad Moments (1)	Madeleine Mono	Floral
Madeleine de Madeleine (1)	Madeleine Mono	Floral
Magnetic (1)	Gabriela Sabatini	Floral - Fruity
Maja	Myrurgia	Oriental
Mare (unisex)	Beth Terry	Marine
Mea Culpa	Rosine Paris	Floral

Michelle (1)	Balenciaga	Floral
Miracle	Lancôme	Floral - Oriental
Miss Balmain(1)	Pierre Balmain	Chypre - Floral Animalic
Moments (1)	Priscilla Presley	Chypre - Floral Animalic
Mon Ange	Princess Elizabeth	Floral
Montana Parfum de Peau (1)	Claude Montana	Chypre - Floral
Moods (1)	Krizia	Floral - Fresh
Moschino (1)	Franco Moschino	Floral - Oriental
Muguet Millésime*	Guerlain	Floral
My Sin (1)	Lanvin	Floral - Aldehyde
Mystère (1)	Rochas	Chypre - Floral Animalic
Nina (1)	Nina Ricci	Floral
Nokomis	Coty	Oriental - Fresh
Nude (1)	Bill Blass	Floral - Aldehyde
Ocean Dream*	Giorgio	Floral
Odalisque (1)	Nettie Rosenstein	Oriental
Oh la la! (1)	Loris Azzaro	Oriental
Petit Guerlain	Guerlain	Floral - Fruity
Prélude (1)	Balenciaga	Oriental - Spicy
Quadrille (1)	Balenciaga	Floral
Quartz (1)	Molyneux	Floral - Fruity
Que Viva*	Escada	Floral - Fruity
Quelques Violettes	Houbigant	Floral
Rare Orchid	Stephanie Powers/Elysee	Floral - Fresh
Relaxing Fragrance	Shiseido	Floral - Fresh
Romeo Gigli (1)	Romeo Gigli	Floral - Fruity
Rose Cardin (1)	Pierre Cardin	Floral - Oriental
Route du Thé	Route du Thé	Citrus
Rumba (1)	Balenciaga	Chypre - Floral Animalic
Sacrebleu!	Patricia de Nicolaï	Oriental
Scaasi (1)	Arnold Scaasi	Floral
Scherrer 2 (1)	Jean-Louis Scherrer	Floral - Aldehyde
Secret of Venus* (new formula) (1)	Weil	Floral - Oriental (old)
Senso (1)	Emanuel Ungaro	Floral - Fruity
Shocking	Elsa Schiaparelli	Oriental
Soir de Paris (Evening in Paris)	Bourjois	Floral
Sparkling White Diamonds*	Elizabeth Taylor/Arden	Floral
Stiletto	Charles Jourdan	Floral
Sweet Courrèges (1)	André Courrèges	Floral - Fruity
Tabac Blond	Caron	Chypre
Tabu	Dana Perfumes	Oriental
Tamango (1)	Léonard	Floral - Aldehyde
Tatiana (1)	Diane Von Furstenberg	Floral
Té (unisex)	Beth Terry	Citrus
Teatro alla Scala (1)	Krizia	Oriental - Spicy
Tianne (1)	Nettie Rosenstein	Oriental - Spicy
Tilleul (♀♂)	D'Orsay	Floral - Fresh
Truly Lace	Coty	Floral - Oriental
Tweed	Lenthéric/FFC	Floral
Ungaro (1)	Emanuel Ungaro	Oriental - Ambery
Vanilla Fields	Coty	Oriental
Vendetta (1)	Valentino	Floral - Oriental
Venus de l'Amour	Vicky Tiel	Floral - Oriental
Verino	Roberto Verino	Floral Oriental
Vice Versa*	Yves Saint Laurent	Floral
Vicky Tiel (1)	Vicky Tiel	Floral
Vivid (1)	Liz Claiborne	Floral
Volupté (1)	Oscar de la Renta	Floral - Oriental
Wind Song	Prince Matchabelli	Floral
With Love* (1)	Fred Hayman/Parlux	Floral - Oriental
Womenswear (1)	Alexander Julian	Floral
Wrappings (1)	Clinique	Chypre - Green
XS Pour Elle	Paco Rabanne	Floral - Fruity
Zibeline (1)	Weil	Floral - Aldehyde
Zut	Elsa Schiaparelli	Oriental

MEN'S FRAGRANCES

FRAGRANCE	HOUSE/DISTRUBUTOR	SCENT TYPE
Antaeus	Chanel	Chypre
Aspen	Coty	Fougère - Fresh
Au Masculin	Lolita Lempicka	TBA
Avatar	Coty	Fougère
Bel Ami	Hermès	Chypre - Spicy
British Sterling	Dana Perfumes	Fougère
Brut	Fabergé	Fougère - Ambery
Burberry	Burberry	Fougère
Candie's	Liz Claiborne	Fougère
Canoe	Dana Perfumes	Fougère
Cerruti Image	Cerruti	Fougère - Fresh
Chevalier d'Orsay	D'Orsay	Citrus
Contradiction	Calvin Klein	Oriental - Woody
Cool Water	Davidoff	Fougère - Fresh
Coriolan	Guerlain	Chypre - Fresh
Curve	Liz Claiborne	Fougère
Dolce & Gabbana	Dolce & Gabbana	Fougère
Eau Savage	Christian Dior	Citrus
Égoïste	Chanel	Oriental - Spicy
English Leather	Dana Perfumes	Chypre
Envy	Gucci	Oriental - Green
Equipage	Hermès	Oriental - Spicy
Escape	Calvin Klein	Fougère
Eternity	Calvin Klein	Fougère
Façonnable	Façonnable	Fougère
Fahrenheit	Christian Dior	Chypre - Green
Gendarme	Gendarme	Green
Giorgio	Giorgio	Chypre - Spicy
Grey Flannel	Geoffrey Beene	Chypre - Green
Happy	Clinique	Citrus
Helmut Lang	Helmut Lang	TBA
Herrera	Carolina Herrera	Oriental - Woody
Jacomo de Jacomo	Parfums Jacomo	Oriental - Spicy
Kipling	Weil	Fougère - Fresh
L'Eau d'Issey	Issey Miyake	Marine
Lauder	Estée Lauder	Fougère - Fresh
Le Mâle	Jean-Paul Gaultier	Oriental - Woody
Navigator	Dana Perfumes	Fougère - Fresh
Obsession	Calvin Klein	Oriental - Ambery
Opium	Yves Saint Laurent	Oriental
Oscar	Oscar de la Renta	Chypre
Pasha	Cartier	Fougère
Pheromone	Marilyn Miglin	Chypre - Fresh
Preferred Stock	Coty	Fougère
Romance	Ralph Lauren	Fougère
Royal Copenhagen	Five Star Fragrances	Oriental - Ambery
Safari	Ralph Lauren	Fougère
Santos	Cartier	Oriental - Spicy
Stetson	Coty	Oriental - Ambery
Tiffany	Tiffany	Oriental - Ambery
Tsar	Van Cleef & Arpels	Fougère - Fresh
Van Cleef	Van Cleef & Arpels	Chypre
Versace	Gianni Versace	Oriental - Woody
Voyageur	Jean Patou	Chypre - Fresh
XS	Paco Rabanne	Fougère
Yohji	Yohji/Jean Patou	Fougère

* Limited edition or discontinued. Some stock may still be available for a period of time.

(1) Profiled in *Fabulous Fragrances I*; may be in limited distribution.

♀♂: Unisex or shared fragrances.

TBA: To be announced—new.

INTRODUCTION

A FRAGRANT JOURNEY

Life is an adventure: When we embark upon a journey, we rarely tread the path we envisioned in the beginning. A forced detour might lead to delightful discoveries—winding roads, circuitous routes, uphill climbs and downhill rides, rainy nights and halcyon days, harried paces and leisurely strolls. Since the first edition of *Fabulous Fragrances* was published, such has been my fragrant journey.

I have always loved to travel, in both the geographic and the metaphoric sense. Planning for a trip is exciting, like giving birth to an engaging new idea. But once the voyage has begun, the tedium can settle in, and there are problems to solve, challenges to meet, heartaches to overcome.

Writers often say that it is far better to have written than to write. I happen to love the process as well as the result, for I love the magic inherent in what I do; I love sharing my passions with others.

In the first edition of *Fabulous Fragrances* I wrote: "For me, perfume always represented the luxurious life, a life to be lived to the fullest, not hoarded away for special occasions and future days. Life was a voyage and perfume was the passage. It was the olfactory key to a glamorous life far beyond the confines of my small town. It was to my senses what books were to my soul: an avenue of escape to a grown-up F. Scott Fitzgerald world, a world where days were pretty and kind and sweet, and nights were sultry and languid and full of mysterious men. A world where each dawning day held the promise of glittering adventure."

Today, six years later, the only difference is that perfume has proved not just the passage, but also the path.

And what a path it has been! Perfume weaves through my life like a silken thread, connecting my childhood fascination with fragrance to my University of Texas and Harvard Business School days, divided as they were between studies and work with Yves Saint Laurent, Giorgio, and Parfums Stern. From management consulting to starting my own business, my passion for writing and perfumery has served me well. How pleased I am to write this sequel to my first book. Who knows what future opportunities lie in wait?

Since the original edition of *Fabulous Fragrances* was published, my days have been busy. Read about the fruit of my fragrant obsession—the creation of my first perfume, Fabulous, in the women's section. I have also organized a web site, www.fabulousfragrances.com, where I share new insights and information. Visitors may post messages on the bulletin board, as well as explore, learn, and shop. It has been a labor of love, and I hope you will visit and say hello. While you're there, be sure to read the excerpt from my next book, a work of fiction tentatively titled *An Elegant Woman* (and yes—it involves perfume!), as well as other books, such as those from my fellow fragrance author, Michael Edwards of Sydney, Australia.

Finally, I have been serving as general manager of my husband's family foundation, the Louis M. and Birdie Halper Foundation, a nonprofit entity organized and endowed by my husband's dear parents to aid charitable causes. Such stewardship brings me deep joy—the opportunity to help others is incomparable.

It remains an honor and a privilege to write and guide readers through the world of perfumery, to reminisce and to laugh, and to share new fragrance finds and old favorite verses. Many of you have become friends, and I read and treasure every letter you write. I appreciate your comments, suggestions, and support. My mission is simple: To bring a spark of happiness to your day. It is with this humble hope that I dedicate this book to you, my dear readers, my friends. To those who are returning and to those new to our circle, I extend the warm welcome of a shared passion.

In itself, a fragrance is an olfactory excursion, evolving through stages or movements. A scent might progress from a fresh opening to a rich heart to a subtle, lingering sillage. Likewise, as one begins to experiment with fragrance, one embarks upon an olfactory exploration, discovering with delight (and sometimes remorse) the scents that evoke magic and memories. I hope you will find joy in the old classics, the new trends, and the different fragrance families. Broaden your horizons; learn how to use scents to define your personality, ignite your passion, and refine the image you wish to project.

In this edition, I have added hundreds of new fragrances. There is a new men's section, too, a streamlined guide to popular men's fragrances. Unisex scents are clearly noted. And finally, the Buyer's Guide now includes helpful web sites, easily accessible for international readers.

Thank you for joining me. And enjoy your own fragrant journey, as I do mine!

Fabulous Wishes,

Countess Joan Moran

PART I

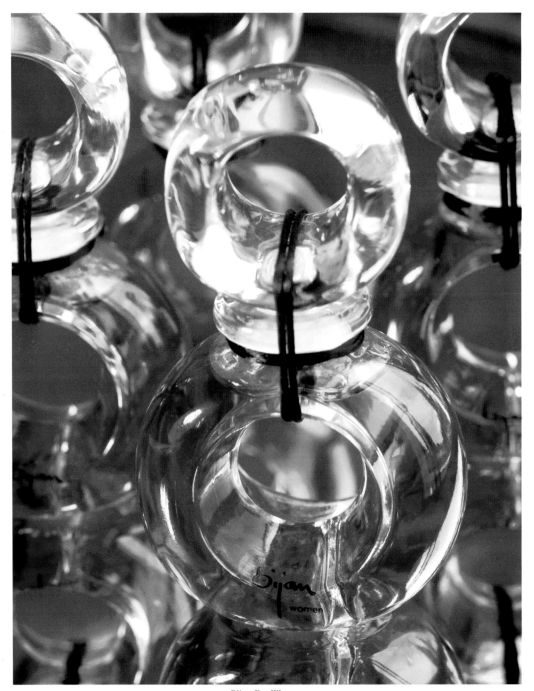

Bijan For Women

PERFUME

—the word conjures up images of romance, sensuality, power, and style. Perfume cloaks a woman with mystery and confidence; it is the transparent veil that turns heads in her wake. The allure of fragrance is legendary. Women from Cleopatra to Empress Josephine to Coco Chanel have treasured its magical powers.

Perfumery brings together the worlds of art and science, creating a compelling medium that magically affects one's state of mind. Happily, it is also a world where one can discover and choose a fragrance that expresses individuality, to say, "This is who I am, my enjoyment, part of my image today." Eighteenth-century philosopher Jean-Jacques Rousseau described this world well, saying, "Smell is the sense of the imagination."

In order to demonstrate how powerful and discerning your olfactory sense is, just close your eyes for a moment and inhale deeply, slowly. Imagine the smell of a fireplace and the vision of an evening spent in front of a fireplace will emerge.

Think of how fireworks smell—does the picture of a celebration leap into your mind? Do you remember the smell of chalk, of baby powder, of a farm, or of the ocean? Evocative memories, rich with scented imagery, may be happy, romantic, or painful. For example, Jean Harlow's husband is said to have drenched himself with her favorite fragrance, Mitsouko, and then, in a fit of despair over their irreparable relationship, shot himself. On a happier note, Aimé Guerlain created the fragrance Jicky in honor of his first true love. But there is much more to finding the right fragrance than simply taking a quick whiff at the perfume counter.

Perhaps the perfume you admire on a friend is horrid on you. Have you noticed that your favorites seem different in winter than in summer? Yet, different still when you are happy or angry, ill or well? These changes are not imaginary—weather, body chemistry, and even mood can alter the effects of fragrances.

Grace De Monaco

How Do I Find the Right Perfume?

It may help to compare the selection of a fine wine with the selection of a fine fragrance. Indeed, there are many similarities—there are even vintages in perfume oils, as there are in wines. Let us paint a mental picture.

First, imagine a snow white, chilly winter's evening, in a cozy cabin high in the Swiss Alps. A fire is roaring in the fireplace, and juicy steaks are broiling in the kitchen. In selecting an appropriate wine for dinner, you will consider the heaviness of the meal, the chill in the air, as well as your own preference. To add balance to the meal, you reach for a full-bodied red wine, say a Bordeaux or Burgundy, and serve it close to room temperature to warm your guests. After dinner, you might serve gently warmed cognac. But what if you do not like red wine, or you are allergic to it? Naturally, you would choose another beverage, while considering its appropriateness.

In selecting a fragrance for the same evening, you would probably want a full-bodied fragrance. Perhaps Bijan, or a spicy scent such as Shalimar, Opium, or Must de Cartier; or a scent with a warm wooded aroma, such as Paloma Picasso or Organza Indécence. Why? When it is cold outside, our bodies do not expend as much energy. Therefore a light floral fragrance might prove to be too fleeting, unless of course, that is the effect you want. A fragrance should always be in sync with your personal preference.

Let us continue the tale. Imagine that early the next morning you board a plane for Acapulco. When you arrive, the temperature is warm and the humidity is high. At lunch time, you opt for a light salad, a delicate, chilled white wine, and clear sparkling water. In the sunshine, you begin to perspire lightly or, as some might say, glow. What fragrance should you wear? The full-bodied scent previously chosen while in the Alps might overwhelm you. Instead, you choose a light, ethereal perfume—something floral, fresh, or fruity, or a sheer, alcohol-free version of your favorite scent. So glad you packed Cristalle, Anaïs Anaïs, Noa, and Acqua di Giò! Perhaps a light veil of body lotion would suffice, or a dusting of powder. That evening, after an afternoon in the sun, you might smooth a glistening emollient body creme over your tender new tan, perhaps a scented creme like Pheromone or Lauren. Then it is back to the beach to sip a chilled Piña Colada and watch the sun slip beneath the horizon.

These vignettes show how you can apply your newly acquired knowledge of perfumery in everyday life. In Part 2, the fragrance profiles will give you the information you need. Enjoy the journey, and enjoy the discovery of the world's most elegant, romantic, and sensual scents.

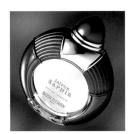

Jaïpur Saphir

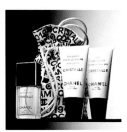

Cristalle

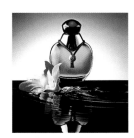

Cassini For Women

FASHIONABLE SCENTS OF THE TIMES

*"Perfume is the unseen but unforgettable
and ultimate fashion accessory.
It heralds a woman's arrival and
prolongs her departure."*

Gabrielle "Coco" Chanel

Perfume reflects the period in which it is
created, like any work of art, literature, or fashion.
From ancient times through today, fragrance has
mirrored the mood of the period. Historical
records show that the Greeks, Romans, Egyptians,
Arabs, Persians, and Asians produced scents for
bathing, religious rituals, banquets, entertaining,
and medicinal purposes.

Modern perfumery began in the seventeenth-
century in the French town of Grasse, where
glovemakers used essences from the region's flowers
and plants to scent gloves. At that time, leather
was cured in a solution that gave it an unsavory
smell. Perfume was used to mask this unpleasant
odor, and scented gloves soon became the rage.

The eighteenth and nineteenth centuries
witnessed expanded fragrance usage. Proper
ladies wore lightly scented, single note fragrances.
Lavender, violet, and rose were favored.
Empress Josephine loved rose water, while Marie
Antoinette went to her scaffold death with two
vials of Houbigant perfume ensconced in her
bosom for courage. Men and women wore similar
fragrances. It was the marketing-savvy merchants
of the twentieth-century who began to promote
fragrances specifically designed for each sex.

The early twentieth-century introduced rapid
technological advances, winds of social change,
and daring new fashions. Heretofore scandalous
multi-floral scents became popular, as did spicy
Oriental blends. In the 1920s and 1930s chemists
experimented with new formulas, using synthetic

ingredients to create classic scents that are still
with us. The mood was expansive. Woolworth
heiress Barbara Hutton, actresses Mary Pickford
and Constance Bennett, and thousands of others
snapped up Joy, which was introduced as the
costliest perfume in the world. Couturiers branded
perfume with their own labels: Coco Chanel, Paul
Poiret, Jeanne Lanvin, Jean Patou, Charles Worth.
Dionne Warwick explains the ongoing success
of designer label perfumes, "Every woman can't
afford a designer dress, but she can wear an
original fragrance."

The late 1940s and 1950s saw a return to
feminine floral fragrances, complementing the
flowing skirts and tiny waists of Christian Dior's
New Look fashions. Estée Lauder sparked demand
in the United States for everyday perfume when
she launched Youth Dew in 1953. Gloria Swanson,
Joan Crawford, Dolores Del Rio, and the Duchess
of Windsor praised the striking Oriental fragrance.
Youth Dew's blockbuster appeal did not go unnoticed
by the large cosmetic and fragrance companies.
The ensuing decades saw larger budgets, mega-
launches, and more designer imprints than ever.

Social upheaval marked the 1960s and
1970s—the sexual revolution, civil rights, and the
women's movement. Fragrance reflected these
changes with bold new scents ladened with musk
and patchouli. The greed-is-good eighties traded
in glitz, intrigue, sex, and money with fragrance
hits like Obsession, Poison, and Opium—distinctive,
heady scents with rediscovered Oriental, or spicy,
essences. The designer race was also ablaze.
Couturier names were recognizable, marketable,
and they also wanted a piece of the action. Carla
Fendi says, "The dream of any design house is
to have its own proper fragrance, because when a
woman gets dressed, the final touch is her fragrance."
Soon, Calvin Klein, Bob Mackie, Bijan, and
Gucci also entered the fray.

The 1990s beheld back-to-basics, return-to-values trends, and softer, subtler scents returned to vogue. Fragrances with names like Realities, Delicious, and Pleasures reflected this attitude. Nineties scents were fresh, light, innocent, natural, fruity, and herbal. Unisex scents established unity between the sexes. CK One, Paco, and the revived Acqua di Parma Colonia gained prominence. Celebrities imparted their sense of style with branded fragrances, from Dame Elizabeth Taylor's Passion and White Diamonds, to Michael Jordan's eponymous fragrances for men.

So what is next on the fragrance horizon? The dawn of the third millennium heralds a return to luxury and glamour, with an emphasis on personal indulgence and individuality. Classic, luxurious fashions from the first half of the twentieth-century have returned. From evening gowns with fish-tail trains, to cashmere shawls, three-quarter sleeves, and Capri pants, designers are embracing classic styles.

Personalization is growing in popularity, as fragrances such as Klein's Truth and Lauder's Pleasures experiment with deconstructing formulas, allowing customers to personalize the experience by wearing or mixing individual fragrance notes. Other houses such as Jo Malone and Annick Goutal encourage customers to layer and mix different scents in their lines to create a unique statement. Still other boutique perfumeries will blend essential oils to the customer's specifications.

Quiet elegance is the new fashion theme, and perfume is keeping pace. Moderation in the key. New perfumes such as Organza Indécence, Christian Lacroix, and Very Valentino have set the trend. Stylish scents with a nod to the past include Lelong Pour Femme and Eau d'Ivoire.

Fragrance, like fashion, continues to evolve. At the forefront of this evolution are perfumers and couturiers eager to interpret the mood of the new millennium. Although scientific advances have revolutionized the perfume industry, perfumery remains an art and, like all art, it is a reflection of the time.

Whether classic or new, perfume projects an image. Scent selections send a message to the world about who we are, or who we wish to be. Why not have fun with it?

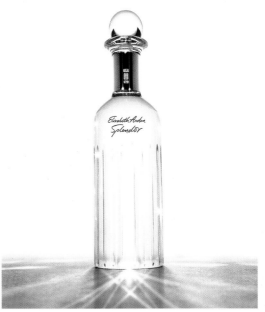

Splendor

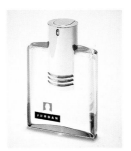

Jordan By Michael

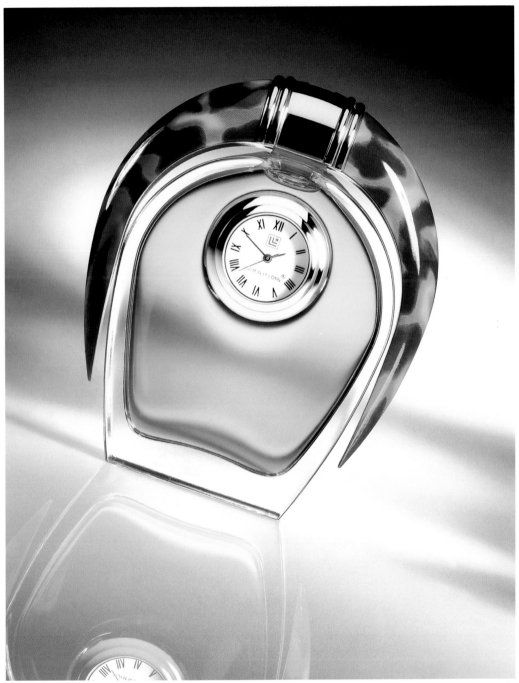

Lelong Pour Femme

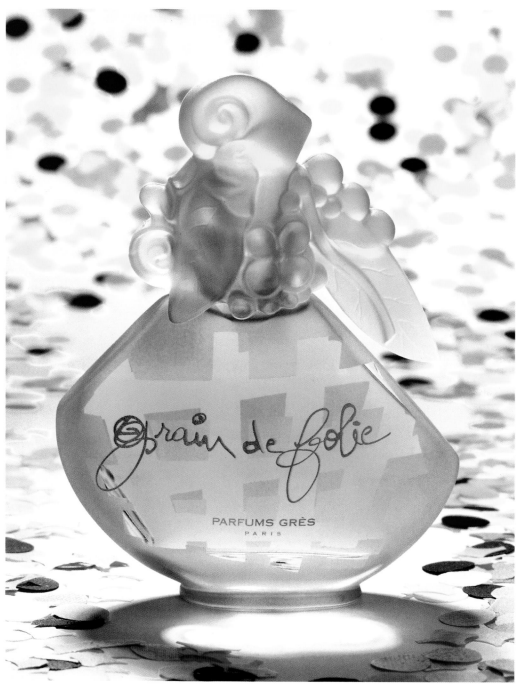

Grain de Folie

INGREDIENTS: THE BUILDING BLOCKS OF PERFUMERY

"The flowers regretfully shed tears of sweet perfume, as they would a treasured secret."
Charles Baudelaire

Fragrances are created from essential oils present in plants, flowers, fruits, bark, roots, and animal secretions. And what precious, pricey substances they are! In Grasse, France, the center of the perfume industry, workers rise early to pick jasmine before dawn. When the sun peeks over the horizon, the flower loses twenty percent of its aroma. A skilled harvester can pick about a pound of flowers in forty-five minutes, or five thousand tiny blossoms. But only a few drops of essence will emerge after processing. Eight hundred pounds of jasmine flowers, or four million flowers, yield just one pound of concentrated oil. And the price for these essences? One pound of this oil, called jasmine absolute, will fetch from $10,000 to $20,000, depending on quality, while rose absolute can cost as much as $6,000 per pound.

There is more. Indian sandalwood must mature for thirty to fifty years before harvesting. Three thousand pounds of bergamot fruit from Calabria, Italy, will yield only two pounds of essence. Now consider that many perfumes have hundreds of different essential oils, and you will realize that the precious artistry and gifts of nature that go into each bottle is staggering.

Keeping a fragrance unchanged over time is a challenge for both art and science. For example, the scent of jasmine differs from field to field and from year to year, depending on climate, rainfall, and soil conditions. The chemist must tweak the formula to compensate for changes in ingredients.

In order to preserve the original perfume formulas, the French have established a library at the Osmathèque near Versailles.

Natural essences are often blended with laboratory-created ingredients from natural or chemical compounds. A synthetic may be created as an imitation of natural aromas or as an entirely new aroma. Synthetics are far from being unworthy substitutes for nature; many are more tenacious and costly than natural ingredients. The aldehydes in Chanel No. 5 are a shining example. And whereas only a few hundred fragrances are available to perfumery from nature, synthetic fragrances offer the perfumer thousands. The combinations available today to the perfumer are virtually unlimited.

When is a rose not a rose? When the perfumer blends several components to give the impression of a rose. It is the essential oil, or combination of oils, that evokes an aroma—be it woody, spicy, floral, or something else.

A floral perfume may contain rose, violet, or sandalwood. Or it may not; perhaps it has been created by a combination of natural or synthetic materials that evokes such an aroma. This is how perfumers re-create the scent of the stubborn violet, which jealously refuses to yield its floral essence. The perfumer uses orris root, which has an aroma similar to that of violet. Apricot is another example. Also re-created synthetically is musk; its source in nature is the male musk deer.

For more guidance on specific ingredients, turn to the back of this book, for Commonly Used Ingredients in Perfumery. For the unusual component not listed, turn to a dictionary or encyclopedia for more information.

COMPOSITION: NOTABLE NOTES

The assembly of ingredients into a perfume is called its "composition." As in music, a fragrance is composed of various notes, which can follow each other or overlap. Most fragrances pass through three phases when used, commonly structured in this way:

Top Note

(or head note;
in French,
note de tete)

Heart Note

(or middle note;
in French, note de coeur)

Base Note

(or bottom or drydown;
in French, note de fond)

The journey of a sensory experience begins in the bottle, where the first whiff is detected. Once applied to the skin, the scent changes—an hour later, it is different still.

The use of musical terms is no accident. In the nineteenth-century, a French master perfumer devised a system whereby each essence was assigned a note based on a tonal scale spanning six and a half octaves. The term "note" can refer to a single ingredient, such as rose or sandalwood, or to a phase, as in top note.

The top note is the initial impression of the scent on the skin and is designed to be fleeting and volatile. It lasts less than a minute. As the fragrance interacts with skin chemistry, the next discernable aroma is the heart note. Several minutes later, the final or base note becomes evident. The base note is enhanced by fixatives, which give the fragrance stability and staying power. As the scent blends with your individual chemistry, only then will the base note emerge, revealing perfume's true personality.

Components are arranged according to their volatility, or how quickly they disperse into the air. Light, fresh ones are usually found in the top note—citrus, greens, aldehydes, and delicate florals. The heart note usually contains mid-range notes of rich florals. Warm woods and fixatives of a high molecular weight are placed in the base: sandalwood, vanilla, musk, vetiver, cedar, balsam, olibanum, incense, and benzoin.

Although perfumes are designed in three phases, the top, heart, and base, a common thread should run through the entire composition. Well-blended perfumes glide from one phase to the next with similar elements, rather than having three distinct phases. Think of a symphony which contains highs and lows, quick and leisurely movements, yet always repeats a theme.

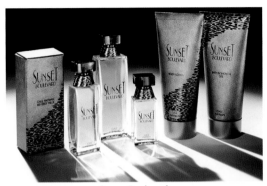

Sunset Boulevard

The various phases occur because ingredients evaporate, or dry down, at different speeds as the alcohol in the perfume evaporates. Fruits, citrus, and greens often dissipate quickly. Therefore, crisp citrus is refreshing and invigorating, ideal for use in brisk top notes and cologne splashes. Animal fixatives are long-lasting, so ambergris, musk, and civet are usually placed in the base to extend the fragrance. When properly blended, these rather pungent animal essences add superb body.

Musk is particularly potent, as French Emperor Napoléon reportedly discovered. Empress Josephine, wife of Napoléon, favored musk. Legend has it that when Napoléon divorced Josephine in 1809 to marry Archduchess Marie Louise of Austria the next year, Josephine doused her apartments with musk in a fit of fury before leaving. On the walls, the upholstery, and the draperies—she marked every room, leaving an indelible imprint, to make her memory inescapable. She vowed that Napoléon would never forget her. Besides, she knew that Marie Louise abhorred the smell of musk and wore only light violet scents. No doubt Josephine had smelled violet on her husband's collar, and Marie Louise had detected musk. It is said the apartments smelled of musk for decades after the unhappy departure.

SCENT TYPES

To bring order to their fragrant pursuits, perfumers divide fragrances into basic categories, or scent types, based on the main theme of the scent. In this book, we use a standard industry system. Noted fragrance firms such as Haarmann & Reimer and industry experts such as fragrance evaluator and author Michael Edwards, also use the same or similar systems. These categories apply to both women's and men's fragrances, as well as to unisex scents. The main categories are:

Floral	*Oriental*
Chypre (also Woody-Mossy)	*Citrus*
Fougère (also Fern)	*Green*
Marine (also Water, Oceanic)	

These categories may be further divided to reflect variations on a main theme. For example:

Floral   - *Green*
         - *Fresh*
         - *Fruity*
         - *Marine*
         - *Aldehyde*
         - *Ambery*
         - *Oriental*

Oriental - *Green*
         - *Fresh*
         - *Fruity*
         - *Ambery*
         - *Spicy*
         - *Woody*

Chypre   - *Green*
         - *Fresh*
         - *Fruity*
         - *Floral*
         - *Floral-Animalic*

In the Part 2 fragrance profiles, you will also discover many category blends, such as Floral - Green, in which the dominant theme is placed first. Other elements might also be present, for example, a hint of greenery in a spicy Oriental blend. Fragrances are usually balanced with ingredients that serve to stabilize or extend the scent, such as woods or mosses, even though the main theme might be a floral or citrus.

Also note that fragrance categorization is highly subjective. Perfumers and evaluators often differ in their opinions. There are no two noses exactly alike; some people may detect more of one note than of another note. Fragrances also vary in their intensity. For a detailed categorization of more than 2,300 fragrances (at last count!) see Michael Edwards's excellent book, *Fragrances of the World*, which is updated annually. (It was formerly entitled *The Fragrance Manual* and *The Fragrance Adviser* in prior editions.) Ordering information may be found in the back of this book on the reply postcard, or visit us at www.fabulousfragrances.com.

(Note: Because of the chemistry involved, the dominant note impressions, not always actual ingredients, are recorded under the composition heading in the fragrance profiles in Part 2.)

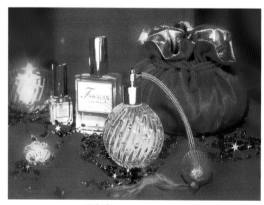

Fabulous By Jan Moran

Now let's look more closely at each scent type:

FLORAL

The largest number of fragrances fall into the floral category. Some are single floral fragrances, although most are rich multi-floral bouquets with various ingredients: jasmine, rose, gardenia, ylang-ylang, hyacinth, honeysuckle, tuberose, lilac, lily of the valley, narcissus, violet, carnation, lavender, orange blossom, and magnolia. These bouquets range from medium strength to high intensity. A few popular floral compositions are: J'Adore, Chloé, Delicious, Fabergé, Beautiful, Salvatore Ferragamo, Jardins de Bagatelle, Joy, Amazing, Sublime, Paris, Tova, White Shoulders, Vivid, Carolina Herrera, White Camellia, Bobbi, and White Diamonds.

Floral - Green

This version of the floral theme has green notes that conjure up images of freshly mown lawns and spring meadows. Green notes can be described as vigorous, crisp, and refreshing, and are made of grasses, leaves, lavender, basil, chamomile, hyacinth, and galbanum. Chanel No. 19, Sabi, Green Tea, Safari, Envy, Jessica McClintock, Tommy Girl, Lizsport, Vent Vert, and Cabotine are green floral blends.

Floral - Fresh

Delicate spring-like freshness characterizes the fresh floral category. Lightness is achieved by the fleeting qualities of florals such as orange blossom and lily of the valley. Citrus fruits of lemon and bergamot are often used to lighten the floral bouquet, while a subtle, powdery trail is another hallmark of this category. Favorite fragrances that fall into this dimension are Anaïs Anaïs, So Pretty, Cashmere Mist, Destiny, Noa, Freedom, So de la Renta, and Amour Amour.

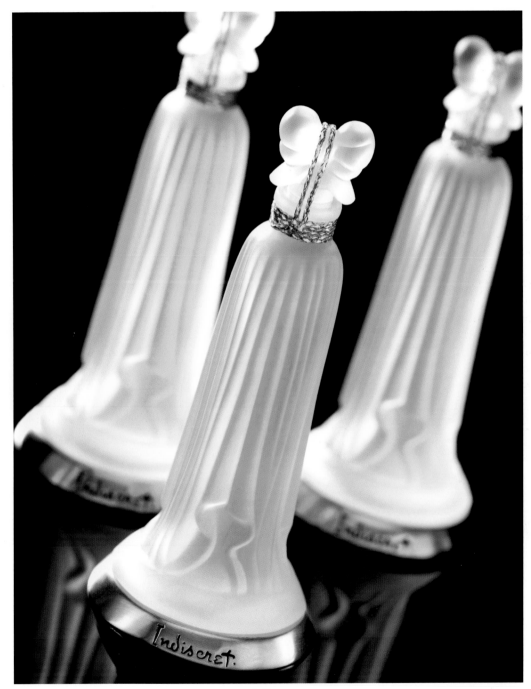

Indiscret

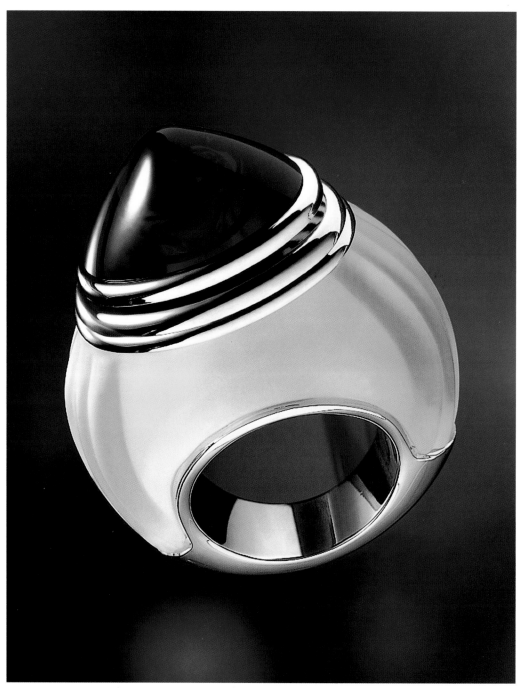

Boucheron For Women

Floral - Fruity

The fruity accented floral theme is known for its succulent radiance and ethereal lightness. Pineapple, mandarin, peach, plum, raspberry, apricot, and apple are often used for their casual freshness. Budding with high demand are fruity floral scents such as Happy, Mariella Burani, Jaïpur, Calyx, Indiscret, Lauren, Birmane, Liz Claiborne, Design, and Amarige.

Floral - Marine

Combining fresh florals and water-themed notes, this category is relatively new in perfumery. Water lily, water hyacinth, lichen, and broom are frequently used to create a marine impression. Cool Water Woman and Fleur de Diva fragrances represent the floral marine theme.

Floral - Aldehyde

Synthetically created aldehydes were popularized in the 1920s, when they were first used in perfumery. Aldehydes represent entirely new fragrances not found in nature and can add unusual characteristics—sparkling, sharp, elegant, or powerful. Chanel No. 5 is perhaps the most famous floral aldehyde and is joined by Arpège, Calandre, Anna Sui, First, Red, Nahema, Liu, Bois des Îles, Calèche, and White Linen. One of our favorite celebrity stories about a floral aldehyde perfume comes from Marilyn Monroe. When the press once asked what type of nightwear she wore to bed, Monroe smiled and answered, "Chanel No. 5."

Floral - Ambery

These are fragrances whose ambery quality adds a heavy, warm sweetness to rich floral compositions. Many fragrances in this category have Oriental ingredients such as vanilla, balsam, and spice. Bijan's DNA, Tiffany, Contradiction, L'Heure Blue, Oscar de la Renta, Caesars Woman, and Galanos de Serene are well-known floral ambery fragrances.

Floral - Oriental

These scents blend exotic floral essences with warm ingredients of spice, balsam, or resin—so named "Oriental" because they were originally found in the Orient. A floral semi-Oriental is a softer version. Popular floral Orientals include: Doulton, Coco, Bijan, Trésor, St. John, Escada, Organza, Vanderbilt, Chloé Narcisse, Byzantine, Realities, Jil Sander No. 4, and Samsara. Boucheron is a floral semi-Oriental.

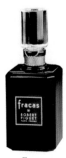

Fracas

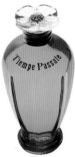

Tiempe Passate

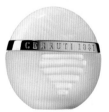

Cerruti 1881 Women

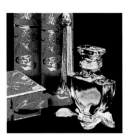
Misuki

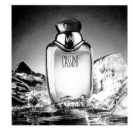
Cassini For Men

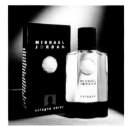
Michael Jordan Cologne

ORIENTAL

Oriental fragrances are those that conjure up images of the Far East—of spices, musk, and resins, of exotic flowers and sweet warm balsam. Actually, Oriental blends are more popular in the Western Hemisphere, due to their highly fragrant nature. Warm and sultry, Oriental fragrances are the heaviest fragrance category, and are ideal for cool weather and evening wear. Guerlain's Shalimar is a particularly memorable Oriental fragrance and was one of the first of its type created. Angel, Hypnotic Poison, Realm, Nuit de Noël, Coquette, and Royal Secret are among other Oriental scent favorites. Popular Oriental fragrances for men include Habit Rouge and Lagerfeld.

Oriental - Fruity

Fruits add a smooth sweetness and light to Oriental compositions, with peach, berry, apple, citrus, and other assorted fruits. Entrants in this relatively new, late twentieth-century category include Wish, Hugo, Jil, and Sun Moon Stars. Green and fresh accords may also be blended to add extra freshness and lift, as exhibited in Boudoir and Nokomis, respectively.

Oriental - Ambery

This fragrance subset puts a citrusy culinary spin on the Oriental theme by blending fresh citrus with amber and vanilla. Sounds almost good enough to eat; but we do not recommend it, even though Scarlett O'Hara gargled perfume to cover the alcohol on her breath in *Gone with the Wind*. Popular scents in this category are Grand Amour, Mania, Roma, Obsession, Must de Cartier, Le Feu d'Issey, Ciara, Dionne, Habanita, and Normandie. Yohji is a close relative; it ranks as an Oriental ambery-fruity.

Oriental - Spicy

A high dose of spice distinguishes this version of the Oriental theme. This type of fragrance may seem familiar to most people because these spices are used in cooking: cinnamon, nutmeg, vanilla, pepper, clove, ginger, coriander, and cardamom. Spicy florals such as carnation and lavender may round out the formulas, which are often blended with musk and dry woods. These spice blends are found in Cinnabar, Opium, and Parfum Sacré. Notable fragrances that are Oriental ambery-spicy blends are Guerlain's Vol de Nuit, Bal à Versailles, Organza Indécence, and Youth Dew, which is said to be one of Madonna's favorites. Old Spice is a classic men's fragrance in this category.

Oriental - Woody

A popular category for men's fragrances, this theme is characterized by spicy Oriental essences blended and balanced with warm woods such as vetiver, patchouli, sandalwood, and cedarwood. Look for Allure Homme, Bijan Fragrance for Men, Escada Pour Homme, and Very Valentino Pour Homme.

CHYPRE

The chypre theme is often described as woody-mossy. The word "chypre" can be traced to François Coty, who created a perfume to mirror the aromas he encountered on the Mediterranean island of Cyprus. He called his fragrance Chypre, which is French for Cyprus. Pronounce it "sheep-ra," with a French accent. Although Coty's Chypre perfume is no longer being made, the name remains; today it is applied to all compositions exhibiting the qualities of the original.

As with other fragrance themes, there are several subsets, yet the main concept is a marriage of fresh citrus and oakmoss. An inedible fruit called bergamot is preferred for its crisp nature, which blends well with earthy oakmoss and the often-used patchouli. The result is natural and foresty, soft, sweet, and warm. Enigma, Guépard, Feminité du Bois, Racquets, and Balmain de Balmain are examples of this category. In the men's arena, Polo, Aramis, and Salvatore Ferragamo are fine examples.

Chypre - Green

As the lightest of the chypre concept, the green theme is made with nature-inspired additions of grasses, leaves, lavender, basil, chamomile, hyacinth, and galbanum. Coniferous notes may include pine, juniper, and fir, while deeper herbal notes are achieved with sage and rosemary. The result is sporty and casual, with a stronger forest aroma than detected in the floral-green theme. Wrappings, Private Collection, and Aliage are green chypre arrangements.

Chypre - Fresh

This lighter variation of the chypre theme highlights the freshness of citrus. Favorite fragrances in this category are Cristalle, 4711 Eau de Cologne, Eau d'Hadrien, and Eau de Rochas.

Chypre - Fruity

A heavier chypre variation is the fruity theme, which imparts mellow warmth to the classic chypre composition, accomplished by the addition of peach. Well-known interpretations include Mitsouko, Femme, Gem, Talisman, Cocktail, and Colony.

Chypre - Floral

A lighter version of the above classification is the chypre floral. Made by downplaying the animal notes and placing rich florals center stage, it is still supported with zesty citrus, green oakmoss, and woody patchouli. Rose and gardenia are the favored florals. To experience this production, try Paloma Picasso, V'E Versace, Eau de Soir, Diva, Chant d'Arômes, Coriandre, and Aromatics Elixir. Cassini is a fine example of the closely related, chypre floral-fruity blend.

Chypre - Floral - Animalic

The fullest interpretation of the chypre theme is achieved through the blending of florals and animal essences. Animal notes include secretions from civet cats and musk deer, whale ambergris and beaver castoreum—though today they are generally synthetic reproductions. Not particularly appealing on their own, these components add magnificent warmth, tenacity, and roundness to fragrance compositions such as Ysatis, Miss Dior, Cuir de Russie, and Jolie Madame.

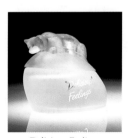

Delicious Feelings

CITRUS

Usually thought of as a male fragrance category, the citrus theme is increasingly popular among women. The citrus concept is one of the oldest themes and dates back to the early eau de cologne. Tangerine, lime, lemon, bergamot, and mandarin are among citrus fruits commonly used today. Often, they are called hesperides. Variations are realized by adding florals, greens, and woods. Generally described as refreshing and exhilarating, citrus compositions can be used by women or men. Acqua di Parma Colonia, Eau de Sud, Eau de Patou, Eau de Guerlain, Eau de Cologne Impériale, Eau de Cologne du Coq, and Eau de Cologne Hermès are citrus favorites.

FOUGÈRE

Another fragrance concept is the fougère theme, which means "fern" in French. Pronounce it "foozh-air." It is a well-balanced interpretation of the fresh green fern, with dominant notes of lavender, citrus, herbs, and oakmoss. Florals, woods, and animal notes often accompany the fresh symphony. Fougère themes are often used in men's fragrances. Guerlain's Jicky, Orange Spice, English Fern, Epicéa, and Royal Water are examples of the fougère theme that are worn by both women and men.

GREEN

This category features dominant green notes: vigorous pine and juniper, dry herbs such as sage and rosemary, and fresh, crisp notes from grasses, leaves, lavender, basil, chamomile, hyacinth, and galbanum. Refreshing sporty scents, these are well-illustrated by the fashionable Pheromone, Reverie, and Sung Spa. For men, Green Irish Tweed and 212 Men are fine selections.

MARINE

A theme also referred to as oceanic, aquatic, or water, the marine category gained popularity in the 1990s. Translucent notes such as water lily and water hyacinth provide the marine theme. Popular entries in the marine category include Polo Sport Woman, L'Eau d'Issey, and Escape. For men, Creed's Erolfa is a fine example.

As you select fragrances, consider the overall scent type or category, as well as the phases, and finally, the individual notes. In Part 2, each fragrance profile will list the Scent Type: Floral, Oriental, Citrus, and so on. The Scent Type is followed by the Composition notes, or ingredients, which are divided into Top, Heart, and Base. Before long you will be able to detect the differences on your own.

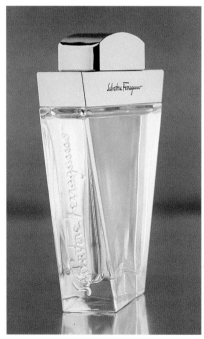

Salvatore Ferragamo Pour Femme

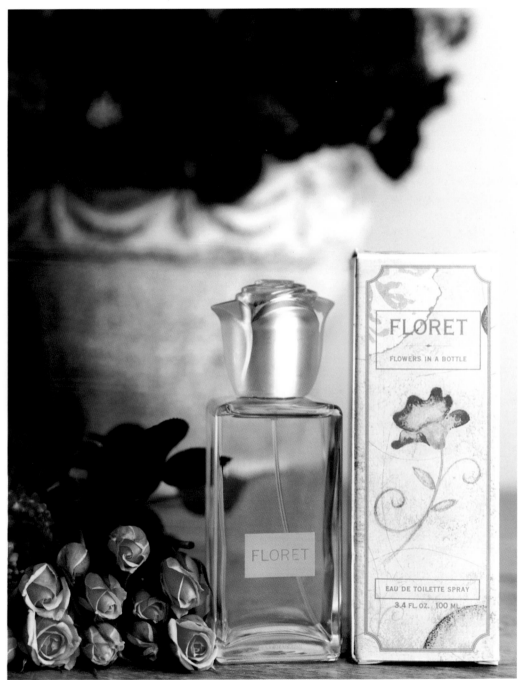

Floret

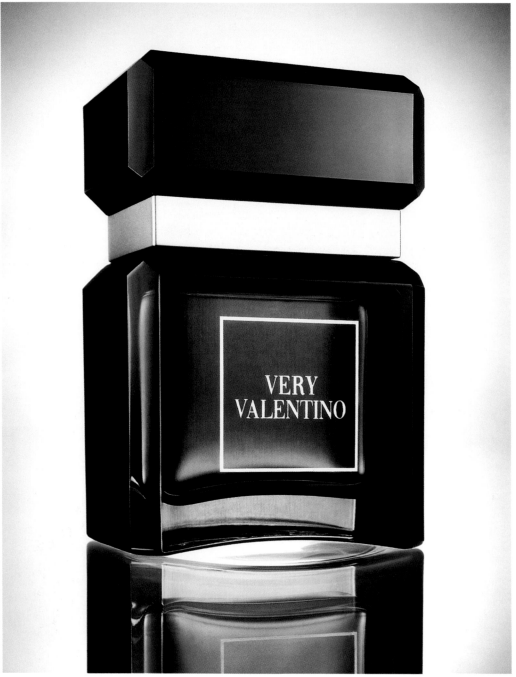

Very Valentino Pour Homme

HOW TO LET FRAGRANCE WORK BEST FOR YOU

Perfume, like glamour, is intangible and magnetic. Now that we have trekked through the jungle of scent types and composition, we are ready to explore the usage of fragrance. Let us look first at skin chemistry, product types and shopping for fragrance. Later you will learn the concepts of layering and wardrobing.

Just as the sound of a symphony varies when performed on different instruments, a fragrance differs when worn by different individuals.

Why? The answer is varying skin chemistry. Diet, acid balance, medication, skin oil, pigmentation, mood, and environmental factors influence how a fragrance develops on the skin as well as its staying power. You may notice a change in the way your favorite fragrances smell if you have changed your diet, moved to a new climate, began taking a new medication, or if you are under more stress than usual. Perhaps you have become so accustomed to your regular perfume that you simply can't detect it. This is called olfactory fatigue. If so, ask friends before you put more on—it may already be strong enough. It might also be time to experiment with new fragrances.

Having a higher proportion of body fat causes one to retain scent longer; fragrance may seem stronger or sharper. Oily or darker skin also retains scent longer than dry or paler skin. You may find that your fragrance is disappearing if your skin is dry, if you are on a low-fat diet with a strenuous exercise regime, or if you live in a cold, harsh climate. What to do? Try using a full-strength perfume, along with bath oils, lotions, and cremes in the same scent family to extend your fragrance. On the other hand, if your skin is dark or oily, or the weather is warm, you may

want to use less fragrance or switch to a lighter scent, especially for daytime or professional wear. Look for fresh or fruity florals, citrus, or green scents. Try an eau de toilette or eau de cologne.

It is wise to use lighter scents in the daytime if you work in a crowded office. Reserve your heady, sensual perfumes for the evening hours when the temperature drops, or for romantic occasions. The general rule is the earlier the hour, the lighter the scent.

Seasons also matter. Many people like a heady floral, heavy spice, or sensual Oriental fragrance in the winter. In the heat of the summer they select a lighter floral, citrus, or green in the form of a soft perfume, a light cologne, or an eau de toilette. This is because more fragrance is emanated as the body perspires.

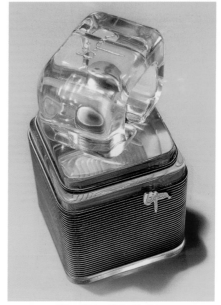

Bijan With a Twist For Men

FRAGRANCE STRENGTHS AND PRODUCTS

Understanding fragrance strengths is crucial to success in buying and wearing scents. Remember that perfume is the most intense form of fragrance, followed by eau de parfum, eau de toilette, and eau de cologne. Some fragrance companies market a light perfume, which is midway between perfume and eau de parfum. Another alternative is an alcohol-free version. Naturally, the more fragrance oils, or compound, used in a formula, the longer the fragrance will last; this also means the retail price will be higher.

Fragrance Strengths

	Percentage of Fragrance Compound
Perfume (also Parfum, Extrait)	15% to 30%
Eau de Parfum	8% to 15%
Eau de Toilette	4% to 8%
Eau de Cologne	2% to 5%

Source: The Fragrance Foundation

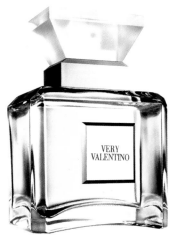

Very Valentino Pour Femme

Designed to be lavished over the entire body, eau de toilette and cologne usually come in large spray or splash bottles. Eau de parfum is a more concentrated version with longer staying power—fine for cooler weather or dryer skin. Usually available in a spray or splash, it should be used with only a little less restraint than an eau de toilette, highlighting the pulse points.

Perfume is generally packaged in a flacon, or perfume bottle, with a tight-fitting cap, to guard against evaporation of the rich, precious compound. Use perfume for maximum impact and long-lasting enjoyment. While the initial investment for a perfume is higher than for a less concentrated form, perfume will last longer and remain truer. Used properly, an ounce of perfume will far outlast the large size eau de toilette that demands frequent application. In France, perfume outsells the less concentrated forms; French women know and value the concentrated perfumes. But many women prefer less concentrated sprays they can use lavishly. It is a matter of personal taste.

When buying perfume, purchase only the amount you will use quickly. Fragrance companies say perfume has a shelf life of twelve to eighteen months after opening, or up to three years if tightly sealed. But test for yourself; we have had fragrances last even longer. Perhaps one-quarter or one-half ounce is a better buy if you use it slowly. Once you open a bottle of perfume, don't save it for special occasions—enjoy it. If you find your fragrance looking thicker or darker, it is spoiling and the scent may be altered. Use it or lose it!

Different strengths in a fragrance line, such as perfume, eau de toilette, and eau de parfum, are usually formulated to give a similar impression, however, since they are unique compositions, they will differ to a degree. For example, an eau de toilette may have a burst of scent and dry down quickly, while a perfume evolves slowly and lasts longer. Experiment to find which product or combination suits you best.

Spray perfume on pulse points to warm and disperse the fragrance most effectively; behind the ears, on the neck, between the breasts, at the bend in elbows and knees—even at the ankles, for fragrance rises. Coco Chanel once said, "Perfume should be sprayed wherever you expect to be kissed."

A spray is better than dabbing perfume with fingers, because your skin oils can enter the bottle and cause the perfume to spoil faster. Spraying fragrance will also result in a finer, more even application. Look for elegant atomizers to preserve your fine perfumes.

Another fragrance-saving tip: Store your fragrance bottles away from direct sunlight and extreme heat. Even though the bottles may be dark colored, the sun can damage delicate fragrance oils. Some women even store their fine perfume in the refrigerator if they do not plan to use it within the year. But be careful, or the butter may begin to take on the scent of your favorite perfume—use a plastic bag!

Bath oil may be used as a substitute for perfume, as well as in the bath. It is usually less costly, and is oil-based rather than alcohol-based. Estée Lauder's Youth Dew is a popular fragrance that was introduced as a bath oil and fragrance. But, as with all fragrances, take care to keep the oil away from your clothing as it may stain.

Many fragrance lines contain a light lotion or moisturizing fluid. For maximum hydrating treatment and a higher concentration of perfume oil, try the rich emollient cremes, usually packaged in jars. These are best applied to slightly damp skin. Top with dusting powder or talc to set the fragrance, just as powder applied to the face sets the foundation base. Lotion and powder alone may suffice for daytime or hot climate wear.

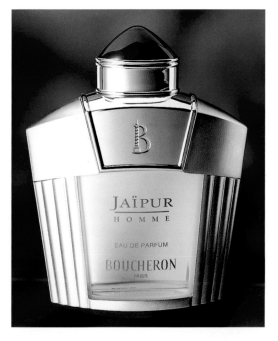

Scented bath products are a wonderful addition to the bathing ritual. But remember, a deodorant soap is designed to kill odors, and unfortunately it might also destroy the aroma of a fine fragrance. Even though a deodorant soap is rinsed off, its lingering residue continues to battle odors for hours, including that of your favorite perfume or body lotion. Solve this by using a mild unscented soap, or a soap from your fragrance wardrobe.

For men, fragrance strengths and application guidelines are the same as they are for women. One important exception is after shave. After shave is designed to be applied to the face, literally "after shaving." After shave balms are soothing formulations, ideal for sensitive skin. Eau de cologne, eau de toilette, and eau de parfum strengths are designed to be applied where a man does not shave; due to their content, they can produce a stinging sensation on freshly shaven skin.

LAYERING FRAGRANCE

Layering several forms of the fragrance together can increase scent staying power. For example, begin with scented soap or bath oil, follow with scented body lotion or creme, dust with scented powder, and for the finale, indulge in a luxurious spritz of the liquid aroma.

Layering results in a more even application of the fragrance, clothing the wearer from head to toe in a cloud of fragrance like an aura. It is perfect for anyone with dry skin who has trouble retaining fragrance, or in cool climates. And remember to carry a small scent flacon, in order to refresh periodically.

Some people create their own fragrances by combining scents. One woman we know, Josette Banzet, the Golden Globe-winning actress from *The Other Side of Midnight* and *Rich Man, Poor Man*, layers the body creme of one scent with the perfume of another. One of her favorite combinations is Shalimar and Must de Cartier. Both are Oriental fragrances, and the result is delightful. This works well with fragrances of the same scent type, but use caution when mixing fragrances from different fragrance families. The key is to try it at home first. Some fragrance lines, such as those of Annick Goutal and Jo Malone, encourage such experimentation.

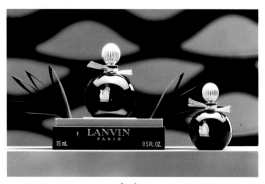

Arpège

SHOPPING FOR FRAGRANCE

We are often asked, "How do I find a perfume that is right for me?" As we have said, experiment! When you shop for scents, limit your trial to three or four fragrances or you will risk overwhelming your sensory perception. Take home samples when they are available, so you can experience it more than once in a variety of settings.

Try this: Sample scents on specific places on your skin, say one fragrance on the back of your right hand and another on the inside of your right forearm, then apply two others to the left side. Jot down what you have tried in each spot, so you will remember what you have applied where. Allow the scents to develop on your skin. Sniff periodically over an hour or two, away from the fragrance-laden cosmetic department. Notice how each fragrance develops differently on your skin as it mingles with your skin chemistry.

When you are shopping you are sure to encounter a myriad of sexy, glamorous ads. While you should not base your perfume purchase on the name or a ten million dollar-plus advertising campaign, elements are often chosen to reflect the fragrance's personality. Fashion and change are fun, but do not be swayed—let your nose be the ultimate authority, regardless of the trend. Select the scents that are best on you and most appropriate for the occasion.

Perhaps you once tried a fragrance, but now you can't find it in a store near you. Don't worry! Most fragrances profiled in this book are carried in fine department stores and Internet retailers. If you have trouble locating a scent, try searching the Internet. Duty free shops and specialty perfume stores are also excellent sources for locating overseas brands, even if they do not normally stock them.

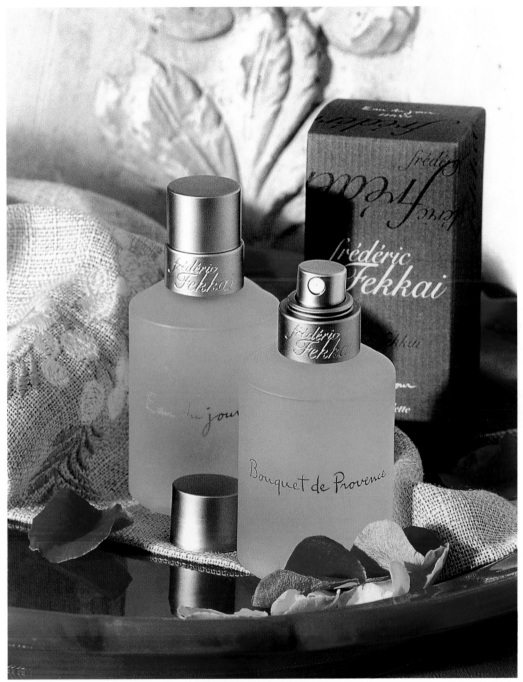

Eau du Jour, Bouquet de Provence

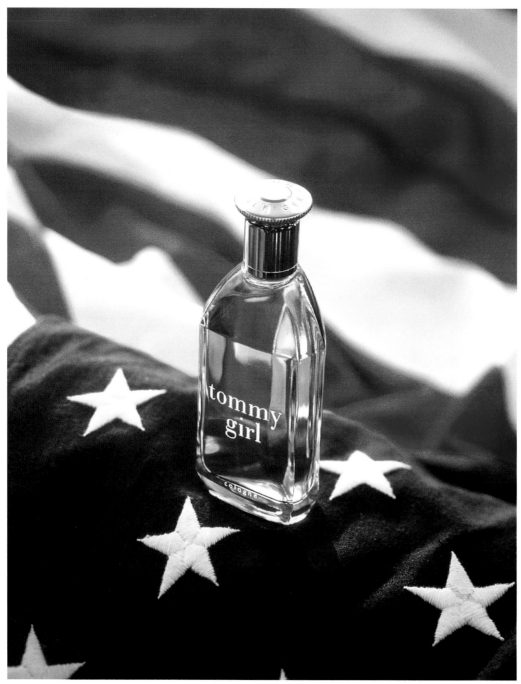

Tommy Girl

If you have to ask the price, and don't we all today?—we are here to help. Here is a quote we thought appropriate from John Dryden, a seventeenth-century English dramatist:

"The sweetest essences are always contained in the smallest glasses."

Since price fluctuates, we have given a price range for each fragrance, based on the per-ounce price for perfume. Of course, less concentrated versions are less expensive.

At the time of writing, perfumes fell into the following price ranges:

	1 ounce Perfume
	(from:)
Mid-range	$125
High range	$200
Top range	$300

(All prices are in U.S. Dollars.)

Some fragrances are not produced in a perfume version. We have classified those according to their range in the fragrance strength produced.

In this book, we selected prestige perfumes found in fine department stores and perfumeries. You may have less expensive favorites, but with so many fragrances on the market, we had to make the cut somewhere! We handpicked hundreds of favorite prestige fragrances for the profiles; many more are included as honorable mentions (HM). That should keep you busy for quite some time... it certainly did us.

Visit our new men's section, where we profiled a select assortment of noteworthy scents. Look for the unisex designations in the women's section, too.

You may also find fragrances that have been discontinued. The world changes so fast around us—classic scents such as Arpège are often revived; distributors drop a fragrance from their stable, only to have it picked up by another distributor later. Some fragrances live on in other countries; others cease production but the fragrance remains on the retail shelf for some time. We included a few old favorites so that you can compare fragrances and perhaps find a suitable replacement. Unfortunately, if we included everything in this book it would be the size of a Manhattan telephone directory!

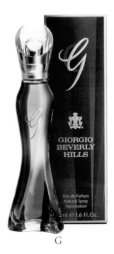

G

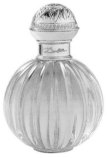

Doulton

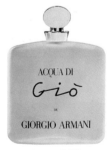

Acqua di Giò

FRAGRANCE WARDROBING

A fragrance wardrobe is like a clothing wardrobe. You will want fragrances for different occasions, moods, and climates. Some people wear just one fragrance, like the Balanchine and Russian ballerinas who were assigned one perfume to wear at all times (and intensely on stage). Most people, however, will enjoy the diversity of wardrobing. Why, even the French King Louis XV was a devout believer in fragrance wardrobes—he insisted his court wear a different perfume for every day of the week.

The Fragrance Foundation, an industry association, suggests a minimum of four scent types to start a wardrobe: a floral, an Oriental, a chypre, and a green. These will carry you through various climates and occasions, and you can enhance your wardrobe from there. To help in your selections, flip to the back of this book to **the Cross Reference by Scent Type.**

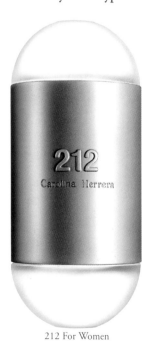

212 For Women

THE MEMORABLE IMPACT OF FRAGRANCE

It is impossible to explore fragrances without also examining how fragrance benefits us. Scientists are discovering that the sense of smell may be the strongest sense we have. Perhaps Oliver Wendell Holmes said it best:

"Memories, imagination, old sentiments and associations are more readily reached through the sense of smell than through any other channel."

Our sense of smell is an automatic memory trigger and is the most direct link to the brain and limbic system, where memories are stored. Consciously or unconsciously, every time we inhale, our brains register smells. Certain scents are stimulating; others are relaxing. Fragrance appeals to our basic instincts, and it is upon this appeal that the fragrance industry was built.

Neiman Marcus fragrance expert Bunni Nance says: "Many times, when a male customer encounters the scent of a perfume once worn by a loved one— mother, wife, girlfriend, grandmother—they are overwhelmed to tears. The memories flood back, and they simply must have that perfume again." Vivid memories evoke powerful feelings.

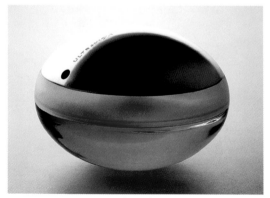

Ultraviolet

AROMA-CHOLOGY AND AROMATHERAPY

*"He set himself to discover what there was
in frankincense that made one mystical;
and in ambergris that stirred one's passions;
and in violets that woke the memory of
dead romances; and in musk that troubled
the brain; and in champak that stained
the imagination."*

Oscar Wilde

Our sense of smell is related to our sense of well-being. Two disciplines are dedicated to this truth, aromatherapy and aroma-chology. The Olfactory Research Fund is an independent, United States tax-exempt, charitable organization, dedicated to the study of the sense of smell and the psychological benefits of scents. It defines aromatherapy as "the therapeutic use of pure essential oils and herbs, the result of which is described by proponents as 'healing, beautifying, and soothing' the body and mind." Aromatherapy uses only pure, natural oils from plants and herbs. The term "aromatherapy" was coined in the 1930s, but this art has been practiced for 5,000 years. It uses only pure, natural essential oils.

The Olfactory Research Fund defines aroma-chology as "a science developed by the Olfactory Research Fund, which is dedicated to the study of the inter-relationship of psychology and the latest in fragrance technology to transmit through odor a variety of specific feelings...relaxation, exhilaration, sensuality, happiness and achievement... directly to the pleasure center of the brain (the seat of emotions, memory, creativity, and sensuality)."

Through tests, psychologists have found that peppermint and lily of the valley are stimulants and actually make students more alert during tests as well as increasing their scores. How much better? About 25% on average. Automobile drivers report a similar improvement in mental alertness when a peppermint air freshener is used.

Many Japanese firms spurt fragrance into the office atmosphere. During one test with keypunch operators, a company found a 21% error reduction with lavender, a 33% error drop with jasmine, and an astounding 54% error reduction with lemon. Plus, operators said they felt better in a fragrant environment. On the other hand, psychologists have discovered that some odors are relaxants. For example, researchers at New York's Sloan-Kettering Cancer Institute have found that the scent of vanilla can relax patients undergoing magnetic resonance imaging (MRI).

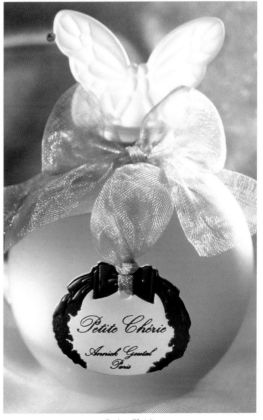

Petite Chérie

Some other scents and their uses are:

	AROMA		AROMA
❧ Relieving Anxiety	*Cedarwood, basil, bergamot*	❧ Invigorating	*Eucalyptus, pine*
❧ Relieving Depression	*Tuberose, fir, osmanthus, hyacinth, neroli, lily of the valley, bergamot, rose, ylang-ylang, nutmeg, basil, tonka bean, geranium*	❧ Relieving PMS	*Chamomile, galbanum, neroli, clary sage, tonka bean*
		❧ Heightening Sensuality	*Hyacinth, musk, jasmine, rose, patchouli, civet, clove, ambergris, ginger, tuberose, sandalwood, ylang-ylang, mimosa, tagetes, neroli, vetiver, tonka bean*
❧ Freshening Air	*Eucalyptus, cinnamon, clove, rosemary, thyme, lemon, bergamot, sage*		
❧ Encouraging Happiness	*Lily of the valley, tuberose, fir, osmanthus, hyacinth*	❧ Stimulating	*Jasmine, lemon, peppermint, lily of the valley, osmanthus, hyacinth*
❧ Curing Insomnia	*Lavender, rose, clary sage, basil, chamomile, tagetes, vanilla, heliotropine, sandalwood*	❧ Reducing Stress	*Rose, tuberose, osmanthus, hyacinth, vetiver, lavender, galbanum, neroli*
❧ Improving Mental Efficiency	*Rose, basil, mint, bergamot, cardamom, grapefruit, pine, juniper, lemon*	❧ Relaxing	*Chamomile, apple spice, lavender, vanilla, lily of the valley, tuberose, fir, hyacinth, rose, orange, geranium*

Sources: The Fragrance Foundation, Olfactory Research Fund, International Flavors and Fragrances, The Complete Aromatherapy Handbook

Note that stimulation and relaxation are not mutually exclusive states. Some essences induce a state of calm vitality by reducing stress yet increase energy and alertness.

Fragrance can also be used to improve moods. A study by the world's largest fragrance manufacturer, International Flavors and Fragrances, found specific psychological effects from certain fragrances. For example, Douglas fir is relaxing, tuberose is relaxing and sensuous, and osmanthus is stimulating and encourages happiness. Hyacinth has a wealth of goodness; it promotes calm vitality through happiness, sensuality, stimulation, and relaxation, while decreasing negative moods.

But wait, there is more. Dr. Susan Schiffman of Duke Medical Center and Hospital tested women and found that the daily use of fragrance lifted their moods—even if they didn't particularly like the fragrance. Tension, anxiety, fatigue, and inertia were dramatically reduced when the women liked the fragrance.

Can fragrance help to lose weight? Schiffman thinks so. Through studies, she found that overweight people want more intense and varied aromas from their food. They have a heightened sensory pleasure in eating. She believes weight loss can be aided by adding strong and varied flavors to a low-fat diet.

For centuries perfume has also been recognized for its aphrodisiac powers. Scents valued for their aphrodisiac qualities include jasmine, clove, ginger, violet, and patchouli. Some people believe rose to be as powerful as a narcotic. Finally, ambergris, musk, and civet are among the most sensually attractive essences.

We recently asked, what does the future in fragrance hold? "In the future, people will be interested in fragrance plus its benefit," says Annette Green, president of The Fragrance Foundation headquartered in New York, an industry association.

"Not only will they purchase fragrance for its aroma, but also for the extra benefits revealed by research in the new science of aroma-chology." Indeed, the trend in aroma-chology inspired products has already begun.

THE ENVELOPE, PLEASE

As you read the fragrance profiles in Part 2, you will find references to The Fragrance Foundation, the nonprofit educational arm of the international fragrance industry. Each year the Foundation recognizes achievement in several categories at an awards ceremony. Incorporating the Foundation's initials, *Beauty Fashion* and *Cosmetic World* publisher John Ledes nicknamed the awards "FiFis." The FiFi Awards, in the fragrance industry, are a coveted honor, considered equivalent to the Oscar Awards.

LET THE JOURNEY BEGIN

As you enter the world of fragrance, consider the exquisite words of Helen Keller, whose sense of smell was paramount:

"Even as I think of smells,
my nose is full of scents
that start awake sweet memories
of summers gone and ripening fields far away."

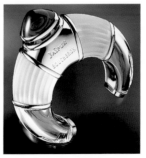

Jaïpur For Women

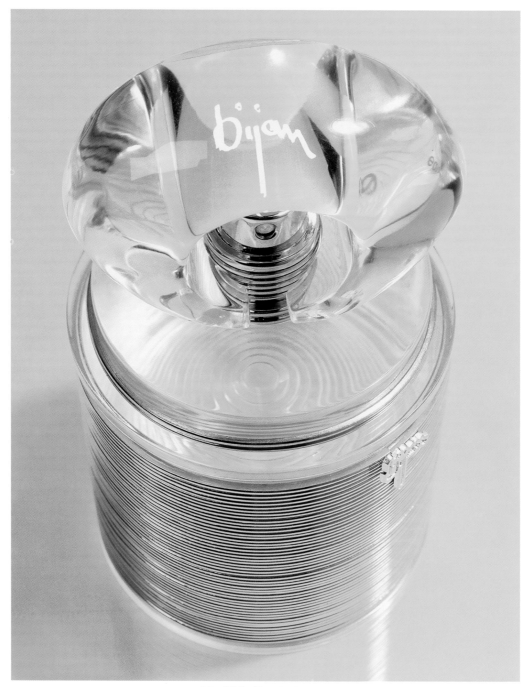

Bijan With a Twist For Women

PART 2

WOMEN'S
AND UNISEX FRAGRANCES

1000

Scent Type	*Floral*
Composition	
Top Notes:	*Greens, bergamot, anjelica, coriander, tarragon*
Heart Notes:	*Chinese osmanthus, jasmine, rose, lily of the valley, violet, iris, geranium*
Base Notes:	*Vetiver, patchouli, moss, sandalwood, amber, musk, civet*

Famous Patrons

Teri Garr	*Jacqueline Kennedy Onassis*
Bianca Jagger	*Andrea Marcovicci*

Jean Kerléo, the in-house master perfumer for Jean Patou, favors the precious essence of jasmine and rose he used in abundance in 1000. The company describes the fragrance as "the essence of extravagance," a costly formula born of mostly natural ingredients.

The addition of violet, iris, and aromatic woods is designed to endow the wearer with an aura of wealth, breeding, and good taste. Wear it to close an important business deal or to a thousand-dollar-a-plate fundraiser—or simply to feel like a million.

Elegant, understated, and refined, it is a first class fragrance that moves gracefully through a variety of seasons and occasions. Another timeless creation from the House of Patou.

Introduced	*1972*
Price	*Top range*

212

Scent Type	*Floral - Fresh*
Composition	
Top Notes:	*Gardenia, bergamot, Queen of the Night cactus flower*
Heart Notes:	*White rosette, lily, lace flower*
Base Notes:	*Sandalwood, satinwood*

New York calling: 212, so named for the New York City area code, is a fresh, hip fragrance from fashion designer Carolina Herrera. She collaborated with her daughter, Carolina Adriana Herrera, and the team of Ann Gottlieb and Puig perfumers, in developing the formula, which they describe as "provocative but well-bred, fresh but refined." Soft fruits and flowers are combined with subtle, powdery woods. A modern scent, 212 is versatile and spirited, designed to carry one through a day with ease and aplomb.

A New York sensibility pervades 212. The clever two-part bottle is a glass and metal cylinder, conceived by bottle designer Fabien Baron. The bottle disengages, yielding two fragrance-filled orbs—one to tote and one to keep at home. A practical luxury, indeed.

Introduced	*1997*
Price	*High range*

24, FAUBOURG

Scent Type	*Floral*
Composition	
Top Notes:	*Orange blossom*
Heart Notes:	*Sambac jasmine, iris*
Base Notes:	*Ambergris, vanilla*

Hermès presents 24, Faubourg, a fragrance of distinction christened for the company's elite address: 24, Faubourg St.-Honoré, Paris. The elegant floral opens with an ethereal whisper of sweet orange blossom, followed by a rich heart of Sambac jasmine from India, warmed with a feminine, sensual accord of ambergris and vanilla. Exquisite and refined, it is ideal for lunch at the Ritz or a grand evening gala.

Presented in a clear rectangular flacon, tasseled, curved, and etched with a design reminiscent of a fluttering Hermès silk scarf. Packaged in shades of Hermès orange and silken yellow.

Introduced   1995
Price   Top range

273

Scent Type   Floral
Composition
   Top Notes: Gardenia, tuberose, jasmine, peach, plum
   Heart Notes: Peach, apricot, ylang-ylang, orris
   Base Notes: Sandalwood, vetiver, amber, spices, cedarwood

Fred Hayman created 273 to reflect the desires of his elegant international clientele. The fragrance takes its name, of course, from the address of Fred Hayman's former store at 273 North Rodeo Drive, Beverly Hills. The Swiss-born Hayman relied on the collective critiques of his store's clientele in developing this scent, which was nearly two years in the making. He created a VIP Fragrance Panel of prominent women to contribute their expertise and opinions.

The fragrance is a velvety floral of more than 250 ingredients—classic rich florals, exotic spices, smoldering amber and earthy woods. Elegant and easy to wear, 273 is a smooth harmony.

The fragrance is housed in a pyramid-shaped bottle, with a stopper encircled by a 24-karat gold band. The entire vibrant yellow presentation captures the sophisticated spirit and fun of sunny Southern California.

Introduced   1989
Price   Mid-range

360 PERRY ELLIS

Scent Type   Floral
Composition
   Top Notes: Melon, tangerine, osmanthus, lily, cool blue rose
   Heart Notes: Lily of the valley, lavender, water lily, sage
   Base Notes: Sandalwood, vanilla, vetiver, amber, musk

From the Perry Ellis fragrance team comes 360, a musky floral blend that re-creates the late American designer's energetic outlook.

Packaging was a collaboration between Perry Ellis design teams and bottle designer Marc Rosen. A silvery ring encircles the round package that the company says is meant to suggest "a crystal ball, a full moon, a perfect pearl." The eau de toilette is held in a sleek cylinder topped with another 360 sphere.

Introduced   1993
Price   High range

4711

Scent Type	*Chypre - Fresh*
Composition	
Top Notes:	*Bergamot, orange oil, lemon, basil, peach*
Heart Notes:	*Bulgarian rose, jasmine, melon, lily, cyclamen*
Base Notes:	*Haitian vetiver, Indian sandalwood oakmoss, patchouli, cedarwood, musk*

This is the original 4711 Eau de Cologne formula first produced in eighteenth-century Germany. Invigorating citrus top notes create a tart, stimulating scent, followed by light florals and warm, exotic woods. It is a refreshing, sporty fragrance worn by women and men. Indeed, many of the herbs used in 4711 have been used historically as external application for headaches and rejuvenation, though we can't vouch for their effectiveness.

The dominant note in 4711 is bergamot, a tangy fresh oil derived from a nonedible citrus fruit. Perfumers tell us the best bergamot trees in the world are in Calabria, Italy. Bergamot is often found in the top notes of fragrances, especially eaux de cologne. An excellent fixative, it is also the prime ingredient in Earl Grey tea.

The history of 4711 is as rich as the fragrance: a Carthusian monk reputedly developed the eighteenth-century formulation. The formula came into the hands of German businessman Ferdinand Muelhens, who began marketing the cologne. When the French descended upon Germany in that century, they renumbered street addresses. The businessman found himself with a new address, Glockengasse No. 4711, Köln, a number he adopted for the cologne. The name and the scent have endured.

The elegantly tooled label remains unchanged. The cologne is housed in a handsome gold-colored bottle, embellished with turquoise lettering. A spritz of history, indeed.

Introduced	*1792*
Price	*Mid-range*

5ᵀᴴ AVENUE

Scent Type	*Floral Semi - Oriental*
Composition	
Top Notes:	*Lilac, lily of the valley, mandarin, bergamot, linden blossom*
Heart Notes:	*Violet, rose, jasmine, ylang-ylang, tuberose, nutmeg, clove, peach*
Base Notes:	*Iris, musk, vanilla, amber, sandalwood*

Elizabeth Arden chose a well-known landmark, the Empire State Building, to launch 5th Avenue. A modern, metropolitan scent with a saucy attitude, 5th Avenue is expertly blended, a classic floral composition with a soft Oriental base of amber, sandalwood, and vanilla. Stylish and sophisticated, a scent to announce that you have reached the pinnacle of success.

The tall, clear, cylindrical bottle is reminiscent of a New York City skyscraper. Sleek, saturated shades of black and gold with a touch of Arden red encase the spirited urban scent.

Ah, 5th Avenue—how we love that singular address!

Introduced	*1996*
Price	*Mid-range*

ACQUA DI GIÒ

Scent Type   *Floral - Fresh*
Composition
    Top Notes: *Sweet pea, sea spray*
    Heart Notes: *Jasmine, freesia, Muscat grape,*
                white hyacinth
    Base Notes: *Musk, woods*

Famous Patrons
    Michelle Pfeiffer   *Lauren Holly*
    Faye Dunaway

Italian fashion designer Giorgio Armani drew inspiration for Acqua di Giò from his aromatic memories of the isle of Pantelleria, his Mediterranean sanctuary. A fresh floral with aquatic marine notes, Acqua di Giò is an elegant, understated composition with a modern Armani edge. The ease of classic Armani design is evident in this easy-to-wear fragrance. Breezy and chic, it is equally suited for a sunset stroll on a remote island, or a busy day in bustling Manhattan.

Armani is known for the spare simplicity of his unconstructed silhouettes designed to drape the body. Acqua di Giò evokes the same style.

The packaging is also pure Armani—the flacon's rounded shoulders are reminiscent of those on his classic unconstructed jackets. Muted seafoam green reflects aquatic marine impressions of sea spray and sweet pea. And the inscription on the bottle? It is Armani's own signature—Giò.

When you ask for it, pronounce it "Joe," as do those who know, for Giò is the diminutive form of Giorgio.

Introduced   *1995*
Price   *High range*

ACQUA DI PARMA COLONIA
♀♂

Scent Type   *Citrus*
Composition
    Notes: *Citrus, verbena, lavender, rose*

Famous Patrons
    Audrey Hepburn   *Isabella Rossellini*
    Ava Gardner   *Sandra Bullock*
    Cary Grant   *David Niven*
    Kate Moss   *Sharon Stone*

Much to the dismay of fragrance lovers the world over, Acqua di Parma Colonia, favorite of the silver screen set and other icons of style, languished for years in the marketplace in relative obscurity. Then, to the delight of many, new ownership breathed renewed life into this magnificent unisex scent. A dynamic trio of style setters—Diego Della Valle of J.P. Tod's, Paolo Borgomanero of La Perla, and Luca di Montezemolo of Ferrari—have revived this popular Italian classic.

Acqua di Parma Colonia, literally translated as "water of Parma," is a brisk citrus cologne with lavender overtones and a rosy heart. It is packaged in apothecary-style bottles ensconced in sunny yellow boxes. Crisp and cool and undeniably sexy, with a streak of chic. Wear it anytime to keep your cool. Imagine yourself in the 1950s, in dark sunglasses and Capri pants, taking a leisurely stroll overlooking the magical Italian coast. That's Acqua di Parma Colonia.

Additions to the Acqua di Parma line include Lavanda Tonica, a lavender formulation for women and men, and Profumo, the company's first fragrance made exclusively for women—an intense potion of eighty percent jasmine. Finally, for aromatherapy aficionados, try the company's Blu Mediterraneo line.

Introduced   *1916*
Price   *High range*

ACTE 2

Scent Type   Floral
Composition
    Top Notes: Tangerine, freesia, rose
    Heart Notes: Peony, blackberry, cinnamon,
        star aniseed
    Base Notes: Amber, incense, vanilla,
        sandalwood

Escada takes center stage with Acte 2, a sheer floral with accents of soft fruits and powdery incense aldehydes. Joyful, energetic, and versatile, the scent is equally at ease in sunny climes and busy offices. Acte 2 is a refined statement, an embraceable scent—and sure to inspire curtain calls.

Introduced   1995
Price   Mid-range

ACTE 2 EN FLEURS

Scent Type   Floral - Fresh
Composition
    Top Notes: Blackberry, clementine
    Heart Notes: Jasmine, honeysuckle, peony, freesia
    Base Notes: Amber, vanilla, myrrh

Escada offers a variation on a theme with Acte 2 En Fleurs. Subtle and understated, the scent yields an easy-to-wear, inviting effect. The fresh formula includes a tapestry of florals and a smooth vanilla-amber base. Preview this Acte 2 sequel: Be on the lookout for white packaging with bright yellow accents and a frosted bottle topped with a swirled, golden cap. Bravo!

Introduced   1997
Price   Mid-range

ADIEU SAGESSE
(See also Jean Patou Collection)

Scent Type   Floral - Fruity
Composition
    Top Notes: Neroli, jonquil, lily of the valley
    Heart Notes: Carnation, tuberose, opopanax
    Base Notes: Musk, civet

Adieu Sagesse is the third fragrance of French couturier Jean Patou's love trilogy, along with Amour Amour and Que sais-je?. Adieu Sagesse was created to commemorate the third stage of love, the moment when the body surrenders to desire. In French, *adieu sagesse* means "farewell wisdom." Patou envisioned this slightly spicy, tart floral for fiery redheads, though anyone can enjoy the melange of light fruity top notes artfully blended with sensual base notes.

Introduced   1925
Price   Mid-range

ADORATION
(See also William Owen Collection)

Scent Type   Floral
Composition
    Top Notes: Freesia
    Heart and Base Notes:
        Apricot blossoms

Famous Patrons
    Diana, Princess of Wales
    Hillary Rodham Clinton

Adoration is a fresh, natural fragrance, resplendent with English freesia and sweet apricot. Fine fragrance purveyor William Owen III describes this scent as "cool and flirtatious, and when worn, the name happens." Perfect for warm weather, daytime, anytime. The effect is subtle, soft, sensuous sophistication, fit for royalty. In fact, English-born Owen created Adoration for Diana, Princess of Wales.

Owen was born into a family of perfumers who have created memorable scents for European royalty for generations. Now residing in Palm Beach, Florida, Owen is a man of many passions, including antique perfume flacons, lavish millinery, vintage Rolls-Royces (including one from the Prince Aga Khan), and a dog named Bertie. His artistry in perfumes has long been recognized by a select group of women who discover his fragrances at the House of Isis in England, by appointment only, of course. Owen scents can also be found at exclusive department stores.

The natural fragrance is ensconced in glamorous packaging, designed by Owen and graced with his elegant drawings. The perfume is beautifully attired in cut-crystal bottles resting amidst silken French brocade. The perfume comes in two versions, one in a plain cut-crystal bottle, the other with sparkling pavé Swarovski crystals from Austria. The "totally jeweled" perfume flacons are to die for—dazzling purse-size containers you'll love using, drenched in crystals and accented with Swarovski *faux* rubies. Beautiful!

Introduced　　　*1991*
Price　　　*Mid- to High range*

AIMEZ-MOI

Scent Type　　　*Floral - Oriental*
Composition
　Top Notes:　　*Freesia, anise, bergamot, mint, violet leaf, caraway, cardamom, magnolia*
　Heart Notes:　*Jasmine, peach, iris, magnolia, heliotrope*
　Base Notes:　*Amber, vanilla, tonka bean, clove, musk*

Founded by perfumer Ernest Daltroff nearly one hundred years ago, the venerable house of Caron continues into the twenty-first century under the stewardship of new owners. Aimez-Moi, literally translated as "love me," is a floral Oriental of classic French tradition. A fresh opening accord does a slow dissolve into an enticing heart of feminine florals, then segues into a movement of rich woods, amber, and vanilla—an exotic finale to a well-orchestrated arrangement that is sure to please even the most discerning nose. With a nod to its heritage, Aimez-Moi is presented in a traditional Caron bottle.

Other additions to the Caron line include Eau Pure, a fresh marine scent, and Eau Fraîche, a sparkling citrus scent. Lovely daytime fragrances, both are suitable for men or women. Caron's offerings are vast; there is a Caron fragrance for every occasion.

Introduced　　　*1996*
Price　　　*High range*

ALCHIMIE

Scent Type   *Floral - Oriental*
Composition
   Top Notes: *Grapefruit, bergamot,*
                 black currant bud
   Heart Notes: *Jasmine, passion flower, acacia*
   Base Notes: *Vanilla, tonka bean, sandalwood*

Alchimie de Rochas is a fragrant tribute to the art of transformation. The name is French for "alchemy," which refers to the Medieval chemical quest to turn baser metals into gold, a science of transmutation heavily influenced by magic. Alchimie is yet another fine fragrance from the French firm that brought the world Femme, Madame Rochas, Lumière, and Byzance, among others.

Created by perfumer Jacques Cavallier of Firmenich, Alchimie weaves its spell with a fruity green opening accord, then transforms into a sensual floral heart, followed by a charmed base of vanilla and wood that lingers 'til the morning light. A whimsical, pumpkin-shaped Cinderella bottle designed by Serge Mansau completes the theme.

Alchimie: For magical days and gothic evenings.

Introduced   *1998*
Price   *High range*

ALEXANDRA

Scent Type   *Semi - Oriental*
Composition
   Top Notes: *Italian iris,*
                 South African marigold
   Heart Notes: *French jasmine, Moroccan rose,*
                 French jonquil
   Base Notes: *Indian sandalwood, Singapore*
                 patchouli, Réunion Island vetiver

A feminine semi-Oriental fragrance from Alexandra de Markoff, Alexandra is composed of rare essences from around the world. A classic scent, surprisingly well-priced.

If you haven't tried the Alexandra de Markoff cosmetic line lately, you're in for a treat. The entire line has been updated, but the perennial favorites remain, such as the feminine Alexandra fragrance and the incomparable Countess Isserlyn foundations. The Hollywood movie community particularly favors these long-lasting, flawless foundations.

Introduced   *1979*
Price   *Mid-range*

ALIAGE

Scent Type   *Chypre - Green*
Composition
   Top Notes: *Greens, peach, citrus oils*
   Heart Notes: *Jasmine, rosewood, pine, thyme*
   Base Notes: *Oakmoss, musk, vetiver, myrrh*

Aliage is a green chypre blend of more than 300 ingredients from Estée Lauder. Reportedly the aroma of fresh palm leaves served as inspiration for the sporty scent, which Lauder created for casual active wear. It is said she was searching for a light fragrance suitable for a midday tennis game.

The remarkable story of Estée Lauder began with a skin treatment creme formula that spawned the signature line of color cosmetics, skin care and fragrance, as well as the Prescriptives, Clinique, Aramis, and Lauder for Men lines, along with a host of acquisitions. Other Lauder activities include the Estée and Joseph H. Lauder Foundation, and the endowment of the Lauder Institute for International Studies at the Wharton School of Business, University of Pennsylvania. The Lauder empire serves as a shining example of what one woman can accomplish.

Introduced   1972
Price   Mid-range

ALLURE

Scent Type   Semi - Oriental
Composition
    Top Notes: Citron, mandarin
    Heart Notes: Rose, jasmine, honeysuckle,
                    water lily, magnolia
    Base Notes: Vanilla, vetiver

The venerable House of Chanel does it again. Allure is a tangy semi-Oriental blend from Chanel's in-house perfumer, Jacques Polge, a scent built around six movements. His expert sleight of hand is evident in this light, yet captivating, Oriental creation.

We previewed it at the Chanel Boutique in Aspen, between ski and après-ski at the Ritz-Carlton. What a way to work! Allure held up well in the cool mountain air, even with the initial cologne-style freshness of citron—the mark of a truly elegant perfume.

The naming of Chanel No. 5 is legend, and Allure follows suit in an uncanny fashion. During Allure's creative development, it seems that fated submission number 819 from the

Chanel laboratory, proved to be the winning Allure formula. Later, upon reflection, it was realized that Mademoiselle Chanel's birthday was August 19, or 8/19. Coincidence? She'd always been fascinated with numerology.

Allure is packaged in chic beige and black, Mademoiselle Chanel's favorite combination. A versatile, multifaceted scent, for the woman with a certain indefinable something, a certain *je ne sais quoi*.

Introduced   1996
Price   High range

AMARIGE

Scent Type   Floral - Fruity
Composition
    Top Notes: Mandarin, neroli, violet leaves,
                    rosewood
    Heart Notes: Gardenia, red fruits, ylang-ylang,
                    acacia farnesiana, mimosa
    Base Notes: Musk, vanilla, tonka bean,
                    woods, ambergris

Amarige is an elegant offering from French couturier Hubert de Givenchy. According to him, it is designed to conjure up images of "Mirages and magic...amorous, marvelous encounters and marriage...a tribute to youthful exuberance."

Amarige is a romantic floral creation, youthful and fresh, lightened by sparkling notes of mandarin and neroli, and followed by rich white flowers embedded in a sensual musk, wood, and vanilla base.

The frosted glass flacon is naturally curved and presented in packaging bearing the familiar Givenchy 4-G imprint. Amarige: A delicately feminine fragrance.

Introduced   1992
Price   High range

AMAZING

Scent Type	Floral
Composition	
Top Notes:	Plumeria, lily of the valley, mandarin flower, cotton flower
Heart Notes:	Hydrangea, mimosa, water lily, linden blossom
Base Notes:	Jacaranda wood, amber, sandalwood, musk

Not only is "Amazing!" one of the favorite expressions of legendary American couturier Bill Blass, now it is the moniker for his fragrant 1999 introduction. Amazing is a delicate, feminine floral bouquet, bursting with unusual aromatic combinations such as cotton flower and pink plumeria. Yielding a fragrance that is crisp, yet stunningly translucent, Amazing is lovely, versatile, ladylike.

The fragrance is housed in an enchanting Japanese lantern-style flacon of black-ribbed, frosted glass. Bottled by Dawson-Messina, blended by International Flavors and Fragrances, styled by Blass. Simply amazing, pure Bill Blass class.

Introduced	1999
Price	High range

AMAZONE

Scent Type	Floral - Fruity
Composition	
Top Notes:	Lemon, orange, bergamot, peach, strawberry, grapefruit, tangerine, galbanum, black currant bud
Heart Notes:	Daffodil, hyacinth, narcissus, black currant bud, iris, jasmine, raspberry, lily of the valley
Base Notes:	Sandalwood, vetiver, cedarwood, neroli, ylang-ylang, oakmoss

Amazone is from Hermès, the Parisian maker of fine leathers, silks, porcelains, fashions, and more since 1837. Amazone is a modern floral bouquet with lively top notes of fruity citrus, most notably orange, lemon, raspberry, and black currant bud. The delicate floral heart is formed with hyacinth, jasmine, and narcissus amid a proliferation of other floral essences. It is ideal for liberal daytime use.

In French, the name refers to a horsewoman riding sidesaddle. Hermès describes Amazone as "tender and impetuous," a playful fragrance, full of romance and charm. The second women's fragrance developed by Hermès, Amazone is packaged in a vivid orange-red box, and nestled in a print silk paper.

Introduced	1974
Price	Top range

AMERICA

Scent Type	Floral - Fruity
Composition	
Top Notes:	Texas ruby red grapefruit, South Carolina lilac, East Hampton freesia, blueberry
Heart Notes:	California nectarine, Mojave yucca flower, honeysuckle, iced tea, lily
Base Notes:	Virginia cedarwood, Hawaiian vanilla flower, California redwood, plum, musk

Paying tribute to the independence of the United States, America for Women from Perry Ellis was launched on the fourth of July. Composed of essential oils from East Hampton to Hawaii, America is a casual scent—as American as blue jeans and apple pie. Supporting the conservation of the natural environment, America is packaged in cartons made of recycled materials. Clear glass bottles feature a proud American eagle in flight. For men, there is America for Men.

Sadly, fashion designer Perry Ellis is no longer with us. But his legacy and inspirational design live on in the company that bears his name. Salute!

Introduced   1996
Price   Mid-range

AMOUR AMOUR
(See also Jean Patou Collection)

Scent Type   Floral - Fresh
Composition
   Top Notes: Bergamot, strawberry,
             lemon, neroli
   Heart Notes: Jasmine, narcissus, rose,
             ylang-ylang, carnation,
             oregano, lily
   Base Notes: Vetiver, honey, musk, civet,
             heliotrope

The first perfume from French couturier Jean Patou, Amour Amour was an instant success in chic 1925 Paris circles. Patou reportedly created this beguiling scent for the smoldering brunettes and dark-skinned women who made his heart beat faster. The name refers to the first moment of love, the instant when the heartbeat quickens. Amour Amour was the first of Patou's love trilogy scents commemorating the three great stages of love, a trio that includes Que sais-je?, meaning "What do I know?" and representing the instant of hesitation, and Adieu Sagesse, or "farewell wisdom," the time of surrender. Amour Amour is a fragrance of comfort and luxury; its seductive multi-floral notes are lightened with a tangy top note of bergamot.

The haute couture House of Jean Patou opened in 1919, catering to the changing trends of an increasingly mobile and active wealthy class. Patou was on the crest of the 1920s introduction of modern sportswear, with his slimming bathing suits and sun products for the newly emerging sun worshippers—tremendous hits across the Mediterranean sands. Always at the forefront of fashion, he was the first to stamp his monogram on his designs, sparking a designer label trend that has spanned decades. In 1925, Patou swept to American shores and enjoyed similar success as the first French couturier to employ American models and design specifically for the American woman.

Patou—classic designs, classic fragrances.

Introduced   1925
Price   Mid-range

ANAÏS ANAÏS

Scent Type   Floral - Fresh
Composition
   Top Notes: White Madonna lily,
             black currant bud, hyacinth,
             lily of the valley, citrus
   Heart Notes: Moroccan jasmine, Grasse rose,
             Florentine iris,
             Madagascar ylang-ylang,
             orange blossom, Bourbon vetiver,
             California cedarwood,
             Singapore patchouli,
             Yugoslavian oakmoss
   Base Notes: Russian leather, musk

Famous Patrons
   Jennifer Aniston   Lisa Kudrow

Anaïs Anaïs is a nostalgic floral blend, delicate, soft, and subtle. French couturier Jean Bousquet, founder of Cacharel, describes his fragrance in these words: "Anaïs Anaïs is a perfume whose essence is romanticism with the scent of lilies. It has been housed in opaque jars reminiscent of the ancient world." The white jars bear a peach floral motif, created by bottle designer Annegret Beier. Anaïs Anaïs is an ideal scent for the young and the young at heart, those who are gentle and feminine in nature.

The innocence of the scent is created by the dominant note of white lilies, called Madonna lilies, cultivated in the south of France, Bulgaria, and the Middle East. Greeks and Romans considered this lily a symbol of purity. Each lily produces a few drops of the precious essence; in fact, one ton of petals produces only one pound of lily oil.

Bousquet clearly takes pleasure in selecting interesting names. He borrowed the name of his company, Cacharel, from the wild ducks native to Provence. And Anaïs Anaïs? The fragrance is named after the Persian Goddess of Love.

Introduced   1978
Price   Mid-range

ANGEL

Scent Type   Oriental
Composition
    Top Notes: Fruits, dewberry, helonial, honey
    Heart Notes: Chocolate, caramel, coumarin
    Base Notes: Vanilla, patchouli

Famous Patrons
    Nicole Kidman   Diana Ross
    Barbara Walters   Hillary Rodham Clinton
    Iman   Josette Banzet
    Joan Chen   Jerry Hall

Futuristic fashion designer Thierry Mugler is wishing upon a star with his first fragrance, Angel. The blue-colored essence is an Oriental composition, with fragrance notes that sound more like dessert ingredients: chocolate, caramel, honey, and vanilla. Mugler says the scent is

meant to stir "innocent childhood memories." Sensual wooded notes provide the adult theme.

Mugler explains his ambition: "I wanted a mouthwatering fragrance that also had strength and punch, just like my designs—my suits can be cut sharp and tight, yet molded to the feminine curve. It's called Angel because angels bring about dreams and the imaginary; they are a mystery; powerful, yet soft."

Angel comes in heavenly packaging. Mugler's personal symbol is the star, evidenced by his star-shaped ring and tattoo. The elongated five-pointed star flacon is produced by glassmaker Brosse in heavy glass of brilliant blue, and is refillable, as well as recyclable.

Catch a falling star with Angel, Mugler's rising star.

Introduced   1993
Price   High range

ANGEL INNOCENT

Scent Type   Oriental - Fruity
Composition
    Top Notes: Bergamot, mandarin, helional
    Heart Notes: Honey, dewberry, black currant,
                  passion fruit
    Base Notes: Sugar almonds, meringue,
                  amber musk

Many fragrance companies of late have sought to extend their lines by capitalizing on the 1990s trend toward sheer scents, offering consumers lighter versions of their most popular brands. Angel Innocent follows this trend. The scent is a sheerer version of the original richly imbued Angel, by designer Thierry Mugler.

A tasty blend, referred to as "gustative" in perfumery, Angel Innocent focuses on sweet, celestial notes, such as dewberry, honey, sugar almond, and meringue. The result is a soaring composition, a cloud-soft Oriental of youthful appeal. Clad in heavenly shades of silver and blue and topped with a stylized star, Angel Innocent is out of this world.

Introduced   1999
Price   High range

ANNA SUI

Scent Type Floral - Aldehyde
Composition
  Top Notes: Apricot, raspberry, bergamot
  Heart Notes: Bulgarian rose, jasmine,
       aqueous flowers
  Base Notes: Tonka bean, sandalwood,
       cedarwood

Fashion designer Anna Sui is known for her nostalgic and often humorous approach to fashion. Therefore, her perfume is no surprise—it is trendy, youthful, and fun. Her signature fragrance is a joyful, inspiring scent, rife with florals and the powdery finish of tonka bean. Funky and feminine, it will remind you of playing dress-up with feather boas and stiletto heels. Look for the Anna Sui scent in a jet-black, filigreed bottle enhanced with brilliant purple accents.

Introduced   1999
Price   Mid-range

ANNÉ PLISKA

Scent Type Floral - Oriental
Composition
  Top Notes: Mandarin, bergamot
  Heart Notes: Jasmine, geranium
  Base Notes: Amber, musk, patchouli

On Valentine's Day in 1987, the romantic signature scent from Californian Anné Pliska was introduced. Blended by Givaudan-Roure perfumers, the natural, expansive floral Oriental opens with sparkling notes of mandarin and bergamot and evolves into an enticing tapestry of jasmine, amber, patchouli, and musk. Hypnotic and mesmerizing, it is an entrance-making fragrance for the feminine, spirited woman. "My fragrance leaves an indelible impression on a man's heart," says Pliska.

The all-American woman served as the inspiration for this unique fragrance—independent, passionate, and optimistic. Indeed, creator Anné Pliska is the embodiment of such a lovely woman. Her boutique line is exclusive to Nordstrom in North America, where she has developed a loyal clientele over the course of many years.

The fragrance is presented in satin-etched crystal bottles and is packaged in shades of California sunset pink, golden hues, and pure cloud white. We love the sparkling body lotion, as well as the dusting powder with the retro-glamour fluffy pink powder puff. Anné Pliska—a rare find.

Introduced   1987
Price   Mid- to High range

ANTONIA'S FLOWERS

Scent Type Floral
Composition
  Notes: Freesia, jasmine, lily of the valley,
      magnolia, fruits

Famous Patrons
  Chynna Phillips Rosie O'Donnell
  Martha Stewart

A delightful bouquet of flowers is gathered in Antonia's Flowers. The delicate composition is based on the fresh scent of freesia and enhanced by a selection of spring flowers and fruits. A light fragrance, Antonia's Flowers is suitable for casual daytime and warm weather wear, afternoon tea, or an evening walk on the beach.

"I imagined a perfume that would evoke the sensation of entering my flower shop," says creator Antonia Bellanca. She selected the dominant note of freesia for its clean, innocent aroma. She first discovered and fell in love with freesia as an art student in France. And now, she has put the flowers in a bottle.

Packaged in rectangular glass flacons, Antonia's Flowers is decorated with pastel watercolor sketches of wildflowers.

Introduced   1985
Price   Mid-range

APRÈS L'ONDÉE

Scent Type   *Floral - Ambery*
Composition
    Top Notes: *Violet, bergamot, cassie, neroli*
    Heart Notes: *Carnation, ylang-ylang, iris, rose, jasmine, mimosa, vetiver, sandalwood*
    Base Notes: *Vanilla, musk, amber, heliotrope*

Famous Patrons
    Ines de la Fressange   *Susan Gutfreund*
    Karl Lagerfeld

A graceful creation by Jacques Guerlain, the company describes Après L'Ondée as "an inspired portrait of the most delicate imaginary flower." Elusively charming, fresh and sparkling, it is a refined floral bouquet with a sweet amber base, suitable for most any occasion. Après L'Ondée is one of more than 300 scents developed by the renowned House of Guerlain.

The House of Guerlain is the world's oldest family-operated fragrance and cosmetic company. Spanning five generations, it was founded in 1828

by doctor and chemist Pierre-François-Pascal Guerlain. The shop was first located on the rue de Rivoli in Paris, then moved to No. 15 rue de la Paix, where young Guerlain created his hallmark—personalized fragrances in sync with the wearer's personality, fragrances that often lived for only one evening or event. Writer Honoré de Balzac commissioned a custom-blended scent during the writing of *César Birotteau*, and Empress Eugénie named Guerlain perfumer to the Napoléonic court, for which many Empire fragrances were created. In fact, Guerlain was appointed perfumer to most of the royal courts of Europe, including those of the Empress of Austria and the Queens of England, Spain, and Romania.

Introduced   1906
Price   High range

AQUA ALLEGORIA COLLECTION

FLORA NEROLIA
Floral - Fruity
HERBA FRESCA
Green (♀♂)
LAVANDE VELOURS
Floral (♀♂)
PAMPLELUNE
Citrus (♀♂)
ROSA MAGNIFICA
Floral
YLANG & VANILLE
Floral

The Aqua Allegoria scents are a fragrant wardrobe from the venerable House of Guerlain. Each scent in the palette is a fresh rendering developed around nature-based accords. For example, Herba Fresca is a green herbal blend, Lavande Velours is a lavender and sandalwood composition, and Pamplelune is a spirited, citrusy grapefruit explosion, tinged with vanilla and patchouli. Ylang & Vanille combines sweet ylang-ylang and smooth vanilla, while Rosa Magnifica is a rose cornucopia smoothed with violet, narcissus, and pink peppercorn. Flora Nerolia is an orange blossom special, enhanced by jasmine and smoky incense. These beautiful scents are ideal for daytime and casual evenings.

Youthful, simple, and carefree, the Aqua Allegoria scents are easy to love—unfettered, yet elegant in their simplicity. The classic Guerlain "bee bottles" are color-coded to identify each scent in the line. An instant fragrance wardrobe, the Aqua Allegoria essences provide a variety of year-round choices for the Guerlain collector.

Introduced   1999
Price   High range

AROMATICS ELIXIR

Scent Type   Chypre - Floral
Composition
    Top Notes: Chamomile, orange blossom,
                    bergamot, coriander, rosewood,
                    aldehydes, greens, palmarosa
    Heart Notes: Jasmine, rose, ylang-ylang,
                    tuberose, orris, carnation
    Base Notes: Sandalwood, oakmoss, vetiver,
                    patchouli, musk, cistus, civet

Famous Patrons
    Glenn Close   Kate Blanchett

Aromatics Elixir is designed to soothe and subtly stimulate, with notes of gentle chamomile and sweet sandalwood set against a classic blend of French florals and aromatic woods. The dominant chypre theme is a natural accord enhanced by juicy citrus and lawn greens.

Introduced   1971
Price   Mid-range

ARPÈGE

Scent Type   Floral - Aldehyde
Composition
    Top Notes: Bergamot, aldehydes, peach,
                    orange blossom, honeysuckle, iris
    Heart Notes: Rose, jasmine, ylang-ylang,
                    coriander, mimosa, tuberose,
                    violet, geranium, genet
    Base Notes: Sandalwood, vetiver, patchouli,
                    vanilla, musk

Famous Patrons
    Diana, Princess of Wales   Martha Stewart
    Princess Grace of Monaco   Rita Hayworth
    Jacqueline Bisset

Arpège is a restoration and reformulation of the original 1927 scent from French couturier Jeanne Lanvin and perfumer Andre Fraysse.

More than sixty natural essences are housed in the classic Art Deco, ball-shaped flacon, or *boule noire*. A black opaque glass bottle houses the perfume, while the eau de parfum resides in a clear glass bottle. A gold-colored image, by artist Paul Iribe, of Jeanne Lanvin and her daughter, musician Marie-Blanche, dressing for a ball is stamped on the glass, just as it was on the original bottles. The fragrance was christened Arpège by Marie-Blanche for its similarity to a musical arpeggio—a tumble of notes in quick succession. The result is an elegant floral composition with a sensual wooded finish.

Lanvin created the popular mother-daughter design concept, in addition to designing evening gowns, bridal wear, and menswear. After her death in 1946, Marie-Blanche, also known as the Comtesse de Polignac, continued the business with Bernard Lanvin.

The relaunch of Arpège coincided with the remodeling of Lanvin's boutiques on the rue du Faubourg Saint Honoré. How we love to see the classics revived. Welcome back, Arpège.

Introduced   1927
Reintroduced   1993
Price   Top range

AZURÉE

Scent Type   Chypre - Floral Animalic
Composition
    Top Notes: Bergamot, aldehydes, gardenia,
                  artemisia
    Heart Notes: Jasmine, geranium, ylang-ylang,
                  orris, cyclamen
    Base Notes: Leather, oakmoss, patchouli,
                  musk, amber

Azurée is a chypre floral melody from Estée Lauder, said to have been inspired by the tangy Mediterranean bergamot fruit, an inedible fruit prized for perfumery.

The fragrance features herbal and aldehydic top notes, dry floral heart notes and woody base notes redolent of warm leather and moss. Azurée is a versatile everyday scent.

Introduced   1969
Price   Mid-range

BAL À VERSAILLES

Scent Type   Oriental - Ambery Spicy
Composition
    Top Notes: Grasse jasmine, Bulgarian rose,
                  Anatolian rose, May rose,
                  Farnesian cassie

Heart Notes: Sandalwood, patchouli, vetiver
Base Notes: Musk, ambergris, gums, resins, civet

Famous Patrons
Dame Elizabeth Taylor

Bal à Versailles is a classic French fragrance from the legendary Parisian perfumer Jean Desprez. More than 350 rare essences were used to create the long-lasting, dramatic fragrance. A rich and feminine Oriental blend, it features floral, amber, spice, and sweet balsamic base notes. Bal à Versailles is ideal for sophisticated day wear and elegant evenings.

In the 1930s, Jean Desprez established his perfumery on the prestigious rue de la Paix in Paris, serving an exclusive clientele. Besides his popular Bal à Versailles, he also created Grand Dame, Étourdissant, and Vôtre Main in 1939, Jardanel in 1972, and Révolution à Versailles. Upon his death in 1973, he was succeeded by his son Denis Desprez and daughter Marie Celine Garnier.

Bal à Versailles is presented in an array of classic fragrance flacons. Our favorite is a round decanter with a label featuring a romantic party scene; no doubt it is from the most famous dance or "ball" of Versailles—the Bal à Versailles. This scene is a miniature reproduction of a Fragonard painting that is part of the Sevres Museum collection. The scene also appeared on a porcelain dish by Madame Ducluzeau known as La Coupe des Sens, or "cup of the senses," featuring miniatures representing the five senses. When Desprez was searching for inspiration, he spied the cup and was intrigued by the Fragonard scene representing the sense of smell. Quel appropos!

Introduced   1962
Price   Mid-range

BALMAIN DE BALMAIN

Scent Type	*Chypre*
Composition	
Top Notes:	*Bergamot, black currant, pepper, galbanum*
Heart Notes:	*Jasmine, May rose, violet, iris*
Base Notes:	*Oakmoss, vetiver, patchouli*

Introduced in 1999, Balmain de Balmain is the first new fragrance since 1979 from the couture house of Balmain. The composition is based on the firm's first fragrance, Élysées, which was created in 1947. In Pierre Balmain's heyday, his designs graced the figures of Katherine Hepburn, Marlene Dietrich, and Brigitte Bardot. He also became the exclusive couturier to Her Majesty Queen Sirikit of Thailand. Although Balmain died in 1982, his company survived, and Oscar de la Renta signed on in 1993 to serve as artistic director of the Paris-based firm.

Balmain de Balmain, blended by perfumer Jean Amic, is a classic chypre composition with an abundance of verve and vivacity. A joyful scent, Balmain de Balmain features a snappy bergamot opening with a dash of pepper, followed by a feminine floral heart and a sensual base of oakmoss and patchouli. The bottle is based on a Balmain design, updated by Xavier Rousseau. The clever 'round-the-corner label is a reflection of the original Balmain design, which is refrained on the cream and gold-toned carton. This well-priced line proves that excellence need not break the purse. Retro glamour at its finest, Balmain de Balmain is undeniably chic.

Introduced	*1999*
Price	*Mid-range*

BANDIT

Scent Type	*Chypre - Floral Animalic*
Composition	
Top Notes:	*Neroli, orange, ylang-ylang, galbanum*
Heart Notes:	*Jasmine, rose, tuberose, leather*
Base Notes:	*Patchouli, mousse de chêne, vetiver, musk*

Famous Patrons
  Marlene Dietrich

Bandit is a classic fragrance developed during World War II for couturier Robert Piguet by Roure perfumer Germaine Sellier. It is a delightfully wicked blend of sultry spices and florals with a long-lasting base of woods and musk, and the interesting of addition of leathery note. This is the original 1944 formula, resurrected in 1999, heretofore unavailable for twenty-five years.

Swiss-born Piguet apprenticed under couturier Paul Poiret in glamorous 1920 Paris. By 1928 he had his own salon, specializing in couture creations for petite, youthful women. He trained the next generation of designers at his salon: Pierre Balmain, Hubert de Givenchy, Castillo, James Galanos. Christian Dior once said that he learned from Piguet "the virtues of simplicity...how to suppress." Piguet is often credited with "the little black dress."

Piguet was a man with a rebel heart, both in design and by action. In 1944, he introduced Bandit in a provocative manner, with runaway models in black bandit masks brandishing toy guns and knives. Remember, this was 1944. During the German occupation of France, Piguet defied Nazi orders to relocate to Berlin, remaining in Paris, in business, for the duration of World War II.

How to catch a Bandit? Look for it dressed in pared-down Piguet black, naturally.

Introduced   1944
Reintroduced   1999
Price   Mid-range

BEAUTIFUL

Scent Type   Floral
Composition
    Top Notes: Bergamot, galbanum, lemon,
                  cassie, fruits
    Heart Notes: Rose, ylang-ylang, lilac, violet,
                  lily of the valley, carnation, sage,
                  geranium, rose violet, narcissus,
                  orange blossom, mimosa, marigold,
                  freesia, chamomile, tuberose,
                  jasmine, neroli, jonquil, magnolia
    Base Notes: Sandalwood, vetiver, musk,
                  vanilla, cedarwood

Beautiful is a romantic scent from Estée Lauder, bursting with a cornucopia of fruit and wildflower essences. The fragrance embodies femininity, softness, and romance, like a goddess floating through a cloud of white. Lauder reportedly received her inspiration for the fragrance from the gardens of Giverny, the same gardens that inspired Monet.

The bottle, from I. Levy-Alain Carré, is a study in classic simplicity, a vessel of clear glass inscribed with the name Beautiful. It rests easily in the hand and travels well. Like wildflowers, Beautiful blossoms in the springtime sun.

Introduced   1985
Price   Mid-range

BELLODGIA

Scent Type   Floral
Composition
    Top and
    Heart Notes: Rose, jasmine, lily of the valley
    Base Notes: Spicy carnation

Bellodgia is a classic 1920s fragrance from the notable French fragrance house Parfums Caron. The fragrance takes its name from a romantic island on Lake Como in Northern Italy. The feminine floral bouquet is distinguished by a rich accord of rose and jasmine accenting the dominant theme of spicy carnation. Bellodgia is a chic, sophisticated perfume.

Parfums Caron was established in Paris in 1904 to introduce fragrances created by master perfumer Ernest Daltroff. Today, Parfums Caron presents its timeless fragrances on the fashionable avenue Montaigne in Paris. The store is a sight to behold—each exquisite Caron fragrance is suspended in Louis XV-style Baccarat crystal flacons, from which customers can draw a desired amount of fragrance. Elsewhere, look for Bellodgia prepackaged in perfume and eau de toilette fragrance strengths.

Introduced   1927
Price   High range

BIJAN

Scent Type   Floral - Oriental
Composition
    Top Notes: Ylang-ylang, narcissus,
                  orange blossom

Heart Notes: Persian jasmine, Bulgarian rose,
                lily of the valley
Base Notes: Moroccan oakmoss, sandalwood,
                patchouli

Famous Patrons

Queen Elizabeth II	Anjelica Huston
Oprah Winfrey	Barbra Streisand
Annette Bening	Bo Derek
Candice Bergen	Natalie Cole
Liza Minnelli	Hillary Rodham Clinton
Whoopi Goldberg	Aretha Franklin
Teri Garr	Lesley Anne Warren

A floral Oriental with soft top notes, Bijan Perfume for Women is the original signature fragrance from Bijan, prominent Beverly Hills menswear couture designer. "The woman who wears my fragrance is certainly not afraid to be noticed," says Bijan. "She is definitive about her personal style and is as sophisticated as she is alluring."

Two-and-a-half years in the making, the fragrance is composed of rich seductive florals poised against exotic woods, creating a refined, feminine statement that whispers of wealth. From kings to presidents to the simply well-to-do, Bijan's clients seek out his inimitable style at his "by appointment only" boutique in Beverly Hills.

The scent is packaged in a round bottle with a hole in the center. Designed by Bijan, the bottle garnered a 1993 Clear Choice Award from the Glass Packaging Institute. So exquisite is the bottle, Bijan created a custom-made chandelier for his Beverly Hills showroom, using more than one million dollars worth of Bijan Perfume for Women bottles. "At night, when the light is on, the perfume in the bottles gives off the most gorgeous amber colors," explains Bijan. "It is magnificent!"

Introduced   1987
Price   Top range

BIJAN WITH A TWIST!

Author's note: At press time, we were excited to hear of a pending arrival, Bijan With a Twist! Although we can't share the details just yet, Bijan says the women's perfume will be "one of the most expensive perfumes in the world." (We understand a men's version is also in development.) Sworn to secrecy, we previewed the work-in-progress. The perfume is joyful, with a real twist; the bottle has a twist of its own. All we can say is, it is sure to become a collector's item.

BIRMANE

Scent Type   Floral - Fruity
Composition
    Top Notes: Peach, freesia, kumquat
    Heart Notes: Jasmine, white rose, red lily
    Base Notes: Cedarwood, tonka bean,
                    white musk

For more than one hundred years, French jeweler Van Cleef & Arpels has enchanted the world with exquisite designs. Today the company dazzles with the treasure of Birmane, meaning "Burmese" in French, which refers to the precious rubies of Burma. The smoothly sophisticated, fruity floral perfume dries down to a feminine accord laced with tonka bean, which is a sweet, nutty bean often blended with musk or vanilla for a powdery effect.

Birmane's multifaceted flacon suggests a treasured gemstone cut from the heart of a Burmese mine. It is fashioned after the "step cut," a nine-faceted cut that features an octagonal contour with a ninth plane in the center, a design used only for the most resilient and pure of gemstones. The rich red carton is flecked with golden hues—perfect for holiday gift giving—especially when paired with a sparkling ruby bauble or two.

Introduced   1999
Price   High range

BLONDE

Scent Type   Floral
Composition
    Top Notes: Green violet, neroli, tuberose
    Heart Notes: Jasmine, orange blossom,
                  daffodil, broom
    Base Notes: Tuberose, woods

Fashion designer Gianni Versace created Blonde in tribute to his sister and muse, the platinum-blonde Donatella Versace, who has recently stepped into the creative shoes of her late brother. Blonde was envisioned as a fragrance for the woman who can do it all, on her own terms. Not for the shrinking violet, Blonde is a heady creation, rife with tuberose, an intensely fragrant white flower that is native to Mexico. Passionate, alluring, and sensual, Blonde is a fragrance that will turn every head.

Introduced   1996
Price   High range

BLUE GRASS

Scent Type   Floral - Amber
Composition
    Top Notes: Aldehydes, lavender, orange,
                  neroli, bergamot
    Heart Notes: Jasmine, tuberose, narcissus, rose,
                  carnation

Base Notes: Sandalwood, musk, tonka bean,
                  benzoin

Famous Patrons
Queen Elizabeth II

Blue Grass from Elizabeth Arden is an enduring, easy-to-wear classic, ideal for casual, professional or daytime wear. Surprisingly well-priced, too.

Elizabeth Arden was an early entrepreneur in the American cosmetics industry. Born Florence Graham in Ontario, Canada, she derived her professional name from a favorite book: *Elizabeth and Her German Garden*. As a nurse, she developed a skin care regime that became popular in her beauty salons, the first of which opened its red door in New York in 1910. Her love of nature and flowers moved her to create fragrance and inspired the name for Blue Grass, after the shimmering view of verdant fields visible from the windows of her Virginia home.

Introduced   1934
Price   Mid-range

BOBBI

Scent Type   Floral
Composition
    Top Notes: Citrus, bamboo leaf, cucumber,
                  ylang-ylang
    Heart Notes: Water lily, jasmine, osmanthus,
                  peony, phlox
    Base Notes: Sandalwood, patchouli, orris,
                  cedarwood

Bobbi is the first fragrance from makeup artist extraordinaire Bobbi Brown, whose company is now a division of Estée Lauder. The initial green lift is an unusual combination of cucumber and bamboo leaf, enhanced by clean, citrusy top notes, which dissolve into a soft floral heart, poised against a subtly wooded finish. Bobbi was designed as a personal, easy-to-wear fragrance—equally at ease on a sunny summer outing or on a heated day at the office. Ideal for hectic days, Bobbi is as comfortable as a pair of worn khakis, a crisp white cotton shirt, and casual loafers—and equally as easy to love.

Introduced	*1998*
Price	*High range*

BOIS DES ÎLES

Scent Type	*Floral - Aldehyde*
Composition	
Top Notes:	*Bergamot, petitgrain, coriander, aldehydes*
Heart Notes:	*Jasmine, rose, ylang-ylang, iris*
Base Notes:	*Vetiver, amber, sandalwood, tonka bean*

In the 1920s, French couturier Gabrielle "Coco" Chanel collaborated with the great perfumer Ernest Beaux to create the Chanel scents that have become legend: No. 5, No. 19, and No. 22. Now, Chanel reintroduces a trio of exhilarating Beaux fragrances from the twenties: Bois des Îles, Cuir de Russie, and Gardénia.

The woody floral blend of Bois des Îles begins with top notes of fresh citrus, spice, and sparkling aldehydes entwined with rich florals and sweet lasting woods. A subtly sensual fragrance, understated and understood.

Bois des Îles, or "wood of the isles," is a welcome return to an era of grace and elegance. Look for it in Chanel Boutiques.

Introduced	*1926*
Reintroduced	*1993*
Price	*Mid-range*

BOUCHERON

Scent Type	*Floral Semi - Oriental*
Composition	
Top Notes:	*Sicilian tangerine, Calabrian bitter orange, apricot, Persian galbanum, African tagetes, Spanish basilica*
Heart Notes:	*Moroccan orange blossom, Grasse tuberose, Madagascar ylang-ylang, Moroccan jasmine, Auvergne narcissus, British broom*
Base Notes:	*Mysore sandalwood, amber, Indian Ocean vanilla, South American tonka bean*

Boucheron is the signature fragrance from the renowned French jeweler Frédéric Boucheron. The delicate, feminine scent is introduced by lively green and fruity top notes, then develops into an intense heart of sensual florals. Underscoring the arrangement are warm, woody background notes, sensual and long-lasting.

Frédéric Boucheron established the first Boucheron jewelry store more than a century ago in the exclusive Palais Royal section of Paris. The store can now be found in the famous Place Vendôme of Paris, as well as in major cities around the world. In 1988, descendant Alain Boucheron moved into the universe of fragrance to create jewelry for the senses. He combined the craftsmanship of the jeweler with the art of the perfumer to produce the fragrance—a scent designed to exude elegance, mystery, and allure, as a reflection of legendary Boucheron jewels.

The fragrance swirls in an oval ring-shaped bottle. The flacons are made in France, carved from rock crystal and ringed with golden orbs, called "gadroons." The fragrant ornament is crowned in deep blue Burmese sapphire. The lovely package echoes Boucheron jewelry designs of soft sculpted curves. In 1989, the fragrance industry honored Boucheron with two prestigious FiFi Awards, one for best packaging and one for best fragrance in its distribution category.

Boucheron...a beautiful, artistic marriage of French perfume and French jewelry.

Introduced	*1988*
Price	*Top range*

BOUDOIR

Scent Type	*Oriental - Green*
Composition	
Top Notes:	*Viburnum, marigold, orange blossom, orris*
Heart Notes:	*Red rose, cinnamon, coriander, cardamom*
Base Notes:	*Amber, vanilla, sandalwood, patchouli*

British fashion designer Vivienne Westwood entices with Boudoir—a pink-potioned Oriental concoction from Dragoco perfumer Martin Gras. The unusual use of viburnum, from the wayfaring tree, a shrub or tree of the honeysuckle family, achieves a rare balance between green, woody, and Oriental notes. English red roses warm to an ambery vanilla base that is as smooth as satin sheets. Boudoir is saucy and racy, a spark of surprise and delight.

The Fabrice Legros-designed bottle is cleverly crowned with Westwood's signature orb, a gold-colored, Saturn-ringed cap topped with a Celtic-styled cross. In intimate shades of rose, mauve, and pink, this beautiful scent belongs in any well-dressed lady's boudoir.

Introduced	*1998*
Price	*High range*

BOUQUET DE PROVENCE

Scent Type	*Floral - Fresh*
Composition	
Top Notes:	*Peach, lemon, black currant*
Heart Notes:	*Rose*
Base Notes:	*Oakmoss, cypress*

Bouquet de Provence is one of Frédéric Fekkai's Parfums de Provence collection and is based on his memories of the sunny south of France region from which Fekkai hails. Says Fekkai: "Bouquet de Provence represents all that is beautiful in Provence—heady afternoons strolling in a garden, bicycling along a country road, or resting in the cool shade of the terrace." Bouquet de Provence, a floral bouquet created by master perfumer Jacques Polge, is composed of the flowers and herbs that grow in profusion in the south of France. Delicate and enchanting, Bouquet de Provence is an enchanting feminine fragrance.

Presented in shades of French blue, with pewter-toned caps and terra cotta accents. Bouquet de Provence: Simply sublime.

Introduced	*1997*
Price	*High range*

BULGARI

Scent Type   *Floral*
Composition
  Top Notes: *Orange blossom, rosewood,*
                 bergamot, ylang-ylang
  Heart Notes: *Prelude rose, violet, mimosa,*
                 Sambac jasmine tea
  Base Notes: *Musk, vetiver, iris*

The signature scent from Italian jeweler Bulgari is a follow-up to Bulgari's Eau Parfumée. Bulgari is a modern floral developed around a jasmine tea note. It is a lovely "Let's do lunch" or evening-out scent. Bulgari is cultured and refined, with a whisper of Italian sensuality.

Thierry de Baschmakoff designed the understated packaging and the frosted, ellipsoidal bottle. The color theme is sunny Italian yellow, like the summer sun of Capri.

Introduced   *1994*
Price   *High range*

BULGARI EAU PARFUMÉE

Scent Type   *Floral*
Composition
  Top Notes: *Italian bergamot,*
                 Spanish orange blossom,
                 Ceylonese cardamom,
                 Jamaican pepper,
                 Russian coriander
  Heart Notes: *Bulgarian Rose, Egyptian jasmine*
  Base Notes: *Green tea, woods*

Famous Patrons
  Alec Baldwin   *Sharon Stone*

World-renowned jeweler Bulgari's first fragrance is Bulgari Eau Parfumée, a unisex formulation. The initial impression is fresh and fruity with zesty bergamot, quickly followed by soft notes of spicy coriander and pepper. After a few minutes, the fragrance develops into a warm floral heart of rose and jasmine. The lingering aroma is a soothing blend of florals with exotic woods and spices, plus an unusual component, the essence of green tea.

The history behind the fragrance revolves around Ming-Le, the philosophy of the Chinese tea ceremony. In Chinese, Ming-Le means "the joy of tea" and, according to Bulgari, denotes "honoring meditation, the time for a break" and "the respect of one's own rhythm," representing "a philosophy of life where understatement and discretion play a leading role." It is based on "the art of living, and the act of giving oneself pleasure, beauty, and joy." Tea symbolizes harmony and purity and is the important base note of the Bulgari fragrance.

The scent is presented in a curved rectangular flacon of pale green frosted glass, in recycled and biodegradable packaging.

The descendants of founder Sotirio Bulgari, an 1879 Greek immigrant to Italy, still manage the artisans who blend the elegant styles of the Mediterranean and Italian Renaissance into fine Bulgari jewelry, noted for its quality, volume, purity, and smoothness.

A footnote: In 1997 Bulgari launched Eau Parfumée Extrême, a concentrated version of Eau Parfumée. The difference? The original version is a 4% formulation, while the Extrême formula is a long-lasting 15% blend.

Introduced   *1993*
Price   *High range*

BURBERRY

Scent Type	Floral - Oriental
Composition	
Top Notes:	Lavender, mint, peach, marigold, bergamot, thyme, black currant bud, green apple
Heart Notes:	Geranium, jasmine, oakmoss, cedarwood
Base Notes:	Amber, tonka bean, sandalwood

British clothier Burberry of London is a prime purveyor of classy classics, well known for understated styles. Burberry is back with its eponymous scent—a sophisticated floral Oriental formulation by Creations Aromatiques. The fragrance is housed in a carton of scarlet and beige Burberry plaid; the classic, curved bottle is designed by Pierre Dinand. Burberry is a well-mannered perfume of impeccable pedigree, a metropolitan scent suitable for dashing 'round merry old London town.

Introduced	1997
Price	High range

BURBERRY TOUCH

Scent Type	Floral
Composition	
Top Notes:	Orange
Heart Notes:	Rose, peach, lily
Base Notes:	Vanilla, cedarwood

Burberry updates its image with Touch, a pink-tinted floral bouquet blended by Quest perfumers. Burberry has revamped its classic clothing and accessory line for the new millennium. Touch is a nod to the sumptuous, tactile fabrics used in the line.

The Touch bottle was designed by Fabien Baron and resembles an inverted shot glass, capped with dark wood. Tucked into beige Burberry plaid boxes, Touch is the ideal accompaniment to a bespoke British wardrobe.

Introduced	2000
Price	High range

BYBLOS

Scent Type	Floral - Fruity
Composition	
Top Notes:	Mandarin, grapefruit, cassie, marigold, bergamot, peach
Heart Notes:	Honeysuckle, gardenia, mimosa, ylang-ylang, lily of the valley, orchid, rose, heliotrope, violet, orris
Base Notes:	Musk, vetiver, pepper, raspberry

Imported from Milan, Byblos is a floral bouquet inspired by the magic of the Mediterranean and its ancient cultures. The memorable scent combines tangy fruits, fragrant florals, fresh greens, and light lingering woods.

Byblos is housed in a bottle of brilliant Mediterranean blue, and crowned with a carved apricot blossom.

Introduced	1992
Price	Mid-range

BYZANCE

Scent Type   Floral Semi - Oriental
Composition
    Top Notes: Citrus, cardamom, spices, greens,
                  mandarin, aldehydes, basil
    Heart Notes: Jasmine, tuberose, Turkish rose,
                  lily of the valley, ylang-ylang
    Base Notes: Sandalwood, vanilla, musk,
                  heliotrope, amber

Byzance is a 1980s creation from Parfums Rochas. Inspired by the meeting between Eastern and Western cultures, the semi-Oriental blend contains rare essences from around the globe.

The initial impression of Byzance is one of soft fruits and fresh aldehydes. Ephemeral and airy, it sets the stage for the delicate floral bouquet. The drydown notes are subtly rendered as refined sandalwood is blended with the tenacity of vanilla and musk. The result is an understated composition with a magnificent trail, that certain something that makes people turn and wonder, "What was she wearing?" Byzance is a tasteful fragrance, suitable for most any occasion, day to evening.

The round flacon, designed by In-House, draws heavily from Baroque art. The crystal decanter is the deepest Mediterranean blue, gilded with a seal that contains the name Byzance thrice sculpted in relief. A fuchsia ribbon encircles the slender neck. One of the most beautiful bottles we've seen, it echoes the opulence, femininity, and sensuality of the fragrance itself.

Introduced   1986
Price   *High range*

BYZANTINE

Scent Type   Floral - Oriental
Composition
    Top Notes: Freesia, mandarin, bergamot,
                  orange blossom
    Heart Notes: Mimosa, lily of the valley,
                  sweet pea, orange blossom,
                  heliotrope
    Base Notes: Sandalwood, vanilla, musk,
                  cedarwood

From France, Parfums Rochas introduces Byzantine, a romantic white floral composition. Fresh citrus fruits are blended with orange blossoms, while the heart sings with white flowers, reaching a bass crescendo with a final wooded accord of warmth and depth. Elegant and worldly, this sophisticated scent is housed in rounded flacons, emblazoned with Byzantine blue labels. A fine tribute to the brilliant Byzantine Empire.

Introduced   1995
Price   *High range*

CABOCHARD

Scent Type   Chypre - Floral Animalic
Composition
    Top Notes: Citrus, aldehydes, fruits, spices
    Heart Notes: Jasmine, rose, ylang-ylang, orris,
                  geranium
    Base Notes: Leather, tobacco, amber,
                  patchouli, musk, moss, vetiver,
                  castoreum

Famous Patrons
    Chynna Phillips

Originally introduced in 1959, the classic Cabochard from the Parisian House of Grès is a delightful chypre blend of citrus, mosses, and dry florals.

Grès was born Alix Barton and became known for her fluid designs that draped the body. Twice she had to close her salon doors during World War II, but in 1946 she reestablished the House of Grès, along with the fashions and the fragrances that remain with us today.

Legend has it that Grès had taken a trip through the Spice Islands and wished to re-create the olfactory experience. In response her perfumer, Omar Arif, produced a scent evocative of fresh island greenery, citrus, herbs, tobacco, and leather. The result was Cabochard, the essence of the Spice Islands.

Introduced	*1959*
Reintroduced	*1972*
Price	*Mid-range*

CABOTINE

Scent Type	*Floral - Green*
Composition	
Top Notes:	*Orange blossom, tangerine, ylang-ylang, peach, plum, greens, cassie, coriander*
Heart Notes:	*Ginger lily, iris, hyacinth, tuberose, rose, carnation, jasmine, heliotrope*
Base Notes:	*Sandalwood, black currant bud, musk, vanilla, amber, cedarwood, civet, vetiver, tonka bean*

From the House of Grès, Cabotine is a green floral harmony with dominant notes of ginger and ginger lily. Delicate florals are balanced with fruity top notes and sensual spicy base notes. Subtle, fresh, and long-lasting.

The exquisite bottle is wreathed with frosted emerald glass flowers and topped with a similar green floral stopper echoing the green fragrance notes. A beautiful flacon, it is destined to be a collector's item.

Wonder what the name means? Cabotine is French for "mischief."

Introduced	*1990*
Price	*Mid-range*

CAESARS WOMAN

Scent Type	*Floral - Ambery*
Composition	
Top Notes:	*Orange blossom, geranium*
Heart Notes:	*Egyptian jasmine, rose, iris*
Base Notes:	*Tibetan musk, sandalwood, patchouli*

Famous Patrons
Carol Channing

From Caesars Merchandising for Caesars Palace hotel and casino comes Caesars Woman, an exotic spicy floral that rests on a bed of precious woods. Introduced by the team of Jim Roth and David Horner, who helped bring the world Giorgio, Caesars Woman is a dramatic, long-lasting scent, designed to evoke the carefree privileged life in ancient Rome. It is ideal for alluring days and opulent evenings.

The fragrance was launched at a celebrity-packed gala that included George Burns, Carol Channing, and models clad as Roman gladiators. Henry Gluck, Caesars chairman of the board, says, "Like everything else we do, we have been careful to create a product which bears the elegance and style associated with our resorts."

Caesars says the fragrance bottle is a "derivative of Lalique and Baccarat styles, imported from France." The scent is packaged in a rich marbleized box, accented with black and gold-colored Roman motifs.

Glamorous. Sexy. As the company states, "The most sensuous fragrance since Caesar invented pleasure." Let the games begin.

Introduced   1987
Price   Mid-range

CALANDRE

Scent Type   Floral - Aldehyde
Composition
    Top Notes: Greens, aldehydes, bergamot
    Heart Notes: Rose, jasmine, lily of the valley,
                   geranium, orris
    Base Notes: Sandalwoods, vetiver, oakmoss,
                   amber, musk

Famous Patrons
    Barbara Bush

Calandre is a classic fragrance from Spanish designer Paco Rabanne, who has dressed stars such as Jane Fonda and Raquel Welch. Barcelona native and Compar president Dr. Fernando Aleu brought together the magic of Paco Rabanne and the Puig family fragrance company to create Calandre. The fragrance is a floral blend with cool greens and mossy woods, fresh, clean, and casual. When it was introduced, it was a shocking departure from heavy, sweet, sensual fragrances of the past, ushering in a new age of fresh, natural scents.

Calandre is French for "the grille of a car" and is intended to signify the modern woman's mobility. Rabanne explains: "Women today are on the move, traveling near and far to pursue careers of every endeavor. What could be a better

symbol of this than the grille of a car?" Of a Ford Model-T, to be exact. This theme is carried through to the bottle, a sleek, modern design of glass and chrome from the talented team of Paco Rabanne and Pierre Dinand. The bottle is a stylized rendition of the grille and the New York United Nations building, selected to symbolize international appeal and cooperation.

Sisters, start your engines.

Introduced   1969
Price   High range

CALÈCHE

Scent Type   Floral - Aldehyde
Composition
    Top Notes: Bergamot, lemon, aldehydes,
                   neroli
    Heart Notes: Gardenia, ylang-ylang, jasmine,
                   rose, iris
    Base Notes: Sandalwood, oakmoss,
                   cedarwood, vetiver, amber, musk

Calèche is a classic floral aldehyde from Hermès, endowed with subtle French floral essences of rose and jasmine languishing on a bed of sweet woods and mosses. Hermès describes Calèche as "vibrant and luminous," a clean fragrance developed for the woman of timeless charm and classic style.

Calèche is housed in a clear glass flacon of simple elegance and wrapped with a yellow silk bow. It is presented in a vibrant spring yellow box, embellished with the proud gold-colored symbol of the House of Hermès, a stately horse-drawn carriage, or calèche, which was the most elegant of nineteenth-century carriages.

Introduced   1961
Price   High range

CÂLINE

(See also Jean Patou Collection)

Scent Type   *Floral - Fresh*
Composition
   Top Notes: *Greens, aldehydes, mimosa,*
                 mandarin, bergamot, basil
   Heart Notes: *Iris, orange blossom, patchouli,*
                 moss, coriander
   Base Notes: *Musk, amber*

Câline debuted in 1964, the year of *My Fair Lady* and the beginning of the Beatles craze. The French house of Patou dedicated this creation to youthful women to celebrate their entrance into society. Câline is a light scent, suitable as a teenager's first serious fragrance, or for the professional woman who wants an ethereal, understated fragrance with a classic pedigree.

Introduced   1964
Price   Mid-range

CANDIE'S

Scent Type   *Floral - Oriental*
Composition
   Top Notes: *Mandarin, bergamot, peach,*
                 grapefruit
   Heart Notes: *Pink peony, violet, ylang-ylang,*
                 lily of the valley
   Base Notes: *Patchouli, black pepper,*
                 sandalwood

Initially, the Candie's brand burst onto the 1970s scene with sexy, high-heeled mules in screaming colors. Now, three decades later, Candie's revives a quirky brand of seventies funk with its patchouli-based scent, wrapped in bright neon shades of yellow and orange. Candie's is a contradiction: a sharp, bright, fruity opening evolves into a flirty, sensual base of woods and spice. Therein lies plenty of zip and zest for energetic teens. Trendy and hip, a fragrance for fun, for kicking back and letting loose.

Introduced   1999
Price   Mid-range

CAROLINA HERRERA

Scent Type   *Floral*
Composition
   Top Notes: *Orange blossom, apricot,*
                 rosewood, bergamot, greens
   Heart Notes: *French and Spanish jasmine,*
                 Indian tuberose, hyacinth,
                 honeysuckle, narcissus,
                 ylang-ylang, lily of the valley
   Base Notes: *Amber, moss, sandalwood,*
                 cedarwood, vetiver, musk, civet

Couture designer Carolina Herrera received inspiration for her signature fragrance from her garden in Caracas, Venezuela. She says, "It was a combination of tuberose and jasmine, which has a very appealing, uncomplicated, and very feminine fragrance...quite elegant and memorable." She describes the brilliant floral with fruity accents as "jasmine fireworks."

Compar President Fernando Aleu, a medical doctor, says Herrera's fragrance was developed after a chance meeting between the two when he complimented her on the scent she was wearing. He asked what it was and she replied: "It has no name. I make it." Aleu and Herrera then set about duplicating the scent with the assistance of the Puig fragrance company.

The fragrance packaging is uplifting; black polka dots on a white background are wrapped with bright yellow "ribbons." Created by Barcelona designer Andre Ricard, it suggests an Art Deco influence. Why polka dots? Herrera explains: "They are reminiscent of the dresses that some dancers wear in Seville. They are visually attractive and happy. In a way, they have become sort of a trademark of my fragrance, and I love them." She's right. Polka dots always give us happy feet.

Introduced   1988
Price   High range

CARTIER
(See Must de Cartier, Panthère, So Pretty)

CASHMERE MIST

Scent Type   Floral - Fresh
Composition
    Top Notes: Bergamot
    Heart Notes: Jasmine, lily of the valley
    Base Notes: Sandalwood, vanilla, amber,
                      musk

Famous Patrons
    Actress Jennie Garth

Fashion designer Donna Karan indulges her desire for luxury with the warmth of Cashmere Mist, a subtle, intimate scent. "Cashmere is the most sensual way to embrace skin," explains Karan. Designed for luxurious use, Cashmere Mist suggests a sueded snuggle in whisper-soft pashmina.

Karan favors highly touchable, tactile fabrics for her clothing designs, from supple suedes and to caressing cashmere. Cashmere Mist captures the aromatic sense of these materials, embodying their sumptuous qualities with a formula of natural ingredients. Voluptuously curved bottles of frosted glass heighten the sensory experience.

Wrapped in shades of creamy beige and white, this is a line to pack for the spa. Canyon Ranch Spa, anyone? Should be on my speed dial.

Introduced   1994
Price   High range

CASMIR

Scent Type   Oriental - Fruity
Composition
    Top Notes: Peach, mango, coconut,
                      bergamot, hesperides
    Heart Notes: Jasmine, lily of the valley,
                      geranium
    Base Notes: Vanilla, amber, sandalwood,
                      patchouli, castoreum, musk

Arriving on the international market is Casmir, a fruity Oriental fragrance from Parfums Chopard. Casmir is described as a fruity Oriental with gourmet ingredients that sound like a feast on a tropical Asian isle. The initial impression is of succulent fruits, evolving into a floral treasure trove. The dominant base note is vanilla, while sandalwood and musk complete the Eastern influence. Soft and smooth as cashmere.

The reach of India envelops Casmir, from the exotic fragrance to the Taj Mahal-inspired bottle. A burgundy lotus flower embellishes the bottle, which is shaped like a graceful lotus flower resting amidst colored packaging of wine red and black.

Casmir is an enchanting fragrance to pack for your next trek through Kashmir and Tibet...or simply close your eyes and let your daydreams whisk you away on the aroma of Casmir.

Introduced   1994
Price   Top range

CASSINI

Scent Type   Chypre - Fruity Floral
Composition
  Top Notes: Mandarin, freesia, osmanthus
  Heart Notes: Jasmine, Bulgarian rose, tuberose,
                        chrysanthemum, carnation
  Base Notes: Mousse de chêne, amber, oakmoss

Cassini is a smooth blend of natural ingredients from Parisian couturier Oleg Cassini. He explains: "This fragrance is my effort to synthesize all that the most beautiful women in my long career did for me. It is a tribute to their beauty and their charm." He calls it "a love affair that never ends" and describes it as having "soft power...not an American blast." The scent is subtle and sophisticated, light enough to be worn even on sultry days and balmy nights.

Oleg Cassini has a rich and fascinating history. He was born a count in Paris; his grandfather was the Russian ambassador to the United States. After apprenticing with Patou in Paris, he embraced Hollywood, dressing countless movie stars for the studios, including Lana Turner, Rita Hayworth, Bo Derek, Victoria Principal, Angie Dickinson, and ex-fiancée Grace Kelly. He has been credited with many design accomplishments, such as the sheath, the A-line, and the military look for women. His White House designs for Jacqueline Kennedy won him international acclaim. But his life is not all work. He is a Doctor of Fine Arts and an accomplished sportsman: Cassini is a 10 handicap golfer, a former top-ranked tennis player and an avid skier. He also competes in professional harness racing, a demanding and dangerous sport. He shares highlights from this exciting life in his 1987 autobiography, *In My Own Fashion*.

One of our favorite stories is that of Oleg Cassini's screen debut, in the 1950 film *Where the Sidewalk Ends*. He played a couturier with leading lady Gene Tierney, who also happened to be his leading lady in real life. He had but one brief line, yet his exquisite touch was seen throughout the film, for he designed the costumes and gowns that his wife wore...the fashions that made him famous the world over. And now he spoils us again, with Cassini the fragrance.

Introduced   1990
Price   Mid-range

CATALYST

Scent Type   Floral
Composition
  Top Notes: Jonquil, tuberose, otto of rose,
                        jasmine absolute, galbanum
  Heart Notes: Black currant bud,
                        lily of the valley, violet,
                        chamomile, herbs
  Base Notes: Vetiver, sandalwood, patchouli,
                        oakmoss, musk

Catalyst is a fragrant creation from the house of the late fashion designer Halston. The potent feminine scent is said to have been created for the woman who has the "ability to cause a reaction, in whatever world she claims as her own."

Halston once commented: "Fashion doesn't stop with clothes. It's a total image...including the fragrance a woman wears. I'm committed to helping evolve that image." Indeed he did, during his many years at the forefront of fashion.

This full-bodied floral bouquet is blended with fragrant woods for a warm, lingering aura. The essence of jonquil is used as the basis of the fragrance, a rare choice because its essence is difficult to distill.

Catalyst is presented in fluid glass flacons, similar in line to a flowing Halston evening gown.

Introduced   1993
Price   High range

CE SOIR OU JAMAIS

Scent Type   Floral
Composition
     Notes: Turkish rose, florals

Ce Soir ou Jamais, French for "tonight or never," is an expansive floral composition from Annick Goutal, and sadly, the last fragrance she personally introduced. The dominant impression of Ce Soir ou Jamais is Turkish rose, or *R. damascena*, yet in actuality, this complex perfume is made up of 160 floral essences.

The packaging for Ce Soir ou Jamais is a departure from the classic Goutal bottles. Brosse created a bottle styled after the cinched pouches frequently used in Goutal's line. Ce Soir ou Jamais is presented in a tasseled hatbox of rich, velvet burgundy. A beautiful idea for thoughtful gift-giving, or for personal indulgence.

Introduced   1999
Price   Top range

CERRUTI 1881

Scent Type   Floral
Composition
     Top Notes: Bergamot, violet, mimosa, freesia
     Heart Notes: Jasmine, orange blossom, geranium, coriander, rosewood, chamomile
     Base Notes: Sandalwood, musk, ambrette

Cerruti 1881 Pour Femme is an elegant floral from Italian fashion designer Nino Cerruti. There is also a man's version, Cerruti 1881 Pour Homme.

An accord that the company describes as "linen *enfleurage*" is embedded within the floral heart, lending a crisp, natural texture to the feminine composition. Captured in a curved, frosted flacon with a marbleized cap in pale coral, Cerruti is both chic and understated.

Introduced   1995
Price   High range

CERRUTI IMAGE

Scent Type   Green
Composition
     Top Notes: Grapefruit, green leaves, black pepper
     Heart Notes: Carbon
     Base Notes: Amber, birch wood, blond wood, leather

Italian designer Nino Cerruti found success with his airy men's version of Cerruti Image. For the woman seeking to update her image, Cerruti envisioned an earthy green fragrance with a spicy accent, developed by Firmenich. A versatile, well-balanced scent with a focus on naturals, Cerruti Image Woman is perfect for active lifestyles.

Designer Thierry de Baschmakoff created the women's presentation, a sleek, clear bottle with a silver-colored cap.

Cerruti Image—for the urban pioneer woman with a busy schedule. Sisters, synchronize your date books.

Introduced   2000
Price   High range

C'EST SI BON

Scent Type   Floral
Composition
    Top Notes: Violet leaves, rose
    Heart Notes: Jasmine, ylang-ylang,
                lily of the valley, plum
    Base Notes: Sandalwood, musk, woods

C'est Si Bon Pour Femme is a floral bouquet, as pretty and fresh as Paris in the spring. C'est Si Bon translates from French as "it's good," or "it's great!" Such exuberance is evident in the feminine floral. Violet and rose burst from the opening accord. A rounded heart of white flowers conveys a sunny disposition, while sandalwood tempers the final impression on the skin.

C'est Si Bon's bottle brings a smile to the face. The bottle is a replica of the Eiffel Tower. We discovered C'est Si Bon firsthand in Paris—that is, in the Paris Hotel and casino in Las Vegas. For men, try C'est Si Bon Pour Homme.

Introduced   2000
Price   Mid-range

CHALDÉE

(See also Jean Patou Collection)

Scent Type   Oriental
Composition
    Top Notes: Orange blossom, hyacinth
    Heart Notes: Jasmine, narcissus, opopanax
    Base Notes: Amber, spices

Famous Patrons
    Suzanne Lenglen

Chaldée is a 1927 Jean Patou fragrance that derives its name from the country of Sumer in Babylonia, where beautiful golden-skinned women once lived.

Inspired by the new outdoor sports of the 1920s, tennis and swimming, French couturier Patou designed Chaldée so that the richness of florals, spices, and amber would be amplified by the sun's warmth. The women at Deauville and the Riviera embraced it, as did tennis champion Suzanne Lenglen. Why not wear it to Wimbledon?

Introduced   1927
Price   Mid-range

CHAMADE

Scent Type   Floral Semi - Oriental
Composition
    Top Notes: Greens, galbanum, bergamot,
                hyacinth, aldehydes
    Heart Notes: Rose, jasmine, lilac, clove
    Base Notes: Vanilla, amber, benzoin,
                sandalwood, vetiver

Famous Patrons
    Princess Grace of Monaco
    Audrey Hepburn   Catherine Deneuve
    Phyllis Diller   Glenn Close

Fifth-generation perfumer Jean-Paul Guerlain formulated this modern classic for the contemporary woman, the bewitching woman of strength, confidence, and liberation. Chamade features green top notes, a spicy floral heart, and a semi-Oriental base of soft woods.

Chamade was created in 1969, partly inspired by Françoise Sagan's novel of the same name. Chamade has dual meaning in French: "the drumbeat of surrender" and "the wild beating of the heart." And according to our dictionary, chamade is a trumpet or drum signal sounded for retreat or parley, discussion, or truce. The bottle resembles an upside-down heart and was supposedly inspired by a woman who turned hearts upside down. Obviously, the woman was a handful....

The long-lived House of Guerlain has created memorable scents that reflect the nature and mood of their times. Guerlain has endured from the Romantic period of the 1800s, through the Napoléonic Empire, the Third Republic, La Belle Époque, World War I, and the Roaring Twenties. During World War II, the factory was twice bombed and abandoned. Guerlain overcame adversity to rebuild and prosper, and remain current with changing styles.

Guerlain suggests Chamade for "an audacious and radiant woman...feminine, seductive, dynamic, and sensual."

Introduced   1969
Price   High range

CHAMPAGNE
(YVRESSE)

Scent Type   Floral - Fruity
Composition
    Top Notes: Nectarine, mint, anise
    Heart Notes: Blue rose, otto rose, litchi
    Base Notes: Oakmoss, vetiver, patchouli

From Parisian couturier Yves Saint Laurent comes Champagne, a sparkling gay concoction of fruits and florals. It is said to be an effervescent mix of "daring and tradition...refined and timeless."

Champagne is corked in a bubbly flacon accented by hammered gold and corkwire, and stored in a black and gold-colored box lined in scarlet red.

Yves Saint Laurent Couture president Pierre Berge commented on the history behind Champagne, reporting that the rights to the name Champagne were acquired from Parfums Caron, the company that registered rights to the name in 1942. However, a French court ruled that Champagne is a name reserved for wine and can't be used for perfume. Saint Laurent was ordered to pay damages to the major Champagne wine makers. As a result, the fragrance is marketed under the name Yvresse in Europe.

À vôtre santé!

Introduced   1993
Price   High range

CHAMPS-ÉLYSÉES

Scent Type   Floral - Fresh
Composition
    Top Notes: Mimosa leaves, rose, herbs, almond flower, cassis berries and leaves
    Heart Notes: Mimosa, buddleia blossom
    Base Notes: Almond bark, amber, hibiscus seeds

Guerlain stakes a prime piece of Parisian real estate with its launch of Champs-Élysées, a modern fresh floral with the intriguing essence of a new mimosa accord. Of the name, Guerlain president Christian Lanis explains: "Our first fragrance came from a factory established in 1828 just paces away from the Arc de Triomphe. Later, Guerlain moved its headquarters to Paris' most chic boulevard, 68 avenue des Champs-Élysées."

Feminine and versatile, Champs-Élysées is a scent that moves with ease from the office to high tea to a spontaneous evening out. A brushed gold-colored carton with pink accents encases the clear flacon, an angular, curvilinear creation that evokes the incomparable *joie de vivre* of Paris.

Introduced   1996
Price   High range

CHANEL NO. 5

Scent Type   *Floral - Aldehyde*
Composition
   Top Notes: *Aldehydes, Grasse jasmine*
   Heart Notes: *Rose, ylang-ylang, iris*
   Base Notes: *Amber, patchouli*

Famous Patrons
   Kate Moss   *Catherine Deneuve*
   Marilyn Monroe   *Andrea Marcovicci*
   Carole Bouquet

Chanel No. 5 was the first fragrance from Parisian couturier Gabrielle "Coco" Chanel, who was one of the first designers to introduce a perfume. According to Chanel, the secret behind Chanel No. 5 is an extraordinary blend of aldehydes—ingredients that defy categorization—combined with rich floral and warm amber notes. A classic fragrance with an effervescent personality, it is versatile enough to be worn for a variety of occasions, winter through summer. Or take a tip from Marilyn Monroe—when the press once asked what nightwear she wore to bed, she smiled and answered, "Chanel No. 5."

With a reputation as one of the world's most sophisticated, elegant fragrances, Chanel No. 5 has been known for years as the epitome of luxury, in keeping with Chanel's fashion vision of simple elegance. But what inspired the numeric name? Chanel once reported that when she asked Ernest Beaux to create a fragrance for her, he presented her with several scents, and she selected the bottle numbered "5." Coincidentally, her couture collection was scheduled for presentation on the fifth day of the fifth month—May 5. Interpreting this as a good omen, she bestowed upon the fragrance the name of Chanel No. 5 and placed it in a sleekly modern bottle. And so, Chanel entered the fragrance industry. Indeed, it was the popularity of the early Chanel fragrances that spawned the designer fragrance industry of today.

And the flacon? Pure and minimal, with pared-down polish in classic rectangular Chanel bottles. As the company states, "True elegance stems from subtlety."

Introduced   1921
Price   High range

CHANEL NO. 19

Scent Type   *Floral - Green*
Composition
   Top Notes: *Greens, galbanum, bergamot*
   Heart Notes: *Jasmine, may rose, iris,*
                     ylang-ylang
   Base Notes: *Sandalwood, oakmoss, vetiver*

Famous Patrons
   Coco Chanel   *Catherine Deneuve*
   Christie Brinkley

Chanel No. 19 was Coco Chanel's personal fragrance, said to have been named, partly, after her birth date of August 19. The fragrance opens with fresh green floral notes, tempered with fragrant mosses and aromatic woods. Chanel No. 19 is a spirited, easy-to-wear scent.

Chanel's designs changed women's fashion forever. From humble beginnings, she founded her first store in Deauville, France, in 1912, and went on to stamp her style throughout the twenties and thirties with the little black dress, bobbed haircuts and a profusion of oversize costume jewelry.

She closed her operation when World War II broke out. After a long hiatus the House of Chanel opened its doors again in 1954, and at the age of 71 she introduced the straight collarless suit that today is synonymous with Chanel.

Coco Chanel's life and romantic liaisons were as remarkable as her designs. She lived to see her life chronicled in a 1969 Broadway musical, *Coco*.

The Chanel company describes Chanel No. 19 in terms that were also applicable to Mademoiselle Chanel, as she was known, who died in 1971: "Forever young, intensely feminine, contemporary, brilliant, witty, outspoken, supremely confident, and completely independent." A lovely, lasting tribute to one of the world's most memorable women.

Introduced   1972
Price   High range

CHANEL NO. 22

Scent Type
  Floral
Composition
  Notes: *White roses, jasmine, tuberose, lily of the valley, lilac, orange blossom*

Famous Patrons
  Catherine Deneuve

Gabrielle "Coco" Chanel designed Chanel No. 22, a melange of white flowers, to shimmer like Champagne bubbles, a small ray of light as the world sank toward the darkness of the Depression. The floral symphony complemented her couture line, known as the White Look, designs

that celebrated the resurgence of joy, romance, and femininity.

No. 22 is a fresh, light blend of delicate florals, soft and sensuous. Decidedly feminine. Roses, jasmine, and orange blossoms dominate the profusion of white flowers. It is an ideal fragrance for daytime and long warm evenings with a special someone.

No. 22 is representative of Chanel's view of style, as she once explained: "In perfume, as in fashion, simple understatement is pure elegance."

Introduced   1928
Price   High range

CHANT D'ARÔMES

Scent Type   *Chypre - Floral*
Composition
  Top Notes: *Mirabelle, gardenia, aldehydes, fruits*
  Heart Notes: *Rose, jasmine, honeysuckle, ylang-ylang*
  Base Notes: *Benzoin, musk, vetiver, heliotrope, moss, olibanum*

Famous Patrons
  Lynn Redgrave   *Shirley Bassey*

Chant d'Arômes, meaning "song of scent" in French, is a light, playful scent designed by Jean-Paul Guerlain. The company says it was created "for the debutantes of life as a first perfume." A floral chypre fragrance, it was partly inspired by poet Saint-John Perse, who "dreamed of an isle greener than dreams." Guerlain imagined the aromas that might be found on such an idyllic island, and the result was Chant d'Arômes, a fragrance of innocence and tenderness, a scent of eternal youth. True to his vision, Chant d'Arômes opens with island-fresh fruits, followed by a spicy floral heart and sweet balsamic background notes tinged with fresh moss.

The House of Guerlain was a court-appointed perfumer to many of the royal courts of Europe. From Queen Victoria of England to Empress Eugénie of France, Queen Isabella of Spain to Empress Sissi of Austria, Guerlain fragrances have graced world's most fashionable and influential women of the last two centuries—as well as those of today. Even the unforgettable Sarah Bernhardt commissioned her own Guerlain scent during the height of La Belle Époque.

Chant d'Arômes is available only in a light eau de toilette. Ideal for daytime, warm weather, office, or anytime a discreet, refined scent is desired.

Introduced	*1962*
Price	*Mid-range*

CHANTILLY

Scent Type	*Oriental - Ambery*
Composition	
Top Notes:	*Fruits, lemon, bergamot, neroli*
Heart Notes:	*Jasmine, rose, orange blossom, spices, ylang-ylang, carnation*
Base Notes:	*Indian sandalwood, moss, vanilla, musk, leather, tonka bean, benzoin*

Chantilly is a classic French blend of florals, Oriental woods and spices with a sweet amber finish, created by Paul Parquet for Houbigant. Chantilly shares its name with the picturesque French town, the pastoral site of championship Thoroughbred horse racing.

Introduced	*1941*
Price	*Top range*

CHLOÉ

Scent Type	*Floral*
Composition	
Top Notes:	*Honeysuckle, orange blossom, hyacinth, ylang-ylang, lilac*
Heart Notes:	*Tuberose, jasmine, narcissus, carnation, orris, rose*
Base Notes:	*Amber, sandalwood, oakmoss*

Chloé is a long-lasting floral bouquet, an enduring modern floral created by designer *extraordinaire* Karl Lagerfeld for the couture House of Chloé. "I love to create fragrance, and Chloé was my first love," he says.

The vivid scent dissolves into a distinctive, delightful floral blend. The sweet notes of tuberose and jasmine are particularly apparent. Chloé is for those who want a heady, entrance-making floral fragrance. A superbly lingering fragrance, you'll still be able to detect it the next morning. Lovely for cool, elegant evenings.

Chloé is packaged in feminine shades of soft peach of frosted glass. The perfume is crowned with a sculpted calla lily stopper, a creation that won the 1975 FiFi Award for packaging from The Fragrance Foundation. Try the rich bath and body products, too. "The bath," says Lagerfeld, "is still one of life's best extravagances." Absolutely.

Introduced	*1975*
Price	*Mid-range*

CHLOÉ NARCISSE

Scent Type   Floral - Oriental
Composition
    Top Notes: Living orange blossom, apricot,
       living red plumeria, marigold
    Heart Notes: Jasmine, rose otto,
       living narcissus, spices
    Base Notes: Sandalwood, vanilla absolute,
       musk, tolu balsam

Famous Patrons
    Queen Elizabeth II

Chloé Narcisse is the younger sibling to the original Chloé fragrance from the Parisian House of Chloé. It consists of a lush bouquet of exotic flowers, touched by tropical fruits and seductive spices for rich, full-bodied allure. A fruity top note introduces the fragrance, which dissolves into an Oriental composition of exotic florals and provocative spices. Chloé Narcisse is a fresh, dramatic blend.

The fragrance is said to have been inspired by a storybook romance between a young woman and her lover. The advertising campaign features passages that are supposedly from her diary, chronicling the sweet affair.

Packaging reflects the romantic, passionate scent; the flacon is a fluid sinuous shape cloaked in vivid tones of citrine green, purple, red and white. A citrine green stopper is the crowning centerpiece.

Introduced   1992
Price   High range

CHRISTIAN LACROIX

Scent Type   Floral
Composition
    Top Notes: Tangerine, neroli, coriander,
       hyacinth, seringa
    Heart Notes: Jasmine, narcissus, lily,
       heliotrope, nasturtium
    Base Notes: Sandalwood, incense, musk,
       moss, vetiver

French couturier Christian Lacroix sought to re-create his fond childhood memories of seashore visits and yuletide celebrations in Provence.

A designer known for his elaborate, detailed designs, Lacroix offers a scent that is a rich, baroque floral, with discreet accents of incense, nutmeg, and clove. The lush, elegant theme is communicated through vibrant red packaging. Sure to delight the eye, the reclining, seashell-shaped flacon made of *Biot* bubble glass was fashioned by a local Provençal artist.

A sensual, full-bodied fragrance of warmth and allure, the scent is ideal for special occasions or, perhaps, a romantic Christmas Eve stroll through the snowy streets of Paris.

Introduced   2000
Price   Top range

CIARA

Scent Type   Oriental - Ambery
Composition
    Top Notes: Vanilla, sandalwood, patchouli,
       cedarwood
    Heart Notes: Herbaceous spices
    Base Notes: Frankincense, balsam, myrrh,
       raspberry

Ciara is a spicy Oriental blend designed to make a bold statement. Dramatic, sweet, and long-lasting, Ciara is not for the shy of heart.

Revlon co-founder Charles Revson created the assertive Ciara for his wife, Lynn. Inspired by Greek and Roman goddesses, Ciara was conceived to typify the "eternal woman." Though the packaging has been revamped, the gold-colored goddess remains on the bottle.

Ciara is also available in three fragrance concentrations: 80, 100, and 200. Think of it as "proof," with 200 being the most potent formula next to the perfume. This system is unique to Ciara.

Reserve the enticing Ciara for strong impressions and cool weather wear.

Introduced	*1973*
Price	*Mid-range*

CINNABAR

Scent Type	*Oriental - Spicy*
Composition	
Top Notes:	*Tangerine, orange blossom, clove, peach, bergamot, spices*
Heart Notes:	*Jasmine, rose, carnation, ylang-ylang*
Base Notes:	*Amber, patchouli, incense, vanilla, vetiver, benzoin, tolu*

Cinnabar is a spicy Oriental fragrance from Estée Lauder. Opening citrus notes add a fresh lift to the sultry, exotic scent.

All Lauder fragrances are closely guarded family secrets. It is said that Estée Lauder always added the final two to five percent of the ingredients to the end of the formula personally, so as to ensure secrecy. One whiff of the balsamic Cinnabar potion and you can just imagine Lauder meticulously measuring those last drops.

Introduced	*1978*
Price	*Mid-range*

CK BE
♀♂

Scent Type	*Oriental*
Composition	
Top Notes:	*Bergamot, mandarin, mint, lavender, juniper berry*
Heart Notes:	*Peach, magnolia, spices*
Base Notes:	*White musk, tonka bean, sandalwood, opopanax*

With his unisex scent CK Be, American fashion designer Calvin Klein advises us to just be. The scent is made up of fruits and spices, with a dominant strain of white musk threaded throughout the composition. Youthful, edgy, and sensual, CK Be is housed in a matte black flask with a silver inscription, suggesting strength and vitality.

Introduced	*1996*
Price	*Mid-range*

CK ONE
♀♂

Scent Type	*Citrus*
Composition	
Top Notes:	*Bergamot, papaya, pineapple, cardamom*
Heart Notes:	*Hedione high cis*
Base Notes:	*Green tea, amber, musk*

The blockbuster scent of Generation X, CK One is the gender-free brainchild of fashion designer Calvin Klein. The unisex scent is a citrus blend with a green tea accord and an unusual heart of hedione high cis, an aromatic material likened to jasmine.

A frosted flask with a silvery screw-on cap houses the pale yellow fragrance. Approachable price points and open-sell displays helped send sales of CK One into orbit. CK One—a scent as perennial as blue jeans.

Introduced   1994
Price   Mid-range

CLAIRE DE NILANG

Scent Type   Floral - Fruity
Composition
  Top Notes: Freesia, coriander, bergamot,
                  kumquat
  Heart Notes: Acacia, cassie, pepper
  Base Notes: Sandalwood, hibiscus, vanilla

Claire de Nilang is a fresh, lighthearted addition to the Lalique Parfums family. The fragrance is composed of sheer flowers, sweet fruits, spices, and woods for added depth and stability. The green note of coriander is reflected in the packaging, with its soft, leafy shades of green. The bottle is a swirl of femininity topped with a green floral cap. A sheer fragrance, Claire de Nilang is lovely for a languid midsummer's eve.

Introduced   1998
Price   Top range

COCKTAIL
(See also Jean Patou Collection)

Scent Type   Chypre - Fruity
Composition
  Top Notes: Greens, bergamot, citrus
  Heart Notes: Jasmine, rose
  Base Notes: Oakmoss

Cocktail is a witty, refreshing splash of citrus fruits and oakmoss, a classic chypre combination.

Created in 1930 by French couturier Jean Patou, it was inspired by the art of original mixing. Crisp and easy to wear, day through evening, Cocktail is a glamorous retro scent enjoying a new lease on life. It's a clever scent to wear with your little black cocktail dress. Anyone for a martini, mimosa, or cosmopolitan?

Introduced   1930
Price   Mid-range

COCO

Scent Type   Floral - Oriental
Composition
  Top Notes: Peach, coriander,
                  Comoros Island orange blossom
  Heart Notes: Spice Island clove bud,
                  Caribbean cascarida,
                  French angelica, Bulgarian rose,
                  Indian jasmine, mimosa,
                  frangipani
  Base Notes: Mysore sandalwood, amber,
                  leather

Famous Patrons
  Gwyneth Paltrow   Vanessa Paradis
  Catherine Zeta-Jones

Coco was created in honor of couturier Gabrielle Chanel. Colleagues called her "Mademoiselle," but her dearest friends knew her as "Coco." The scent that bears the affectionate nickname is said to embody "the spirit of Chanel...a microcosm of youth, desire, daring, sensuality, force, and fragility."

A warm spicy fragrance, Coco develops around a major amber chord. Mellow fruits, heady florals, and exotic spices are balanced against woods and leathers, creating a rich, smooth balsamic blend. Artfully composed, it is as flamboyant as it is understated. Coco is a dramatic, classy fragrance that can be worn for a variety of occasions and seasons. It is wonderful for career days that stretch into elegant evenings, and is equally at ease in long black velvet or the barest of sundresses on a Mediterranean cruise.

The perfume comes in the familiar rectangular flacon favored by Chanel, while other strengths are sold in sleek black and gold-colored lacquered bottles that pack and travel well.

As Coco Chanel once said, "Elegance is not possible without fragrance."

Introduced　　　*1984*
Price　　　*High range*

COLONY
(See also Jean Patou Collection)

Scent Type　　　*Chypre - Fruity*
Composition
　　Top Notes:　　*Pineapple, bergamot*
　　Heart Notes:　*Ylang-ylang, iris, carnation, opopanax*
　　Base Notes:　*Oakmoss, leather, musk, vetiver, vanilla*

In 1938, the debonair French couturier Jean Patou introduced Colony, a fragrance inspired by early French colonial holdings with sun-drenched ports, lush vegetation, exotic spices, and tropical sands. Imagine Catherine Deneuve in the film classic, *Indochine.*

Voluptuous fruits and jungle flowers are combined with woods and leathery notes to produce a chypre composition. Such blends are characterized by the marriage of fresh citrus and velvety moss, and are classic, easy to wear fragrances.

In the 1930s and 1940s, Colony was a favorite bon-voyage gift for many a high sea journey. Why not reminisce, and pack the retro-glamour Colony for your next summer cruise?

Introduced　　　*1938*
Price　　　*Mid-range*

COMPTOIR SUD PACIFIQUE COLLECTION

From France, the firm of Comptoir Sud Pacifique specializes in simple yet elegant fragrances, inspiring the loyalty of many customers. Established in 1976 by Pierre Fournier, the company specializes in tropical scents. One of its most popular fragrances is Vanille, a soothing, sweet bend of Tahitian vanilla. As in all Comptoir Sud Pacifique fragrances, the emphasis is on scents that are rich and true to life.

Once your eyes rove over those shiny aluminum bottles, you'll find it difficult to stop with just one. If you like vanilla, try these on for size: Vanille-Café, Vanille-Amande, Rose-Vanille, and Vanille-Abricot (that's not a misspelling—it's French, you know). Other house favorites include Turquoise, Opoponax, Harmonie Creole, Fruits Savages, and Pamplemousse, which is one of Michelle Pfeiffer's favorites. Then there are Tiare, Thè, Amour de Cacao, Chensylang, Motu, and Cristal de Musc. Men's favorites include Vetyver Haiti, L'Homme, Eau des Tropiques, and Barbier des Iles.

The perfect touch with sarongs and sandals—pack a couple for your next lazy holiday. After all, how can you love just one?

Introduced　　　*1975*
Price　　　*High range*

CONTRADICTION

Scent Type   *Floral - Ambery*
Composition
    Top Notes: *To-yo-ran orchid, eucalyptus,*
        pepper flower, seringa
    Heart Notes: *Jasmine, peony, rose,*
        lily of the valley
    Base Notes: *Tonka bean, sandalwood,*
        tambouti, satinwood

Calvin Klein's Contradiction is a modern floral with ambery Oriental notes, a scent with a sexy, cosmopolitan attitude. The composition is a contradiction in terms: A very modern, almost masculine theme with sharp, precise, aromatic accords is blended with fragrant, feminine florals. Eucalyptus and pepper flower occupy the opening accord, classic florals make up the middle accord, and exotic woods complete the final accord. The ultramodern packaging is by bottle designer Fabien Baron, a brushed aluminum sheath that covers three-quarters of the bottle. Very cool, very Calvin Klein.

Introduced   *1997*
Price   *High range*

COOL WATER WOMAN

Scent Type   *Floral - Marine*
Composition
    Top Notes: *Citrus, pineapple,*
        honeydew melon,
        black currant bud
    Heart Notes: *Water lily, lotus blossom, jasmine,*
        rose, lily of the valley, quince
    Base Notes: *Sandalwood, peach, amber, orris,*
        mulberry, vetiver

Cool Water for men dates back to 1984 and has enjoyed a long run on the bestseller list. Cool Water Woman is a highly anticipated companion to the aromatic men's version from Lancaster. Perfumer Pierre Bourdon created both formulas.

Cool Water Woman is housed in an ocean-blue bottle, styled after a *culot*, a mineral water bottle. One cool customer, this soft floral composition is built around aquatic, botanical, and ozonic notes. It is enhanced with fresh fruits, a heart of marine notes, and a tropical rainforest base. Reportedly inspired by natural bodies of water, such as the languid pools of Kauai, the lakes of Scotland, and the warm waters of the South Pacific.

An excellent choice for daytime and sportswear, Cool Water Woman is designed to remind one of a day at the beach, of sultry sunshine and the gentle lapping of waves. After all, it was launched in the Cote d'Azur.

Introduced   *1996*
Price   *Mid-range*

CORIANDRE

Scent Type   *Chypre - Floral*
Composition
    Top Notes: *Coriander, aldehydes,*
        orange blossom, angelica
    Heart Notes: *Rose, geranium, lily, jasmine, orris*
    Base Notes: *Sandalwood, vetiver, musk,*
        oakmoss, patchouli

A classic French fragrance from Jean Couturier, Coriandre is an enchanting blend of rich rosy florals, warm woods, and sultry spices. Literally translated, Coriandre refers to a highly fragrant, sweet and slightly peppery herb of the parsley family, in Latin, *coriandrum sativum*. Presented in malachite green cartons with gold-colored accents.

Reminds us of a Linda McCartney tune, "Coriander, coffee too...I'm the cook of the house." But this is one spicy number that may keep you out of the kitchen.

Introduced   1977
Price   Mid-range

CRÉATION

Scent Type   Chypre - Fresh
Composition
  Top Notes: *Black currant bud, mango, passion fruit, peach, bergamot, lemon, mandarin, galbanum*
  Heart Notes: *Gardenia, jasmine, tuberose, narcissus, rose, ylang-ylang, carnation, lily of the valley*
  Base Notes: *Amber, oakmoss, musk, sandalwood, patchouli, vanilla, civet*

The original fragrance from designer Ted Lapidus is Création, a fresh chypre that opens with citrusy bergamot and green notes. A light floral heart follows, set against a warm woody backdrop of oakmoss, amber, and lingering musk.

Born in Paris in 1929, Ted Lapidus launched his women's designs in the 1960s with the unisex and menswear looks. At first a men's designer, he dressed industrialists and heads of state, including President Harry Truman, then went on to suit up women such as Brigitte Bardot. Today his boutiques dot the globe.

Introduced   1985
Price   High range

CREED COLLECTION

AMBRELLE CANELLE
Semi - Oriental (♀♂)
BOIS DE CÉDRAT
Citrus (♀♂)
EPICÉA
Fougère (♀♂)
FANTASIA DE FLEURS
Floral
FLEURISSIMO
Floral (see Fleurissimo)
FLEURS DE BULGARIE
Floral
IMPÉRATRICE EUGÉNIE
Floral
IMPÉRIAL MILLÈSIME
Marine (♀♂)
ORANGE SPICE
Fougère (♀♂)
ROYAL DELIGHT
Semi - Oriental
ROYAL ENGLISH LEATHER
Chypre (♀♂)
ROYAL WATER
Fougère (♀♂)
SANTAL IMPÉRIAL
Oriental (♀♂)
SILVER MOUNTAIN WATER
Marine (♀♂)
SPRING FLOWER
Floral
TABARÔME
Semi - Oriental (♀♂)
TUBEREUSE INDIANA
Floral
VANISIA
Oriental

VETIVER
Chypre (♀♂)
ZESTE MANDARINE
Citrus (♀♂)

The House of Creed dates from 1760, when founder James Henry Creed established his firm in London. Soon Creed fragrances were accepted into the inner circles of society, including the French, Spanish, English, and Austro-Hungarian courts. In 1854, the House of Creed moved to Paris and continued to flourish under the tutelage of Creed descendents. Today, more than two hundred fragrances later, sixth-generation master perfumer and president Oliver Creed proudly carries on the family business. Creed custom designs scents for the firm's private clientele, and offers thirty-two specialty fragrances to the public. (We've included a partial list, just to get you started.) All fragrances are handmade using a traditional infusion technique.

Creed's custom commissions remain exclusive to the client for five years, then the fragrance may be sold to the public. So who has indulged their fragrant passions? Fleurissimo was created for Princess Grace of Monaco's wedding day, Spring Flower was blended for Audrey Hepburn, and Impérial Millésime went to the King of Saudi Arabia. Royal English Leather was made for King George III, Orange Spice was created for Oscar Wilde, Tabarôme was made for Winston Churchill, and Royal Water was being developed for Diana, Princess of Wales, before she died. Custom blends require four to six months of labor, and start at about $20,000.

Creed eaux de toilette and eaux de parfum are housed in classic Creed signature bottles of varying hues, while the cartons carry the Prince of Wales crest.

Creed: Fragrances for discriminating women and men.

Introduced   Since 1760
Price   Top range

CRISTALLE

Scent Type   Chypre - Fresh
Composition
  Top Notes: Greens, mandarin, lemon, basil, bergamot, galbanum, lavender
  Heart Notes: Rose, hyacinth, honeysuckle, jasmine, peach, lily of the valley, ylang-ylang, iris, mosses
  Base Notes: Woods, santal, musk, fruits, sandalwood, oakmoss

Cristalle is a fresh, fruity chypre blend that was originally developed as a single-strength eau de toilette to be lavished all over the body. In addition to the eau de toilette, a new strength was introduced in 1993, a richer eau de parfum version with a few changes.

"A respect for one's roots and an attachment to the origins of Cristalle were the foundation of the new scent," says Jacques Polge, director of the Chanel Perfume Laboratories.

The eau de toilette version of Cristalle has a tangy top note of lemon, more citrus, and brighter green herbal notes. It is a light energetic scent, perfect for sporty summertime wear. The eau de parfum is a richer composition with a few twists. Fruity mandarin replaces zesty lemon, jasmine is emphasized while greens and herbs are de-emphasized, mellow lily of the valley is added, and iris and woods are increased for new warmth and depth.

Both versions are dynamic fragrances that remind us of Mademoiselle Chanel, whose unconstructed clothing designs were suitable for sporting activities—a radical concept in the early part of the century. These exhilarating, exuberant scents are the perfect mates to the Chanel sportswear lines of yesterday and today.

Introduced   1977
Price   Mid-range

CUIR DE RUSSIE

Scent Type   *Chypre - Floral Animalic*
Composition
    Top Notes: *Orange blossom, bergamot,*
        mandarin, clary sage
    Heart Notes: *Iris, jasmine, rose, ylang-ylang,*
        cedarwood, vetiver
    Base Notes: *Balsamics, leather, amber,*
        vanilla

Cuir de Russie is a 1993 reintroduction of an elegant 1920s fragrance from Chanel. Introduced in conjunction with two other twenties scents, Gardénia and Bois des Îles, Cuir de Russie is reminiscent of a glamorous bygone era.

Cuir de Russie, or "Russian leather," is a vibrant leathery floral composition by master perfumer Ernest Beaux, enhanced by a lingering balsamic aura of woods, amber, and vanilla. An inviting chypre classic; the perfect accent for a special evening at New York's Russian Tea Room restaurant.

Look for Cuir de Russie in Chanel Boutiques.

Introduced   *1927*
Reintroduced *1993*
Price   *Mid-range*

CURVE

Scent Type   *Floral - Fresh*
Composition
    Top Notes: *Grapefruit, mandarin,*
        ylang-ylang, dewberry, bergamot
    Heart Notes: *Pink peony, water lily, orchid,*
        freesia, rose, cassis
    Base Notes: *Musk, iris, cedarwood,*
        sandalwood, mahogany,
        violet wood

The Liz Claiborne company is committed to staying ahead of the curve with its new fragrance for women. Curve for Women is a fresh, fruity floral that appeals to the young and hip generation.

Curve is presented in silvery, apothecary-style bottles with apple-green accents, packaged in matching reusable tins. And for the man in your life, there's Curve for Men.

Introduced   *1996*
Price   *Mid-range*

DAZZLING GOLD

Scent Type   *Floral - Fruity*
Composition
    Top Notes: *Passion flower, fig*
    Heart Notes: *Orchid, plumeria*
    Base Notes: *Amber, vanilla, sandalwood, woods*

Dazzling Gold is one of a dazzling duo of scents introduced by Estée Lauder in 1998. An alchemist's delight, the fragrance is as rich as liquid gold. The rich floral mixture is composed of intense white flowers and smooth woods. Like a fiery golden sunset, Dazzling Gold is warm and radiant.

Introduced   *1998*
Price   *Mid-range*

DAZZLING SILVER

Scent Type   *Floral - Green*
Composition
    Top Notes: *Wild lotus, sunshine flower, lily,*
        greens, purple vanilla orchid
    Heart Notes: *Passion flower, rose, sunset orchid*
    Base Notes: *Ginger, amber, mahogany*

Dazzling Silver represents the other fragrant element of the Dazzling equation from Estée Lauder. Exotic flowers, such as passion flower and orchid, rest upon a bed of woods and spice. A green note adds a sharp, bright contrast to the tenacious floral composition, like a shimmery veil of platinum silk cast over a floral bouquet.

| Introduced | 1998 |
| Price | Mid-range |

DECI DELÀ

Scent Type Composition	Floral - Fruity
Top Notes:	Freesia, raspberry, peach, melon, boronia
Heart Notes:	Hazelnut, freesia, May rose
Base Notes:	Cypress, patchouli, myrrh, tonka bean, oakmoss

From Nina Ricci, the French firm that brought us L'Air du Temps, comes Deci Delà, a French saying that means "Now here, now there."

Frisky fruited notes are reflected in the sherbet colors of the opalescent bottles: raspberry, peach, and cherry. Matte gold-colored shoulders and caps complete the playful arrangement. A casual, lighthearted scent for the young and young at heart, Deci Delà is ideal for a sun-kissed holiday on the French Riviera.

| Introduced | 1995 |
| Price | High range |

DELICIOUS

Scent Type Composition	Floral
Top Notes:	Narcisse, mimosa, mandarin, boronia, neroli, black currant bud
Heart Notes:	Rose, jasmine, tuberose, lily of the valley, ylang-ylang, angelica
Base Notes:	Sandalwood, patchouli, musk, orris

Famous Patrons

Jackie Collins	Jill St. John
Barbra Streisand	Barbara Walters
Raquel Welch	Shirlee (Mrs. Henry) Fonda
Shakira (Mrs. Michael) Caine	

Gale Hayman, creator of the original Giorgio fragrance, brings forth Delicious, a floral fragrance of classic proportion.

Gale Hayman reports: "When I tried this fragrance on my friends, they all said it was delicious. Delicious named itself. Very feminine, Beverly Hills energy, glamour, a bit sexy, yet classic and elegant at the same time." How does this uplifting floral scent compare with Giorgio? "Delicious represents the maturing of my sensibility, my sense of style," she says. "Giorgio is the energy of the eighties. Delicious is a classic, durable fragrance of the nineties, the Giorgio of our time."

Hayman worked with a French perfumer to create the scent, using almost entirely natural ingredients. Created in a subtle fashion with an opening accord of soothing fruits and gentle florals, Delicious develops an intense heart of rare flowers, including rose and jasmine, ylang-ylang, and tuberose. The symphony is underscored by sensual musk and woods, and highlighted by orris, one of the most expensive and treasured ingredients in perfumery. Orris absolute is obtained from iris and has an aroma remarkably close to that of violets in bloom. The resulting composition is refined, elegant, understated, yet very long-lasting and sensual. In fact, in December, 1993 *Consumer Reports* magazine ranked it third out of sixty-six fragrances they tested for quality and integrity.

The fragrance is captured in Hayman's signature reclining leopard bottle, meant to represent sensual, powerful grace—then swathed in peach to reflect the softer scent. Enjoy Delicious for sophisticated days and alluring evenings. It is, indeed, Delicious.

Introduced	*1993*
Price	*Mid-range*

DESIGN

Scent Type	*Floral - Fruity*
Composition	
Top Notes:	*Peach, orange blossom, jasmine, tuberose*
Heart Notes:	*Gardenia, lilac, honeysuckle, carnation*
Base Notes:	*Black currant bud, musk, sandalwood, civet*

Famous Patrons
   Artist Sara Eyestone

Design is a white floral bouquet from Paul Sebastian. Dominant notes of orange blossom, lilac, gardenia, and musk create a soft, feminine effect. A company spokesperson says Design was created to personalize itself to the wearer, drying down differently on each individual according to body chemistry. Some people may detect more florals, while others may experience a fruity aroma, or perhaps even a powdery finish—it's unique to you.

Introduced	*1986*
Price	*High range*

DESTINY

Scent Type	*Floral - Fresh*
Composition	
Notes:	*Calla lilies, white rose, fo-ti-tieng, osmanthus, karo karunde, white orchid, narcissus*

Destiny is an ethereal floral fragrance from Marilyn Miglin of Chicago, who also offers a fine line of cosmetics and skin treatments.

Her mother, Helen, and her daughter, Helena, join Marilyn Miglin in the business. A trio of brainy beauties, the women are glamorous, sophisticated, and accomplished. Destiny reflects the qualities these women share. The light, sparkling fragrance is created with pure white flowers, essences known for their "calming, energizing, and aphrodisiac qualities," says Miglin—essences of inspiration, confidence, and inner harmony.

In perfumery, the fragrance strength of a flower and its color are related. The lighter the blossom, the more fragrant. Therefore, white flowers such as those used in Destiny are among the most prized for their fragrance.

Miglin speaks of her inspiration for Destiny: "I was in Switzerland in 1984, vacationing with my family. We were in a hot-air balloon slowly drifting over the Alpine mountains. The white flowers on the mountaintops portrayed a pure, beautiful and serene energy against the clear blue sky. They sparked in me a sense of awe and wonderment about being alive. I decided that there had to be a perfume that captured that ethereal quality and it should be called Destiny."

Even the bottle is designed to reflect an "upward movement of energy," says Miglin. In this vein, Miglin has established a mentorship program for women, called Women of Destiny. The women selected serve as mentors to others. She explains, "I believe the best way for women to make that journey is by helping other women achieve their destinies." For more information, contact the Marilyn Miglin offices in Chicago.

Introduced   1990
Price   Mid-range

DIONNE

Scent Type   *Oriental - Ambery*
Composition
    Top Notes: *Rose, bergamot, orange blossom*
    Heart Notes: *Rose, jasmine, lily of the valley,*
        patchouli, sandalwood,
        cedarwood
    Base Notes: *Moss, amber, vanilla, musk,*
        benzoin, tonka bean

Famous Patrons
    Dionne Warwick
    Talent agent Joan Mangum
    Lyricist Carol Conners
    Designer Kathleen Baughman

Singer Dionne Warwick hadn't planned on launching her own fragrance when she asked Linda Marshall, president of Elysee Scientific Cosmetics, to help her create a fragrance. "I simply wanted my own distinctive perfume," she says. Warwick and Marshall worked together to create Dionne, a scent that Marshall says is the very essence of Warwick. Next, Warwick gave samples to her close friends at her birthday party and the scent turned out to be a hit. At Christmas she surprised her friends with signed crystal flacons of her fragrance, and suddenly she found herself in the perfume business.

It's not surprising that along with her hit records she now has a hit fragrance, for she worked with the perfumer the way she creates music—combining notes to create unique fragrance chords.

The sumptuous Oriental bouquet carries an unusual top note, created from the finest floral essences. The green floral heart is enhanced by sweet mossy amber, the lingering aromatic theme.

Warwick advises lavish use of the heady fragrance: "Wearing perfume is like loving. You can't be stingy. You have to give yourself abundantly, not just a little here and there."

Introduced   1986
Price   Mid-range

DIORELLA

Scent Type   *Chypre - Fresh*
Composition
    Top Notes: *Sicilian lemon, greens, basil,*
        Italian bergamot, melon
    Heart Notes: *Moroccan jasmine, rose,*
        carnation, cyclamen
    Base Notes: *Oakmoss, vetiver, musk,*
        patchouli

Diorella is an ethereal chypre blend from Christian Dior. Diorella splashes on with cool citrus and greens, followed by radiant light florals and a mossy base. The fragrance is a superb example of the classic citrus-moss chypre blend, so named after the Mediterranean island of Cyprus where many of the ingredients are found.

Christian Dior apprenticed in Paris at the atelier of Robert Piguet before opening his own salon in 1946. His timing was perfect, and his feminine New Look collection of swirling skirts, tiny waists, and glamorous gowns became the rage in postwar Paris. Dior's classic suits set the trend in the fifties until his death in 1957. The reins then passed to a twenty-one-year-old named Yves Saint Laurent, who headed the company until 1960 when he left to serve in the Algerian war. Today the House of Dior still leads the way with artful creations in fashion and fragrance.

Introduced   1972
Price   High range

DIORESSENCE

Scent Type   Oriental - Spicy
Composition
   Top Notes: Aldehydes, greens, fruits
   Heart Notes: Jasmine, geranium, cinnamon,
                carnation, tuberose, ylang-ylang,
                orris
   Base Notes: Patchouli, oakmoss, vetiver,
                benzoin, vanilla, musk, styrax

Dioressence is a sophisticated Oriental blend of florals and spices from the House of Christian Dior, a voluptuous, opulent fragrance for women of confidence. Dioressence is beautiful for cool symphony evenings under a layer of mink or cashmere.

Introduced   1980
Price   High range

DIORISSIMO

Scent Type   Floral - Fresh
Composition
   Top Notes: Greens, bergamot, calyx
   Heart Notes: Lily of the valley, jasmine, lilac,
                boronia, rosewood, ylang-ylang
   Base Notes: Sandalwood, civet

Famous Patrons
   Naomi Campbell   Amanda Harlech

The second fragrance (after Miss Dior) introduced by Christian Dior was Diorissimo. The dominant note is the light, ethereal essence of lily of the valley. Diorissimo is a delicate floral, very feminine, fresh, innocent, and romantic, stylish and mannered in the Dior tradition.

Master perfumer Edmond Roudnitska, who is said to have relied upon dreamlike springtime images to create Diorissimo, developed the serene fragrance. He described Diorissimo, saying, "This is a pure lily of the valley scent that also has the odor of the woods in which it is found and the indefinable atmosphere of springtime." Thus the airy, celestial quality of the fragrance. Always right, never overpowering.

Introduced   1956
Price   High range

DIVA

Scent Type   Chypre - Floral
Composition
   Top Notes: Mandarin, ylang-ylang,
                Indian tuberose, cardamom,
                bergamot, coriander, aldehydes
   Heart Notes: Honeyed Moroccan rose,
                Turkish rose, Egyptian jasmine,
                Florentine iris, narcissus,
                carnation, orris
   Base Notes: Patchouli, ambergris, oakmoss,
                sandalwood, vetiver, musk, civet,
                honey

Diva is a rich chypre blend from high fashion designer Emanuel Ungaro. The fragrance opens with fresh fruit tones, followed by rosy floral notes underscored by exotic woods. Indulgent, romantic, and sensual—a diva embodied.

Emanuel Ungaro worked under Balenciaga and Courrèges before opening his own business in Paris in 1965. Today he is known for his use of vivid color and soft fluid lines in designs that are sophisticated and elegant, as mirrored in his fragrance packaging. In fact, the Diva bottle is fashioned after an Ungaro dress, featuring soft drapes that meet in the center of the flacon.

Introduced   *1983*
Price   *High range*

DIVINE FOLIE
(See also Jean Patou Collection)

Scent Type   *Oriental - Ambery*
Composition
     Top Notes: *Neroli, ylang-ylang*
     Heart Notes: *Orange blossom, styrax, iris, rose,*
                      jasmine, vetiver
     Base Notes: *Musk, vanilla*

Rich, intense, warm, and subtle: French couturier Jean Patou used these words to describe Divine Folie, his 1933 fragrance named after the excessive parties thrown despite the depths of the Great Depression.

Patou wanted the perfect accompaniment to the long white satin and silk bias-cut dresses he designed to fit svelte women like a second skin. Seemingly simple, such a gown often required two to three fittings to achieve such simplicity. Patou created the bias-cut dresses in response to Chanel's little black cocktail dress, a style he reportedly found boring. The flowing, sensual style soared when Woolworth heiress Barbara Hutton selected one for her religious ceremony wedding gown for

her first marriage to Prince Alexis Mdivani. She bought thirty-five other ensembles from Patou for her trousseau, and purchased many of his designs over the years.

Hutton befriended Patou and his assistant, café society woman Elsa Maxwell, and the threesome attended one another's parties—their own *divine folies*—around the globe, from Paris to Biarritz to Morocco.

Divine Folie—after all these years, it's still ready for a grand party.

Introduced   *1933*
Price   *Mid-range*

DKNY

Scent Type   *Floral*
Composition
     Notes: *Orange, vodka*

Donna Karan teamed with beauty pros at Estée Lauder to produce her third fragrance for women. Following fragrances Donna Karan and Cashmere Mist comes DKNY. A hip scent with a New York attitude, DKNY is cutting-edge, or as Karan explained, "a hit of energy." The bar is open, with an unlikely impression of orange and vodka that splashes from the urban bottle. For Manhattan moods and skyscraper style, have a swig of DKNY.

Introduced   *2000*
Price   *High range*

DNA

Scent Type Floral - Ambery
Composition
Top Notes: Rosewood, minty geranium, ylang-ylang, bergamot
Heart Notes: Jasmine, lily of the valley, tuberose, clove, osmanthus
Base Notes: Myrrh, oakmoss, sandalwood, vetiver, vanilla, benzoin, amber

Famous Patrons

Daisy Fuentes	Aretha Franklin
Julia Roberts	Cameron Diaz
Bo Derek	Nancy Wilson

DNA Perfume is the creation of internationally celebrated designer Bijan. DNA incorporates the initials of his children, Daniela, Nicolas, and Alexandra. Certainly gene-inspired. Bijan states, "The sexy type of attitude is about reality and family."

DNA Perfume, which the company describes as a "floramber naturelle," begins with the mellowness of rosewood, quickly followed by tangy bergamot and geranium. The fragrance evolves to a feminine floral bouquet resting amidst a subtle earthy blend of greens, spices, and amber. A soft, romantic and sensual fragrance that ultimately responds to—what else?—your personal deoxyribonucleic acid, or DNA.

The fragrance is packaged in a bottle shaped like intertwined spiral strands of DNA. Bijan enthuses: "Our senses remind us we are alive. Celebrate!"

Introduced 1993
Price Top range

DOLCE & GABBANA

Scent Type Floral - Oriental
Composition
Top Notes: Tangerine, basil, ivy, freesia, petitgrain
Heart Notes: Bulgarian rose, marigold, lily of the valley, orange blossom, red carnation, jasmine, coriander
Base Notes: Sandalwood, tonka bean, vanilla, musk

The signature fragrance from the fiery, dynamic Italian design team, Domenico Dolce and Stefano Gabbana. Dolce & Gabbana is a smooth floral Oriental blend, with spirited top notes of tangerine and freesia. It was honored with the 1993 International Award from the Italian Accademia del Profumo for best women's fragrance.

Dolce and Gabbana had a hand in the overall package design, a composition in hues of deep ruby red and velvety gold. The bottle is a study in right angles, from the rectangular glass flask to the gold-colored collar and crowning stopper. Finally, the entire ensemble is swathed in red velvet.

Dolce and Gabbana designs are attracting the attention of some of the world's most interesting women. Isabella Rossellini and Sherilyn Fenn happily agreed to appear in Dolce and Gabbana ads, while Madonna rang them for help with her 1993-94 Girlie Show tour costumes. Dolce and Gabbana complied, and Madonna and her dancers pranced through the show wearing many of their designs.

Dolce and Gabbana say they created the scent with strong-willed women in mind and that they drew their inspiration from Italian actresses Sophia Loren, Gina Lollobrigida, and Anna Magnani. Beautiful, strong-willed women indeed.

Introduced 1993
Price Top range

DOLCE VITA

Scent Type   Floral - Fresh
Composition
   Top Notes: Lily, rose, magnolia
   Heart Notes: Peach, apricot, cinnamon
   Base Notes: Heliotrope, sandalwood, vanilla

Perfume is an art, and most artists create works that reflect their times. Once again, the French house of Christian Dior is in sync with the times with Dolce Vita. A fragrance of joy and delight, its name means "sweet life" in Italian. Dolce Vita reflects the celebratory mood prevalent at the end of the twentieth century—an age of dawning hope for the new millennium.

Dior perfumer Maurice Roger and Fragrance Resources perfumer Pierre Bourdon created this versatile, easy-to-wear fresh floral composition. Serge Mansau designed the bottle, which is a study in circles, from the rounded flacon to the circular, dimple-dotted facets that sparkle in candlelight. Of course, in *la dolce vita*, everyone kisses by candlelight. But you knew that, didn't you, darling? Dolce Vita: An inspiring, uplifting, life-affirming fragrance.

Introduced   1996
Price   High range

DONNA KARAN

Scent Type   Floral
Composition
   Top Notes: Casablanca lily, apricot
   Heart Notes: Rose, cassia, ylang-ylang,
                          jasmine, heliotrope
   Base Notes: Suede, amber, sandalwood,
                          patchouli

Leading trade magazine *Beauty Fashion* reports that this signature scent is based on a few of Donna Karan's favorite things: "Casablanca lilies, the warmth of cashmere, and the skin scent of suede." The fragrance was born of a three-year collaboration between Karan and her husband. She calls it a sexy day-to-evening scent, designed for subtle sophistication. Soft Oriental chypre notes of leathery suede, amber, and patchouli accent the predominantly floral composition.

Karan's husband and business partner, artist-sculptor Stephen Weiss, designed the black bottle that is destined to be a collector's item. The swirls reflect the graceful silhouette of a woman's form, and hand-painted 24-karat gold accents match the gold-colored tea paper packaging. Weiss says, "The bottle is a gift to my wife, to women, to today, and to life."

Introduced   1992
Price   Top range

DOULTON

Scent Type   Floral - Oriental
Composition
   Top Notes: Melon, plum
   Heart Notes: Lily of the valley, narcissus, lily
   Base Notes: Sandalwood, amber, musk,
                          patchouli

The Royal Doulton history begins in 1815, when John Doulton established a pottery business in England. By 1901, King Edward VII had granted a royal warrant to the company, enabling the use of the name Royal Doulton. Today, the firm produces a variety of luxury goods, most notably fine china and crystal—its Royal Albert "Old Country Roses" bone china is one of the world's best-selling patterns.

Doulton is a modern fragrance with an Old World lineage. It is composed of rich florals, brightened by the modern freshness of melon and plum, rife with the ripe warmth of an English summer day. Wooded base notes speak of tradition and elegance. Doulton is a refined fragrance with top-drawer breeding.

It is only natural that a company so well versed in the art of presentation would offer a fragrance in tastefully designed, timeless packaging. Drawing inspiration from the deep sapphire blue of the Royal Doulton "Oxford Blue" china pattern, the sparkling, Brosse-designed, rounded bottle rests in a satiny package of the richest blue. The Royal Oxford design is embossed on the silver-colored cap, upon which is inscribed Sir Henry Doulton's signature, in his flowing nineteenth-century script.

Expertly rendered, Doulton is a smooth, mannered scent of classic proportions, a luxury suitable for feminine daytime wear as well as the most romantic of evening occasions. Have it packed for your English country estate visits, milady.

Introduced   1998
Price   High range

DREAMS
(See Sui Dreams)

DUENDE

Scent Type   Floral
Composition
    Top Notes: Bergamot, melon, linden, mandarin
    Heart Notes: Mimosa, ylang-ylang, jasmine
    Base Notes: Sandalwood, thyme, cedarwood

Duende is a floral symphony from Spanish fashion designer Jesus del Pozo. Duende, Spanish for "soul of a women," is a feminine fragrance with soft, fruited notes. The curved bottle fits easily in the hand, while the spiraling stopper is reminiscent of perfume flacons from the early part of the twentieth century. *¡Que bonita!*

Introduced   1994
Price   High range

DUNE

Scent Type   Floral - Marine
Composition
    Floral Notes: Lily, wallflower, peony
    Marine Notes: Amber, broom, lichen

Dune hails from the house of acclaimed French couturier Christian Dior. Dior describes Dune as a floral oceanic, or marine blend, a relatively new olfactory category. The effect is fresh and natural—ideal for summer, daytime, sports, or anytime a light soothing scent is desired.

The House of Dior says Dune is "the perfume of serenity [that] tells the story of woman and nature intermingled...a place for serenity, meditation, and harmony." A haven from stress, Dune is described as an understated composition with natural roots, like flowers strewn on the sand. And in an environmental effort, Dior donated $350,000 to the Nature Conservatory Foundation, for its "Protect the Dunes" program.

The fragrant concoction is housed in a fluid apricot-hued flacon tucked inside a box of Persian orange, the color of the sun setting over sand dunes.

Introduced   1992
Price   Mid-range

E BY HRH
PRINCESS ELIZABETH

Scent Type   *Floral*
Composition
   Top Notes: *Mandarin, bergamot,*
                lily of the valley
   Heart Notes: *Orange blossom, jasmine, iris,*
                hyacinth
   Base Notes: *Amber, myrrh, musk, vanilla,*
                woods

In 1941, when Her Royal Highness Princess Elizabeth was four years old, her family, the royal family of Yugoslavia, was forced into exile after a military *coup d'état* during the Nazi invasion. The youngest daughter of Prince Paul and Princess Olga, Princess Elizabeth found herself in an unusual position. She had been brought up to serve a country, but as an exile she had no country to serve. For years she trotted the globe, living in Greece, London, Peru, and finally New York. She married and had three children: actress Catherine Oxenberg, who appeared on *Dynasty*, writer Christine Oxenberg, and son Nicholas, a businessman. At last, her heritage caught up with her, and she returned to her roots on a mission of service. In 1990, she founded the Princess Elizabeth Foundation to raise funds for Yugoslavian relief efforts.

Her cherished memories of her grandmother, the Grand Duchess Helen of Russia, or Elin as she was known, prompted Princess Elizabeth to create a fragrance in her honor, which she entitled simply E. Based on her grandmother's custom formula, the princess re-created the scent, a spirited white floral composition. A touch of sweet mandarin enlivens the bouquet, while sensual undertones of amber and myrrh add elegance.

The result? E is a scent of history, mystery, and romance—a scent to stir the soul.

The princess collaborated with Merv Griffin to produce the elegant line. She makes frequent appearances on television's QVC channel. A percentage of the profits is donated, through her foundation, to relieve suffering in her war-torn homeland. There the princess personally oversees the distribution of medical goods and other aid. Since the success of E, Princess Elizabeth has introduced a second fragrance called Mon Ange, a sheer, white floral.

The lovely Princess Elizabeth is indeed a woman of grace, courage, and talent.

Introduced   *1997*
Price   *Mid-range*

EAU DE CAMILLE

Scent Type   *Floral - Green*
Composition
   Notes: *Honeysuckle, ivy, grass, seringa*

Famous Patrons
   Andrea Marcovicci

Created by Renaissance woman Annick Goutal—former concert pianist and model, and accomplished perfumer.

This fragrance was named in honor of her daughter, Camille. One day her daughter opened a window in their home in France, and Goutal was inspired by the scents wafting through, the smell of ivy and vines and fresh-cut grass, of honeysuckle and other fresh florals. This spirited green floral is available in a light eau de toilette and a concentrated eau de toilette.

For a true delight, visit the Goutal boutique on the rue de Castiglione in Paris' elegant Seventh

Arrondissement. Goutal said of her creative endeavor: "Nature and all her wonders guide me. Emotions find expression in fragrance. Fragrance is the music of my dreams. Fragrance is my inspiration."

Introduced   1986
Price   High range

EAU DE CHARLOTTE

Scent Type   Floral - Fruity
Composition
    Notes: Mimosa, black currant bud,
                  cocoa, lily of the valley

A warm, mellow blend of fruits and florals, Eau de Charlotte is a delightful, easy-to-wear fragrance, available in several strengths.

Eau de Charlotte is packaged in curved, ribbed glass flacons crowned with gold-colored caps. The concentrated eau de toilette and perfumes are housed in rounded opaque bottles, topped with Goutal's signature golden butterfly. For women on the go, some natural sprays and butterfly bottles are presented in a gold lamé purse.

Introduced   1986
Price   High range

EAU DE COLOGNE DU COQ
♀♂

Scent Type   Citrus
Composition
    Top Notes: Hesperides, lemon,
                  bergamot, neroli
    Heart Notes: Lavender, jasmine, patchouli
    Base Notes: Moss, sandalwood

Eau de Cologne du Coq hails is a creation of the Guerlain empire founder, Jacques Guerlain. This century-old classic is a dry, crisp citrus splash. Available only in cologne, it is packaged in the distinctive "bee bottle," a flacon created in honor of the Napoléonic court.

Eaux de cologne are often classified as "hesperides," meaning that they are made from the fruit of citrus trees. We found a romantic history behind the term, too. In Greek mythology, Hesperides were garden nymphs who guarded the wedding gift of golden apples from Gaea to Hera. Hesperia was also the ancient Greek name for Italy and the Roman name for Spain.

Most of these hesperides, or citrus eaux de cologne, are worn by both sexes. They are perfect for sporty active wear, hot humid days, or high-pressure offices.

Introduced   1894
Price   Mid-range

EAU DE COLOGNE IMPÉRIALE
♀♂

Scent Type   Citrus
Composition
    Top Notes: Hesperides, orange blossom,
                  bergamot, neroli, lemon
    Heart Notes: Lavender
    Base Notes: Rosemary, tonka bean, cedarwood

Famous Patrons
    Empress Eugénie   Cary Grant
    Paul Newman   Marcello Mastrionni
    Sir Alec Guiness   George Segal
    President Ronald Reagan

Eau de Cologne Impériale is a timeless, invigorating citrus scent that has been used by men and women for well over a century. The citrus blend is lightened with orange blossom and minty rosemary. A stimulating, subtle blend, it can be worn anytime.

As the name suggests, Eau de Cologne Impériale is a fragrance of royalty. Master perfumer Pierre-François-Pascal Guerlain, the founder of the House of Guerlain, created the fragrance for the Empress Eugénie and placed it in a flacon known as the "bee bottle" to honor the Empire. The bee was a symbol of the Royal Court and of the industriousness of the Second Napoléonic Empire. Today, the French imperial crest is still prominently displayed on the bee bottle.

Empress Eugénie was born in Spain and became the wife of the second Louis Napoléon, also known as Napoléon III. Noted for her beauty, she favored fragrances from the House of Guerlain and gowns from the House of Worth. Due to her patronage and enjoyment of fine fragrances, the House of Guerlain made rapid advances among its well-to-do clientele. Eau Impériale remains one of the most enduring fragrances of our time. It is available in cologne and eau de toilette.

Introduced   1853
Price   Mid-range

EAU DE GIVENCHY

Scent Type   Floral - Fruity
Composition
    Top Notes: Bergamot, spearmint, tagetes,
                    greens, fruits
    Heart Notes: Jasmine, lily of the valley, rose,
                    cyclamen, orris
    Base Notes: Musk, cedarwood,
                    sandalwood, moss

Eau de Givenchy is a light, fresh floral created by the House of Givenchy for a youthful clientele. The mild floral bouquet is accented with greens and fruits. Available only in an eau

de toilette, it is perfect for active summer days and nights.

Hubert de Givenchy was just twenty-five years old when he opened his own couture salon in Paris 1952. His clean, youthful lines garnered immediate praise. Today, the House of Givenchy continues its women's couture, along with fragrance, ready-to-wear, menswear, accessories, and other innovative ideas.

Introduced   1987
Price   Mid-range

EAU DE GUERLAIN

Scent Type   Citrus
Composition
    Top Notes: Lemon, bergamot, basil,
                    petitgrain, fruits, caraway
    Heart Notes: Thyme, mint, lavender,
                    jasmine, carnation, patchouli,
                    rose, sandalwood
    Base Notes: Moss, amber, musk

Famous Patrons
    Bridget Fonda

Eau de Guerlain is a fresh, sparkling *eau fraîche* composed by Jean-Paul Guerlain, an invigorating scent worn by women and men.

In eighteenth-century England, the Victorians assigned meaning to flowers, herbs, and plants. While some of these terms are merely romantic, others are quite fitting. For example, in the Victorian language of flowers, lemon blossoms signify zest, and thyme is the symbol of activity, an appropriate description for this herb with its pine-like vigor. Eau de Guerlain, with dominant notes of lemon and thyme, mint and lavender, is a modern, sporty scent, fresh and stimulating. It is available in one strength, the eau de toilette.

Introduced   1974
Price   Mid-range

EAU DE PATOU

♀♂

Scent Type   Citrus
Composition
    Top Notes: *Sicilian citron, Guinea oranges,*
        Grasse petitgrain
    Heart Notes: *Tunisian orange blossom,*
        pepper, nasturtium,
        honeysuckle, ylang-ylang
    Base Notes: *Musk, moss, amber, civet,*
        labdanum

From the French company of Jean Patou comes a crisp citrus scent that is perfect to splash on before a heated game of tennis or a hot business deal. An eau de cologne that is enjoyed by both sexes, it features juicy top notes balanced by a fresh floral heart and cool drydown notes.

Look for it packaged in ringed frosted glass flacons with sporty accents of marine blue and white, ready to pack for your next ocean voyage. Yachting, anyone?

Introduced   1976
Price   Mid-range

EAU DE ROCHAS

Scent Type   Chypre - Fresh
Composition
    Top Notes: *Sicilian lime,*
        Calabrian mandarin,
        bergamot, tangerine, grapefruit
    Heart Notes: *Wild rose, mountain narcissus*
    Base Notes: *Mysore sandalwood,*
        Croatian oakmoss, amber

Eau de Rochas is a refreshing eau de Cologne from the House of Rochas. An earthy natural, the cool chypre scent begins with tangy citrus notes, often called hesperides, tangy and uplifting. A floral heart adds depth, while woods, oakmoss, and amber combine to create a lingering aura of deep green forest.

The bottle is shaped like rock crystal and nestled in a box clothed with the cool colors of a fast-running stream—images reflective of the shimmering fragrance.

Introduced   1970
Price   Mid-range

EAU D'HADRIEN

♀♂

Scent Type   Chypre - Fresh
Composition
    Notes: *Sicilian lemon, grapefruit,*
        citron, cypress

Famous Patrons
    Nicole Kidman   *Madonna*

Eau d'Hadrien is crisp and tart, refreshing and refined, a fragrance that can be worn by women and men. The vibrant scent from Annick Goutal is available in a light eau de toilette, as well as a more concentrated eau de toilette. It is a zesty scent, perfect for daytime and sporty active wear.

Eau d'Hadrien was Goutal's personal morning scent, the fresh fragrance she splashed on and wore at home in the early hours. As the day progressed, she recommended layering other fragrances from her collection right over it. In fact, the entire Goutal line is made to be mixed and layered for unique interpretations.

Introduced   1986
Price   High range

EAU D'HERMÈS

♀♂

Scent Type   Citrus
Composition
    Top Notes: Cardamom, herbal lavender,
                 petitgrain lemon, cinnamon, cumin
    Heart Notes: Jasmine, Bourbon geranium,
                 vanilla, tonka bean, labdanum
    Base Notes: Sandalwood, cedarwood,
                 flamed birch

Eau d'Hermès is a noble unisex fragrance created by master perfumer Edward Roudnitska. A celestial blend of citrus, spice, and florals, it is subtly enhanced with a touch of woods. It was recently relaunched on the 150th anniversary of the House of Hermès.

Another classic fragrance from Hermès Paris, Eau de Hermès is a fresh, invigorating blend suitable for both men and women. Ideal for daytime, summer, active wear—anytime a fresh scent is preferred. Perhaps right after a sunrise canter on your trusty horse with the Hermès saddle, your favorite silk Hermès scarf flying in the breeze behind you. Ah...we live for luxuries. Packaged in a rectangular crystal bottle, suitable for engraving—a thoughtful gift.

Introduced   1951
Price   Top range

EAU D'IVOIRE

Scent Type   Floral - Fresh
Composition
    Top Notes: Freesia, mandarin, bergamot
    Heart Notes: Ylang-ylang, rose
    Base Notes: Oakmoss, musk, vanilla

In 1979, French couturier Pierre Balmain introduced the original Ivoire—a sophisticated, seductive green floral. While Eau d'Ivoire is based on selected notes from the original formula, such as mandarin and bergamot, rose and oakmoss, the addition of freesia lightens the bouquet. Fresh and classically elegant, Eau d'Ivoire is designed for the youthful, free-spirited woman who resides in us all.

Introduced   2000
Price   High range

EAU D'ORANGE VERTE

♀♂

Scent Type   Citrus
Composition
    Top Notes: Peppermint, mandarin
    Heart Notes: Sweet orange
    Base Notes: Petit grain lemon,
                 orange tree leaves

A scent for men and women, Eau d'Orange Verte from Hermès is a crisp citrus blend that is energizing and refreshing. The inclusion of peppermint adds freshness and vigor, while sweet orange and mandarin are blended with petit grain lemon for a fruity-woody drydown. Sporty and chic, Eau d'Orange Verte is housed in a tall green bottle. It is an ideal choice for steamy city days and beach-front evenings.

Introduced   1979
Price   High range

EAU DU CIEL

Scent Type   *Floral*
Composition
    Notes: *Brazilian rosewood, iris, violet*

Eau du Ciel derives its name from French for "sky" or "heaven." Annick Goutal created this tender scent, christening it "a hymn to balmy summer days recalling the special delights of childhood."

Annick Goutal often aided her olfactory memory with a notebook in which she recorded thousands of fragrance combinations, along with her personal associations, such as "the candies in the green bakery," or "the dunes on the Ile de Ré," one of her favorite vacation spots. The latter became the basis for a scent she created for her husband, called Sables, to which she added a dash of bergamot and sandalwood.

The world is indeed a sweeter-smelling place thanks to the artistry of Annick Goutal.

Introduced   *1986*
Price   *High range*

EAU DU JOUR

Scent Type   *Citrus*
Composition
    Top Notes: *Lemon, orange, rosemary,*
                         tea tree, clary sage
    Heart Notes: *Neroli, jasmine, rose*
    Base Notes: *Cedarwood, moss*

From Frenchman Frédéric Fekkai comes Eau du Jour, a unisex scent made from natural ingredients indigenous to the south of France. Fekkai collaborated with legendary French perfumer Jacques Polge to create Eau du Jour. The citrusy, floral blend is based on the aromas Fekkai recalled from his Provençal childhood. "My memories of growing up in Provence always include its beautiful scents," says Fekkai. The scent of neroli, or orange blossom, is a pleasing, sophisticated addition. Neroli is so named for the Duchess Orsini de Neroli, who popularized the essence during the seventeenth century. Eau du Jour is a sunny, easy-to-wear, daytime scent, ideal for a stroll through the streets of Grasse.

Style-setter Fekkai made his mark as a hairdresser to the rich and famous. He is a multi-talented artist whose careful caress is evident in Eau du Jour. Eau du Jour is packaged in a simple bottle of frosted glass and is housed in a carton of Fekkai French blue.

Introduced   *1997*
Price   *High range*

EAU DU SOIR

Scent Type   *Chypre - Floral*
Composition
    Top Notes: *Bergamot, citrus*
    Heart Notes: *Florals*
    Base Notes: *Amber, musk*

The family-owned French cosmetics firm of Sisley offers a noble fragrance created by a noble couple, the Count Hubert d'Ornano and his wife, the Countess Isabelle d'Ornano. The floral chypre blend opens with crisp citrus top notes before dissolving into a refined heart of floral, amber and musk. The classic rectangular bottle is crowned with an artistic touch—a woman's face rendered in 18-karat plated matte-gold, designed by artist Bronislaw Krzysztof.

For a brisk, herbal experience, try the firm's Eau de Campagne. Herbs, lemon, basil, and green tomato leaves impart a zesty, aromatic personality.

Introduced   *1990*
Price   *Top range*

EAU DU SUD

♀♂

Scent Type	Citrus
Composition	
Top Notes:	Mandarin, bergamot, grapefruit, lemon
Heart Notes:	Mint, basil
Base Notes:	Vervain

Perfumer Annick Goutal sought to re-create summer memories of Provence and Tuscany, of sun-kissed days and southern evening breezes. "I had an irresistible need for the sun," Goutal explained. Citrusy fruits star in the lively, luminous composition. Eau du Sud refreshes with mint, green basil, and herbal vervain—a welcome reprieve as one glides into warmer weather. A versatile formula, Eau du Sud may be worn by either sex. The only prerequisite is a summery frame of mind.

Introduced	1997
Price	High range

EAU FRAÎCHE BY CARON

♀♂

Scent Type	Citrus
Composition	
Top Notes:	Lemon, grapefruit, bergamot, tangerine, basil, thyme, artemisia, galbanum
Heart Notes:	Rose, jasmine, nutmeg, patchouli
Base Notes:	Oakmoss, musk

The legendary French house of Parfums Caron offers a fresh, sophisticated, citrusy unisex scent. Eau Fraîche may be worn with equal ease by women or by men. Hesperides and herbs are blended with florals, spices, and musk, yielding a crisp, energizing scent. The clear bottle is embossed with a shower of miniature water droplets, reminiscent of a soft summer rain. Invigorating, yet relaxing, ideal for a stroll in summery Provence.

Introduced	1999
Price	Mid-range

ELIZABETH TAYLOR'S PASSION

Scent Type	Floral Semi - Oriental
Composition	
Top Notes:	Gardenia, jasmine, lily of the valley, ylang-ylang, rose
Heart Notes:	Spices, musk
Base Notes:	Indian patchouli, Indian sandalwood, incense, cedarwood, moss

Passion was the first fragrance from one of the best-loved actresses of all time. A feminine formula of white flowers and spicy, exotic background notes produces a very wearable, memorable scent, a fragrance for passionate living. Dame Elizabeth Taylor is a passionate woman, dedicated to charity work—most notably her tireless devotion to relieve AIDS suffering, for which the Queen of England knighted her in 2000.

Taylor was personally involved in the creation of the scent and describes Passion saying: "It has a scent of mystery, slightly effusive, kind of smoky and sweet. There is ylang-ylang in it, which gives it a wonderful hint of tangy, crisp freshness, and lilies of the valley... brides use this in bouquets, that's probably why I'm so attracted to it!"

What inspired the name Passion? "Passion is not just a word that indicates lovemaking or lust," she explains. "I think it's passion that's made me a survivor. If you care about other people, it becomes a passion. If you can reach a natural high that is bliss...that's passion. I have a passion for life and loving."

Passion is packaged in an elegantly styled diamond-faceted flacon with a plunging "V" neckline, cast in the violet shade of Taylor's magnificent eyes, and accented with gold-colored highlights. A striking addition to any dressing table.

Introduced	*1987*
Price	*Mid-range*

ELLEN TRACY

Scent Type   *Oriental*
Composition
    Top Notes: *Peach, cinnamon*
    Heart Notes: *Rose, jasmine, carnation, freesia*
    Base Notes: *Sandalwood, tonka bean, cedarwood*

Replacing the 1992 Ellen Tracy fragrance, Ellen Tracy is the reformulated year 2000 version from the ready-to-wear line of the same name.

The peach-colored, Firmenich-blended scent is a symphony of spices, florals, and woods, immensely wearable and intensely romantic—the ideal accoutrement for Ellen Tracy clothes. Marc Rosen designed the bottle, which is styled like an A-line shift with a white rolled-pillow cap. A well-dressed fragrance, indeed.

Introduced	*2000*
Price	*Mid-range*

EMPORIO ARMANI SHE

Scent Type   *Floral - Oriental*
Composition
    Top Notes: *Angelica, cardamom, mandarin, bergamot*
    Heart Notes: *Heliotrope, jasmine*
    Base Notes: *Vanilla, musk, cedar*

Fashion designer Giorgio Armani offers Emporio Armani She, a classic, sophisticated floral, created by perfumer Sophie Labb for International Flavors and Fragrances. Entitled simply She and referred to as Elle in France, it goes native in several other languages as well.

European chic and sensuality is clearly evident, as the scent unfolds around a romantic heart of heliotrope, which is a sunny, fragrant white or purplish flower with hints of almond. The champagne-colored, soft-touch aluminum outer sleeve conceals the fragrance in an unbreakable, cleverly activated spray bottle. Emporio Armani She is portable, a cosmo-to-go. Understated Armani chic, designed to take you everywhere in spare, elegant style.

Introduced	*1998*
Price	*High range*

ENIGMA

Scent Type   *Chypre*
Composition
    Top Notes: *Aldehydes, greens, bergamot, coriander, pimento, herbs*
    Heart Notes: *Jasmine, rose, carnation*
    Base Notes: *Amber, woods, spices, patchouli, oakmoss*

Enigma is a warm, sophisticated fragrance from Alexandra de Markoff. Crisp aldehydes, greens, and citrus introduce the smooth chypre blend, which evolves into a woody herbal base. Sweet amber and patchouli complete the sensual aroma. Enigma is a refined fragrance of classic proportion.

Introduced 1972
Price   Mid-range

ENVY

Scent Type Floral - Green
Composition
 Top Notes: Hyacinth, magnolia, vine flower
 Heart Notes: Violet, jasmine, lily of the valley
 Base Notes: Musk, iris

The Gucci brand is energized with a healthy dose of Envy. Creative director and native Texan Tom Ford aided in the development of Envy, a transparent floral with—well, what else?—green accents. Simply pea green with envy, as one might say. Oh, do forgive us. Envy is hip and modern, a sexy scent, true to Gucci's fashion-forward Italian roots.

Housed in a model-thin bottle, encased in a transparent plastic container, Envy is an easy target. Perfect for black-clad, long-legged strolls across wide, big-city boulevards. A sharp, shimmery, daytime scent, designed to inspire you-know-what. Not that there's a jealous bone in our body. Oh, there we go again.

Introduced 1997
Price   High range

ESCADA

Scent Type Floral - Oriental
Composition
 Top Notes: Bergamot, hyacinth, peach, coconut
 Heart Notes: Orange blossom, jasmine, iris, carnation, frangipani flower
 Base Notes: Vanilla, musk, sandalwood

Escada is the signature fragrance developed by Margaretha Ley, the supremely elegant international fashion designer from Sweden, who was widely noted for her inspirational use of vibrant color.

Escada borrowed its name from a champion Thoroughbred whose name is Portuguese for "staircase." With top notes of fresh, fruity florals, the scent is versatile enough to be worn during the day, yet sophisticated enough for the evening.

Two years in the making, the complex scent from Margaretha Ley and husband Wolfgang is presented in classic Escada design: a voluptuous sculpted glass heart, topped with gold-colored filigree swirls, nestled in Escada red packaging. The scent won a FiFi Award bestowed by The Fragrance Foundation.

In addition to the signature Escada fragrance, the company also introduces an annual seasonal scent. Once a year, a new fragrance is introduced with the company's current Spring/Summer theme. The special eau de toilette is available from April through September of each year. The heart-shaped bottle remains the same, but sports different finishes and colors. Charming! Of course, Escada's original fragrance in the signature red heart is a mainstay, available year-round.

Escada—let it capture your heart.

Introduced 1990
Price   High range

ESCAPE

Scent Type   Marine
Composition
    Top Notes: Mandarin, apple,
                    black currant bud, chamomile,
                    apricot, melon, peach, plum
    Heart Notes: Jasmine, rose, coriander,
                    clove, carnation
    Base Notes: Sandalwood, musk, cedarwood,
                    oakmoss, amber

American designer Calvin Klein compels us to travel, to get away from it all, with his fragrance Escape.

The marine-themed scent begins with a sheer twist of apple, chamomile, and black currant bud, then gives way to a spiced floral bouquet enveloped in lasting sandalwood and musk. Easy to wear, it is perfect for light daytime enjoyment.

The bottle looks as though it will slip comfortably into your suitcase. It was inspired by an antique perfume bottle and comes with a silver-hinged flip-top cap. It travels suited in green moiré and parchment.

Escape...oh yes...just a moment, the valise is almost packed...one-way ticket please...somewhere with a deserted beach...and toned, muscled men.

Introduced   1991
Price   Mid-Range

ESTÉE

Scent Type   Floral
Composition
    Top Notes: Peach, raspberry, citrus oils
    Heart Notes: Rose, lily of the valley, jasmine,
                    carnation, ylang-ylang, honey,
                    orris
    Base Notes: Cedarwood, musk, moss,
                    sandalwood, styrax

Famous Patrons
    Nancy Reagan   Pat Buckly
    Duchess of Windsor

Estée Lauder's namesake fragrance is a sparkling floral composition for the confident woman. Versatile and sophisticated.

Ethereal aldehydic fruity top notes are balanced with sweet florals and a finale of powdery woods and sensual musk. Estée is a fragrance as memorable as the famous women who wear it.

Introduced   1968
Price   Mid-range

ETERNITY

Scent Type   Floral - Fresh
Composition
    Top Notes: Mandarin, freesia, sage
    Heart Notes: Narcissus, lily of the valley, rose,
                    marigold, white lily, jasmine
    Base Notes: Sandalwood, patchouli, amber,
                    musk

The second fragrance in the string of bestsellers from Calvin Klein, Eternity is a blend of sweet white florals, topped with the fresh citrus note of mandarin, and warmed by Oriental background essences of sweet woods and amber. A fresh casual fragrance, Eternity is equally suitable for a busy career day, or a leisurely bike ride on a sunny beach. Packaged in classic bridal white.

Introduced	*1988*
Price	*Mid-range*

EVELYN

Scent Type   *Floral*
Composition
    Top Notes: *Roses*
    Heart Notes: *Rose, lily of the valley, peach*
    Base Notes: *Woods, musk*

Evelyn is the first eau de parfum from Crabtree & Evelyn. The company describes the fragrance as "sophisticated and refreshing." The composition was developed around a multitude of roses. Though the singular impression is of roses, more than eighty-five ingredients were blended to achieve this effect.

Expert rose grower David Austin of Wolverhampton, England, toiled over the fragrance for eight years with master perfumers Mane of Grasse, France. Together they employed new "headspace technology" to exactly re-create the scent of Evelyn roses. The result is superb.

The pink liquid is showcased in a clear flacon inspired by nineteenth-century dressing table bottles. A silver cap sets off the romantic creation.

Introduced	*1993*
Price	*Mid-range*

EXTRAVAGANCE

Scent Type   *Floral*
Composition
    Top Notes: *Green mandarin, rose,*
                     pink peppercorn
    Heart Notes: *Jasmine, violet, orange blossom*
    Base Notes: *Sandalwood, cedarwood,*
                     black iris, musk

Uninhibited, free, and flirty, are apt descriptions of Givenchy's addition to the original Amarige line. Extravagance d'Amarige is a sexy, youthful version of the classic Amarige formula. Warm, spirited notes of green mandarin, pink peppercorn, and black iris add a dash of spice and smoldering sensuality—it's oh, so very, very French. Imagine the South of France in sunny August.

The topsy-turvy, tilted type on the curved bottles and outer packaging reflects a youthful vigor and *joie de vivre*. Amarige red links the lines, and together the two scents enhance any wardrobe with what's naughty and nice. Do we detect a bit of Givenchy fashion designer Alexander McQueen's influence? *Mais oui*—happily, yes.

Introduced	*1998*
Price	*High range*

FABERGÉ

Scent Type	*Floral*
Composition	
Top Notes:	*Neroli, orange flower, ylang-ylang, bergamot, greens*
Heart Notes:	*Rose, jasmine, carnation, violet leaves, clove*
Base Notes:	*Sandalwood, musk, patchouli*

The launch of Fabergé was planned to coincide with the Metropolitan Museum of New York's retrospective on renowned Russian crown jeweler Peter Carl Fabergé. The perfume line is fashioned after Fabergé's Imperial Czarevitch Egg and uses several of the same design elements, such as laurel leaves and crowns, with the color scheme of sapphire blue and 22-karat gold plate.

The Fabergé fragrance is a romantic floral scent, regally rendered and exquisitely feminine. Classic notes of rose and jasmine are delicately combined with a fresh opening accord. The smoothness and sensuality of spices, sandalwood, and musk spark the remembrance of bygone days, of Russian lore and a time forever lost. Fabergé: A romantic fragrance of imperial proportion.

Introduced	1996
Price	Top range

FABLE

Scent Type	*Floral - Oriental*
Composition	
Top Notes:	*Bergamot, ylang-ylang, rosewood, ivy*
Heart Notes:	*Plum, jasmine, pimento*
Base Notes:	*Amber, white musk, sandalwood*

Shrouded in mystery, the fabled Hope Diamond is the most valuable diamond in the world. Currently residing at the Smithsonian Institute, the gemstone has adorned many an aristocrat and was once possessed by Evalyn Walsh McLean. Her great-grandson, Joseph Gregory, drew upon this family history in creating Fable, a floral fragrance of rich ancestry, blended by Quest perfumer Claude Dir.

Fable is an opulent, romantic fragrance, with an opening of ivy and fruit. The heart is smoothed with an accord of *crème brûlé*, while the finale is a sensual sonata of amber, musk, and woods. Designer Marc Rosen created the curved bottle with platinum-hued shoulders and capped it with a deep blue, *faux* gemstone—the enchanting color of the Hope Diamond. A beautiful scent that is best worn with diamonds, even, to quote songwriter Paul Simon, with "diamonds on the soles of her shoes." Or, at least, with a diamond frame of mind.

Introduced	1999
Price	Top range

FABULOUS BY JAN MORAN

Scent Type   *Floral - Oriental*
Composition
     Top Notes: *Italian bergamot, raspberry,*
                         mandarin, orange oil
     Heart Notes: *Jasmine, rose, tuberose, basil,*
                         clove, carnation
     Base Notes: *Amber, ylang-ylang, sandalwood,*
                         cedarwood, musk, vanilla,
                         benzoin, patchouli

Famous Patrons
     Princess Françoise Paleologo
     Actress Josette Banzet, Marquise de Bruyenne

For a lifelong fragrance aficionado, what could possibly ignite a desire for even more? Writing a book on fragrances, as this author discovered. The path I embarked upon with the first edition of *Fabulous Fragrances*, published in 1994, has led me on an incredible journey.

At every book signing and appearance, people would ask, "You're the expert—when do you plan to introduce your own fragrance?" So when the opportunity to create my own perfume presented itself, the idea was simply too much to resist.

And what a fragrance I had in mind!

My grandmother Eva had a perfume developed especially for her in Grasse, France, in the 1930s. She passed away when I was in my teens, but the antique essence was emblazoned upon my memory. Although the formula had been lost, I had always dreamed of re-creating the fragrance, or a series of scents based on the elements of this magical aroma.

Through Bijan, I came to know Michel Mane and Richard Panzarasa of V. Mane Fils and Mane, U.S.A., one of the oldest family-owned French fragrance manufacturers in existence. I shall never forget my first creative session with Panzarasa.

When I produced a list of essential oils I felt my fragrance must contain, he was astonished—so seldom do clients detail their exact desire.

Over the course of two years, I worked with Panzarasa and second-generation perfumer Marvel Fields to perfect the formula.

Creating my own perfume was the culmination of a dream, a tribute to the women in my family, and a personal journey to the inner soul of creativity.

How shall I describe the perfume so dear to my heart? Indeed, it is like describing the depths of my heart, of all I cherish and yearn to become.

We selected the natural ingredients as an artist selects the elements of a composition. As we developed the formula, I concentrated on ingredients that possess almost magical powers in aroma-chology. For the fresh opening accord I chose bergamot to calm and uplift the spirit, and orange oil for happiness, then added a sprinkling of mandarin and raspberry. For the heart I chose jasmine for its sensuality and blended it with rose, a superb anti-depressant, to increase optimism and self-confidence. A sprig of green and a dash of spice completed the full-bodied, harmonious heart.

The base began with ylang-ylang, an essential oil known to raise one's spirits. We combined vanilla, a relaxing aroma, with sandalwood, a subtle aphrodisiac, then added a gentle balance of woods and musk. Finally, we blended in one of my favorite essences: Amber is a tree resin, warm, balsamic, and tenacious, valued for its healing power in certain cultures and believed to enhance and strengthen the soul. A soothing note, amber imparted an exquisite, elegant finish to the composition.

At last, our work was complete. I felt satisfied that my perfume was a long-lasting, rich scent of subtle sophistication, and suitable for year-round wear. It was hauntingly sensual, confident and elegant, reminiscent of the glamour era of yesteryear.

But, I pondered, what shall I name it?

As I was testing the fragrance—in various climates and altitudes—my husband frequently exclaimed, "Ah, you smell fabulous!" "Fabulous" has always been one of my favorite expressions—and who doesn't want to be thought of as fabulous? I explored the word. *Random House Dictionary* defines "fabulous" as "astonishingly incredible… marvelous or superb…told or known through fables or legends." It was exactly what I desired. Thus I chose the name of my treasured perfume: Fabulous by Jan Moran® Beverly Hills.

Then I wondered, how must I clothe and accessorize my creation?

Once again, I listened to my heart. I have a deep appreciation of fine jewelry; I love to design and collect unusual pieces, especially antique works. Perhaps this, too, can be traced to my grandparents. My grandfather proposed marriage to Eva by depositing the gemstones intended for her engagement ring in her crystal perfume bottle, and to this day I associate gemstones with romance. I was thus inspired to immerse gemstones in my own fragrance, a rainbow assortment of purple amethyst, yellow citrine, blue topaz, and red garnet. Suitable for setting, each faceted stone is approximately one carat and is accompanied by a certificate of authenticity. I continued the jewel theme, creating opulent red satin and gold lamé jewelry pouches (which I also use as evening bags).

Every item in the Fabulous line is designed to be reused or recycled. My favorite is the 3.4-ounce eau de parfum, presented in a round, Brosse-designed, French crystalline flacon and crowned with a gold-colored, tasseled bulb atomizer.

Fabulous is my personal perfume, a reminder of Old World elegance, a gift to my beloved friends and family. Enjoy it, with my fabulous wishes!

Introduced	1997
Price	High range

FACE À FACE

Scent Type	Floral - Fresh
Composition	
Top Notes:	Coriander, rose, marigold
Heart Notes:	Iris, lily of the valley, jasmine
Base Notes:	Cedarwood, patchouli, amber, labdanum

Face à Face is the first women's fragrance from Façonnable and is the counterpart to the men's version by the same name. The scents were created in tandem, so they can even be worn together to form a third, synergistic fragrance experience. Hers, his, or ours—what's your preference?

A refreshing floral, Face à Face has an opening marine accord. Packaged in an apothecary-style bottle, it has an effect that is crisp, cool, and green. Face à Face is a fine choice for the confident, cool, casual woman of today.

Introduced	1997
Price	Mid-range

FASCINATION

Scent Type	Floral
Composition	
Top Notes:	Cassis, lily of the valley, greens
Heart Notes:	Jasmine, orange blossom, Chinese osmanthus
Base Notes:	Woods, amber, musk

Fascination is a Holzman & Stephanie fragrance, a refined floral perfume with a heart of white flowers, including the rare Chinese osmanthus. As the all-natural scent develops on the skin, a subtle *sillage* weaves a romantic spell.

Holzman & Stephanie fragrances are still made by hand in the traditional fashion of yesteryear. Chic handmade, black and gold, Holzman-designed boxes and cylinders complete the elegant theme of this exclusively distributed line; a perfume designed to capture your fascination.

Introduced   1990
Price   High range

FATH DE FATH

Scent Type   Oriental
Composition
  Top Notes: Peach, black currant, bergamot, orange blossom, marigold
  Heart Notes: Rose, violet, jasmine
  Base Notes: Cinnamon, vanilla, tonka bean, sandalwood, vetiver, patchouli

French couturier Jacques Fath was well known for his feminine suits, glamorous evening dresses, and elegant wedding gowns. He designed for an exclusive clientele, as well as for Hollywood studios. His designs were showcased in the 1948 classic film *Red Shoes*, based on the Hans Christian Andersen story, starring British ballerina Moira Shearer.

The House of Fath continues today, and the Oriental composition Fath de Fath is reminiscent of Fath's Oriental design period of the 1920s. Fresh, zesty fruits introduce the classic floral bouquet of Fath de Fath. Spicy base notes of cinnamon and vanilla are blended with woods for an effect that is sensual and elegant, like Fath couture designs of yesterday and today. Its diamond-faceted bottle, encased in a golden-hued carton, is the epitome of luxury.

Introduced   1995
Price   Top range

FEMME

Scent Type   Chypre - Fruity
Composition
  Top Notes: Peach, plum, bergamot, lemon, rosewood
  Heart Notes: Ylang-ylang, jasmine, May rose, clove, orris
  Base Notes: Musk, amber, oakmoss, vanilla, patchouli, benzoin, leather

Famous Patrons
Mae West

Femme is a full-bodied fragrance from Parfums Rochas, a fragrance as rich in history as in scent. The distinctive composition was created for the House of Rochas during World War II by the noted perfumer Edmond Roudnitska of Cabris, France. When once asked about his olfactory gift, Roudnitska replied, "The capacity to create is essentially the ability to imagine." To the perfumer, the fragrance is a composition, as evocative as a Monet masterpiece.

Marcel Rochas opened his couture salon in Paris in 1924 and quickly became known for his broad-shouldered suits, bustiers, and elaborate designs. Femme was originally available only by strict invitation. Rochas sent a letter to his clients, allowing them to purchase a limited-edition, numbered bottle. Imagine the demand he created! The next year when he made Femme available to the public, he had an instant hit.

The legendary Femme explodes with Mediterranean fruits, mingled with intoxicating floral aromas, and underscored with lingering balsamics and moss. Femme is a brilliant, recognizable fragrance.

The bottle, designed by René Lalique, is a sensuously curved crystal flacon, symbolic of a woman's graceful silhouette. The voluptuous Mae West, who was a personal friend of Lalique and a valued client of Rochas, inspired the bottle. Our favorite Mae West quote is: "Between two evils, I always pick the one I never tried before."

Femme—created to embody femininity.

Introduced   1944
Price   High range

FENDI

Scent Type   Chypre - Floral
Composition
    Top Notes: Bergamot, aldehydes, rosewood,
                  fruits
    Heart Notes: Jasmine, rose, ylang-ylang,
                  geranium, carnation
    Base Notes: Patchouli, musk, leather,
                  sandalwood, cedarwood, spices,
                  amber, vanilla

Fendi is the original signature scent from the noted Italian design firm of Fendi, known for its remarkable fashions, leather goods, and household designs.

The warm, subtly blended chypre floral is housed in a sleek modern rectangular flacon from Pierre Dinand. Fendi is a harmonious fragrance with a passionate Italian heart.

Introduced   1987
Price   High range

FERENTINA

Scent Type   Floral
Composition
    Top Notes: Fruits
    Heart Notes: Jasmine, rose
    Base Notes: Amber, musk, woods

From Caesars World comes Ferentina, named for the Roman goddess who presided over water and nature. A rich floral with a classic heart of jasmine and rose nestled in a musky base, Ferentina is an expansive, long-lasting fragrance. Sure to delight any modern-day goddess, it is presented in shades of imperial purple and antiqued gold, in a round bottle, or *boule*.

Introduced   2000
Price   Mid-range

FERRÉ

Scent Type   Floral - Fruity
Composition
    Top Notes: Orange blossom, bergamot,
                  ylang-ylang, butterbush
    Heart Notes: Rose, mimosa, peach, passion
                  fruit, violet, cassia, moss,
                  lily of the valley
    Base Notes: Vanilla, sandalwood, spices,
                  amber, iris, vetiver, musk

From the extraordinary Italian fashion designer and architect, Gianfranco Ferré, comes a complex fragrance, a melange of Italian elegance, humor, and sensuality.

The prominent notes are derived from delicate white flowers, giving it a sweet, feminine persona. It comes in a bottle telling of Ferré's architectural design, a flacon of sculpted crystal, black and gold-colored, and topped with a faceted crystal stopper.

Introduced	1992
Price	High range

FIDJI

Scent Type	Floral
Composition	
Top Notes:	Galbanum, hyacinth, lemon, bergamot
Heart Notes:	Carnation, orris, ylang-ylang, jasmine, rose
Base Notes:	Vetiver, musk, moss, sandalwood

Fidji was introduced by fashion designer Guy Laroche. The fragrance borrows its name from the Fiji Islands in the South Pacific. Appropriately, the fragrance opens with fresh tropical notes, evolving into a radiant floral heart. A mild base of fragrant woods produces a soft powdery drydown. It is a perfect fragrance for island adventures or warm weather daydreaming.

Introduced	1966
Price	Mid-range

FIRST

Scent Type	Floral - Aldehyde
Composition	
Top Notes:	Aldehydes, mandarin, black currant bud, peach, raspberry, hyacinth
Heart Notes:	Turkish rose, narcissus, jasmine, lily of the valley, carnation, orchid, tuberose, orris
Base Notes:	Amber, tonka bean, oakmoss, sandalwood, vetiver, musk, honey, civet

First is a fabulous floral bouquet from world-renowned Parisian jeweler Van Cleef & Arpels. The aldehydic note adds a brilliant jewel-like sparkle to the rich classic scent, a rush of fragrance that softens into a sweet amber and wood base.

First is housed in a lovely curved glass bottle bearing a gold-colored pinafore inscribed with the name, and capped with a rounded, easy-to-grasp stopper.

Before you adorn yourself with your Van Cleef & Arpels jewels, be sure to cleanse and soften your skin with First body and bath products. Gives a whole new meaning to the concept of layering, *n'est-ce pas?*

Introduced	1976
Price	High range

FLEUR DE DIVA

Scent Type	Floral - Marine
Composition	
Top Notes:	Freesia, water lily, black currant bud
Heart Notes:	Rose, lily of the valley, water hyacinth
Base Notes:	Sandalwood, musk

Flowers permeate the collections of fashion designer Emmanuel Ungaro, who gained recognition in the fragrance world with the creation of Diva. Fleur de Diva is an abundant floral bouquet, developed around watery, translucent marine notes. A joyful exuberance marks Fleur de Diva, as evidenced by the liberal use of rose, Ungaro's favorite flower. Blossoms bloom gracefully on the petaled carton of the pale, green-bottled scent. Flaunt Fleur de Diva and proudly proclaim the prima donna in you.

Introduced	1997
Price	High range

FLEUR D'INTERDIT

Scent Type   *Floral*
Composition
    Top Notes: *Raspberry, peach, melon*
    Heart Notes: *Gardenia, rose, lilac, cyclamen,*
                      iris, lily of the valley, violet leaves
    Base Notes: *Sunflower, sandalwood, vanilla*

The gentleman of French couture, Hubert de Givenchy, appeals to the younger customer with Fleur d'Interdit. The scent is a youthful, lighthearted version of the popular classic L'Interdit, created for Audrey Hepburn.

A sheer, radiant floral, Fleur d'Interdit is a celebration of fruits and white flowers, with an unusual base note of sunflower. Packaging is beautiful, with an elegant simplicity. A frosted apple blossom motif is delicately carved on the tall bottle, reminiscent of nature's springtime jewels inherent in the composition. Fleur d'Interdit radiates gaiety and spontaneity. Wear it for sheer joy.

Introduced   *1994*
Price   *Mid-range*

FLEURISSIMO

Scent Type   *Floral*
Composition
    Notes: *Tuberose, violet, rose, iris*

Famous Patrons
    Princess Grace of Monaco
    Jacqueline Kennedy Onassis
    Queen Elizabeth II   Cindy Crawford
    Madonna   Rita Wilson

The Paris-based House of Creed has created masterpiece perfumes for royalty, dignitaries and celebrities from around the world, including the courts of England, Spain, and France, since 1760. In 1972, while awaiting his marriage to American actress Grace Kelly, Prince Rainier of Monaco commissioned from Creed a perfume for his bride to wear on their wedding day. Thus was born Fleurissimo, the perfume created for Her Serene Highness Princess Grace of Monaco.

A fragrance fit for a princess, Fleurissimo is a subtly intoxicating bouquet of delicate white flowers. Feminine and beguiling, versatile and easy to wear, the pedigreed eau de parfum exudes privilege, wealth, and a world of infinite possibilities. Presented in a 2.5-ounce classic Creed bottle, Fleurissimo is a majestic scent, once worn exclusively by a legendary woman of international acclaim.

Introduced   *1972*
Price   *Top range*

FLEURS DE ROCAILLE

Scent Type *Floral*
Composition
  Top Notes: *Lily of the valley, clover*
  Heart Notes: *Rose, violet, lilac, jasmine, iris*
  Base Notes: *Sandalwood, musk, civet*

Fleurs de Rocaille is another timeless scent from the great Parisian perfumery of Caron. It is an enduring, sublime floral blend—a classic arrangement. It was introduced in an upturned glass bottle, tied with a gold-colored ribbon beneath a crystal stopper. Sophisticated simplicity.

In addition, Fleurs de Rocaille enjoyed a Hollywood walk-on role in the movie *Scent of a Woman*, with Al Pacino. Pacino portrays a rough-hewn military man who has lost his sight and his will to live. At the end of the movie, when he finally decides to choose life, he meets a woman and is enchanted by her, as well as her fragrance—Fleurs de Rocaille. With one deep breath he identifies the scent, and to him it represents the captivating scent of a woman.

The power of the movies...in just one scene, an entire new generation became acquainted with the classic Fleurs de Rocaille.

Introduced *1933*
Price *High range*

FLIRT

Scent Type *Floral - Green*
Composition
  Top Notes: *Pomegranate, greens*
  Heart Notes: *Magnolia, ginger flower*
  Base Notes: *Iris, tambouti wood,*
    cashmere woods

Prescriptives targets the coquettish soul with Flirt, the company's first fragrance since the 1986 Calyx. The tale is told of a Chinese princess who shed tears of sorrow when forced to marry against her will. These tears splashed upon the humble ginger root, endowing the subsequent flower with an incomparable scent of infinite sweetness.

The feminine, Givaudan Roure-blended scent developed around the fragrant white ginger flower is described as *avant-garde*. Modern and sexy, Flirt communicates an amorous attitude, a naughty, haughty aura. Flirt is presented in a capricious shade of vibrant purple.

Introduced *1998*
Price *Mid-range*

FLORE

Scent Type *Floral - Fresh*
Composition
  Top Notes: *Greens, lily of the valley*
  Heart Notes: *Jasmine, iris*
  Base Notes: *Iris, sandalwood, musk*

From the elegant Venezuelan clothing designer, Carolina Herrera, comes Flore, which means "flower" in Spanish. Flore is composed of powdery iris, with white flower notes of jasmine and lily of the valley. A sprig of green adds lift and freshness, while the sandalwood and musk base contributes a smooth sensuality to the floral composition. Delicate and feminine, Flore appeals to the romantic at heart.

Flore's bouquet-shaped stopper and clear glass bottle are Andre Ricard designs. Shades of coral and yellow give Flore a youthful countenance, setting it apart from the signature Herrera scent.

Introduced *1994*
Price *Top range*

FLORET

Scent Type   Floral
Composition
  Notes: Sweet pea, lily of the valley, tuberose

Floret is the second fragrance from East Hampton florist and entrepreneur Antonia Bellanca, whose first fragrance, Antonia's Flowers, has built a devoted clientele since its 1985 introduction.

Floret is an airy floral, though richer than the lighthearted, freesia-themed Antonia's Flowers. A subtle nuance of fruit adds verve, without an overwhelming fruity accord. The sensual essences of tuberose, lily of the valley, and sweet pea are interwoven like the threads of a fine silken tapestry. Boxed in a flower-strewn carton designed by Dan Rizzi, Floret is presented in a clear, understated bottle topped with a petaled cap.

For a rich, indulgent experience, try Bellanca's 1999 Tiempe Passate, too—a nostalgic, warmhearted fragrance.

Introduced   1995
Price   Mid-range

FOLAVRIL

Scent Type   Floral - Fruity
Composition
  Notes: Jasmine, mango

Annick Goutal's Folavril bursts with naturally fresh, exotic floral notes, smoothed with tropical mango. In French, Folavril loosely translates as "fool's folly," a fun interpretation. Perfect for casual, fun-filled day wear.

Try blending Annick Goutal fragrances to create your own interpretations. For example, give Folavril a crisp top note through a marriage with Goutal's citrusy chypre Eau d'Hadrien, or warm it with the deeper notes of other Goutal favorites. Experiment!

Introduced   1986
Price   High range

FOR EVER

Scent Type   Floral - Fruity
Composition
  Top Notes: Melon, raspberry, pineapple
  Heart Notes: Iris, violet, jasmine,
            lily of the valley
  Base Notes: Oakmoss, sandalwood, vetiver

Jean Kerléo, resident perfumer for Jean Patou, brings forth For Ever. A floral bouquet with fruity top notes and a powdery heart, For Ever is a versatile scent for the romantic soul.

For Ever is presented in a clear flacon, topped with a burgundy cap and ensconced in a gold-colored, burnished box. A perfume of eternal love.

Introduced   1999
Price   High range

FRACAS

Scent Type   Floral

Composition

Top Notes: Bergamot, mandarin,
                        hyacinth, greens

Heart Notes: Tuberose, jasmine, orange flower,
                        lily of the valley, white iris,
                        violet, jonquil, carnation,
                        coriander, peach, osmanthus,
                        pink geranium

Base Notes: Musk, sandalwood, orris, vetiver,
                        tolu balsam

Famous Patrons

Princess Caroline of Monaco

Kim Basinger   Madonna

Courtney Love   Amanda Harlech

Morgan Fairchild   Carolina Herrera

Blaine Trump   Stella Tennant

Beverly Sills   Martha Stewart

Sarah Michelle Gellar

Fracas, by Parisian couturier Robert Piguet, is a classic French floral bouquet, bursting with the white flowers for which Grasse is famous. Fracas, meaning "violet noise" in French, is a cacophony of tuberose, an expansive white floral. The tuberose flower has a scent so intense, a single stalk will drench a room with intoxicating, sensual scent. Free-spirited female perfumer Germaine Sellier created the Fracas formula for Piguet, which was launched just after World War II.

Piguet was known for his designs of simple elegance. During World War II, Nazi orders directed the top couture houses to relocate to Berlin. Piguet rebelled and resisted, and rode out the war in occupied Paris, continuing his work in fashion

and fragrance. During this period he developed Fracas and Bandit, fragrant points of light in a dark time of history. Today, after a lengthy absence, both fragrances have been formulated according to their original versions. Fracas and Bandit have become cult favorites of the celebrity crowd.

Heady, mysterious, frank sensuality—the hallmarks of Fracas are obvious. Look for Fracas in a black glass cube with simple pink accents. Retro-glamour at its finest.

Introduced   1948

Reintroduced   1996

Price   Mid-range

FRAGILE

Scent Type   Floral

Composition

Top Notes: Tuberose, sweet orange,
                        raspberry leaves

Heart Notes: Pink pepper, pimento berry,
                        capsicum seed

Base Notes: Violet wood, musk, cedarwood

Jean-Paul Gaultier's Fragile breaks tradition with a snow-globe flacon (no, we're not kidding). Shake it, and golden-glittered snow swirls round the bare shoulders of a female figurine clad in evening black. How to use? Simply press on the globe and the base emits a spritz. The scent is heady tuberose. Lana Turner would've loved it—tuberose was her favorite scent, or so says her hairdresser, Eric Root, and hairdressers know all, the darlings.

Fragile: Best shaken, not stirred. Oh, how could we resist?

Introduced   1999

Price   High range

FRANGIPANI

Scent Type	*Floral - Fresh*
Composition	
Top Notes:	*Orange blossom, aldehydes*
Heart Notes:	*Frangipani, ylang-ylang, rose, lilac*
Base Notes:	*Sandalwood, benzoin*

In the sunny, Florida Keys, time moves at a languid pace, and mother nature is the queen of her surroundings. The flowers found on these tropical isles possess magical aromas that entice and ensnare. Here, the frangipani tree is revered for its fragrant white blossoms, which have an intoxicating, expansive aroma similar to that of jasmine. Key West Aloe, founded on Key West in 1971, is dedicated to bottling these haunting aromas.

Frangipani is a fresh floral, redolent of moonlit beaches and hypnotic waves. Hints of fruits, spices and woods give body and fullness to the white floral bouquet. For variety, try other Key West Aloe scents: White Ginger, White Orchid, Hibiscus and Black Coral. For men, try Key West Gold, 1000 Portholes, and Lighthouse.

Why not slip into a Key West frame of mind and dangle those pedicured peds from the pier, with a tall, cool drink in your hand?

Introduced	*1985*
Price	*Mid-range*

FREEDOM

Scent Type	*Floral - Fresh*
Composition	
Top Notes:	*Citrus, watercress, quince*
Heart Notes:	*Asian ginger, cucumber blossom*
Base Notes:	*Satinwood*

Freedom for Her is American fashion designer Tommy Hilfiger's second women's fragrance. While Hilfiger's first women's scent, Tommy Girl, is geared for the teen market, Freedom is envisioned for women in their twenties and beyond. The scent is designed to appeal to the adventurous, independent, and free-thinking woman. And for the man in your life, there is Freedom for Him. In Freedom, the fresh green note of watercress bridges notes of crisp citrus and watery quince. The heart of Asian ginger is a common thread between the men's and women's versions. The result is an easy-to-wear scent, fluid and free, soaring like an eagle. Freedom is "All-American" at its best.

Packaging is simple, bold and translucent. In tribute to femininity, the women's version is gently molded in clear and frosted glass, and slipped into a red plastic sheath. Think casual Friday, or wear it anytime you want to declare your own independence day.

Introduced	*1999*
Price	*Mid-range*

G

Scent Type   *Floral - Fruity*
Composition
    Top Notes: *Peach, pineapple, cantaloupe, pink tea*
    Heart Notes: *Golden Sundust orchid, water lily, jasmine, peony, magnolia, ginger lily*
    Base Notes: *Amber, vetiver, frangipani, assam wood*

G, just G, hails from Giorgio Beverly Hills. From the world famous Rodeo Drive boutique, mecca for shoppers from around the world, comes G, a delectable, vibrant, fruity floral bouquet.

The fragrance menu opens with a tasty fruit salad and pink tea accord—zesty and invigorating. The heart contains the rare Golden Sundust orchid, a delicately scented flower that blooms only once every few years. A delightful, lingering base of woods and white Tahitian frangipani flower inspires thoughts of languid island evenings. The lavender-tinted liquid is held in a slender spray, vaguely reminiscent of the classic Giorgio bottle, or of a draped couture gown. G is a grand choice geared for a new millennium of Giorgio fans.

Introduced   *2000*
Price   *High range*

GALANOS DE SERENE

Scent Type   *Floral - Ambery*
Composition
    Top Notes: *Ylang-ylang, pear, apple*
    Heart Notes: *Freesia, gardenia, rose, osmanthus*
    Base Notes: *Sandalwood, tonka bean, musk, vanilla, benzoin, olibanum*

Designer to first ladies, stars, and celebrities, American couturier James Galanos returns to the fragrance scene with Galanos de Serene. The floral scent opens with a fruit accord, then dissolves into a sheer floral heart with subtle Oriental undertones. Serene and elegant, Galanos is a fragrance of classic style, like an impeccably tailored Galanos creation. The scent is housed in a carton that features a sleek Galanos fashion illustration. Galanos de Serene is a fine choice for the beautifully attired woman.

Introduced   *1996*
Price   *High range*

GARDÉNIA

Scent Type   *Floral*
Composition
    Top Notes: *Absolutes of jasmine, gardenia, orange blossom, tuberose*
    Heart Notes: *Clove, sage, pimiento*
    Base Notes: *Musk, patchouli, sandalwood, vetiver*

Coco Chanel's twenties version of Gardénia is a polished floral blend enhanced by a spicy accord and supported by sweet, powdery wooded notes. Created by perfumer Ernest Beaux, Gardénia bursts with the unforgettable essence of the finest French garden.

Perfect for tea in a spring garden, or a two-Evian power lunch. We imagine Chanel slipped Gardénia in her suitcase for her frequent French Riviera vacations. Look for it in Chanel Boutiques.

Introduced   *1925*
Reintroduced   *1993*
Price   *Mid-range*

GARDÉNIA PASSION

Scent Type   *Floral*
Composition
    Notes: *Gardenia*

Famous Patrons
    Oprah Winfrey   *Rosanna Arquette*

Talented French perfumer Annick Goutal is the genius behind Gardénia Passion. The scent is a heady harmony of pure gardenia. An intense, dramatic, unforgettable composition that is beautiful for afternoon tea, garden parties, walks in the park...or any place you want to sprinkle a little sunshine.

Goutal packaging is pure glamour: A limited-edition Louis XVI Baccarat flacon may be filled with a choice of Gardénia Passion or Eau d'Hadrien. The bottle is hand decorated with delicate gold-colored flowers, topped with an old-fashioned atomizer spray, and beautifully presented in a velvet jewelry box with gold-colored cord accents. Exquisite!

Introduced   *1990*
Price   *Top range*

GEM

Scent Type   *Chypre - Fruity*
Composition
    Top Notes: *Peach, plum, myrtle, cypress, cardamom, coriander, rosewood*
    Heart Notes: *Tuberose, jasmine, rose, clove, iris, ylang-ylang, carnation, orris*
    Base Notes: *Patchouli, vanilla, moss, amber, civet, vetiver*

Famous Patrons
    Actress Josette Banzet, Marquise de Bruyenne

The second fragrance offering from Van Cleef & Arpels, Gem is a rich chypre melange of rare floral essences, fresh fruits, and exotic spices. Succulent fruits and spices create a distinctive, top-drawer top note that gives way to a rich floral heart enhanced by spicy clove and carnation. Lingering base notes of sweet vanilla, patchouli, and amber complete the feminine, dramatic fragrance.

Wish all of our gems came from Van Cleef & Arpels. Ahh...if only it were so....

Introduced   *1988*
Price   *High range*

GFF

Scent Type   *Floral - Fruity*
Composition
    Top Notes: *Orange, bergamot, lemon, osmanthus*
    Heart Notes: *Jasmine, rose*
    Base Notes: *Sandalwood, patchouli*

From Italian designer Gianfranco Ferre comes a fragrance bearing Ferre's initials. Brisk hesperides create an exhilarating opening accord, which dissolves into a radiant heart of florals and woods, as uplifting as Lake Como at sunrise.

The artistically structured bottle is evidence of Ferre's architectural training. Sleek and statuesque, the cylindrical bottle is topped with silver- and gold-toned metals formed into the shape of an antique pump. Easy to wear, fresh and transparent, GFF is a surprisingly well-priced Italian import.

Introduced   1996
Price   Mid-range

GIANFRANCO FERRÉ

Scent Type   *Floral*
Composition
    Top Notes: *Hyacinth, bergamot, fruits,*
                        greens, coriander, orange blossom
    Heart Notes: *Tuberose, jasmine, rose,*
                        honeysuckle, narcissus,
                        lily of the valley, orchid
    Base Notes: *Musk, spices, moss*

The first fragrance for women from the Italian fashion designer and architect Gianfranco Ferré is a sprightly floral bouquet. Green herbal notes give a fresh lift, while musk, spices, and moss warm the composition. An easy-to-wear floral fragrance, the effect is quiet and mannered, like a mountain-top stroll through the fragrant Italian gardens of Villa d'Este.

Introduced   1984
Price   Mid-range

GIORGIO

Scent Type   *Floral*
Composition
    Top Notes: *Bergamot, mandarin, galbanum,*
                        greens, fruits
    Heart Notes: *Jasmine, rose, carnation,*
                        ylang-ylang, orris,
                        lily of the valley, hyacinth
    Base Notes: *Sandalwood, cedarwood, musk,*
                        moss, amber

Famous Patrons
    Nancy Reagan   Jacqueline Bisset
    Grace Robbins
    Former Vogue model Aly Spencer

Gale and Fred Hayman found immediate success with Giorgio, named after their internationally famous boutique on Rodeo Drive in the heart of Beverly Hills. The heady, exotic floral fragrance is a glamorous long-lasting scent. One of the best-selling fragrances of all times, it is dramatic and lavish, saucy and full of sexy verve... a fragrance to impress.

Giorgio set the stage for blockbuster fragrance hits of the 1980s and 1990s. The distinctive line, in its yellow and white striped packages, was unveiled at a million-dollar party. It was originally available only at the Rodeo Drive boutique and through mail order. Now, this bestseller can be found virtually worldwide. It is often copied, but never duplicated.

After years of hard work, entrepreneurs Gale and Fred Hayman sold the Giorgio Beverly Hills company for a handsome profit when they divorced. But the fragrance remains, true to their vision.

Introduced   1982
Price   Mid-range

GLAMOUR

Scent Type   *Floral - Oriental*
Composition
    Top Notes: *Ylang-ylang, lily of the valley,
                    water lily, violet leaves*
    Heart Notes: *Carnation, jasmine, gardenia,
                    rosewood*
    Base Notes: *Amber, sandalwood, vanilla,
                    musk*

Giorgio Beverly Hills co-founder Gale Hayman has enjoyed a string of successes, from the blockbuster Giorgio fragrance, which *Newsweek* dubbed "the scent of the century," to Delicious and Sunset Boulevard.

Glamour is one of a pair of perfumes Hayman introduced in 1999. Glamour is a rich floral Oriental composition, ideal for evening wear. Its counterpart, Style, is a floral scent with green highlights, suitable for daytime use. Formulated with common essential oils, the two may also be worn together for a new, creative experience.

Glamour's rich, seductive personality is mirrored in its ruby red, columnar bottle, which is accented with a gold-colored collar and lettering. The scent epitomizes Beverly Hills glamour. And, as we all know, glamour never goes out of style.

Introduced   *1999*
Price   *Mid-range*

GODDESS

Scent Type   *Floral - Oriental*
Composition
    Top Notes: *Peach, apricot, bergamot, plum,
                    apple, pineapple, passion fruit*
    Heart Notes: *Nutmeg, clove, lily, lilac,
                    violet leaves, iris, heliotrope*
    Base Notes: *Amber, sandalwood, vanilla*

Goddesses of love—Venus and Aphrodite, Freya and Ishtar—have intrigued through the ages, imprinting history with legend and lore. Beauty expert Marilyn Miglin created Goddess, *le nectar des dieux*, or "nectar of the Gods," for all goddesses, past, present or future.

Goddess opens with a subtle, soft accord of sun-warmed fruits. A spicy heart, splashed with watery florals, is tempered with a mesmerizing blend of amber, vanilla, and sandalwood—as tantalizing as Venus. Simple, clean packaging belies the sweet notes within. It is a lovely, versatile scent, created for the goddess in every woman.

Introduced   *1999*
Price   *Mid-range*

GOLCONDA

Scent Type   *Floral*
Composition
    Notes: *Floral essences*

An exotic floral fragrance whose name reaches back into history, Golconda is truly "an American in Paris." It hails from the elite Paris shop, Jars on Place Vendôme, a rare gem of a store owned by American jeweler Joel Rosenthal.

Rosenthal christened his scent Golconda after the ancient Indian province whose supply of the world's finest pink diamonds was depleted at the end of the seventeenth century. Golconda is presented in a Baccarat crystal bottle, a design inspired by a Golconda diamond belonging to Shah Jahan, an Indian ruler. The exotic letters carved in the bottle are similar to characters carved into the Shah's diamond, while the stopper is a copy of a rough pink Golconda diamond.

This work of art is crated and cushioned in dried Indian roses as though it had just made the ocean voyage in the bowels of a tall-masted ship, swept through time by the trade winds of our imagination. Perfect for your next voyage.

Introduced	*1988*
Price	*Top range*

GOOD LIFE

Scent Type   *Floral - Oriental*
Composition
   Top Notes: *Bergamot, pineapple, black currant*
   Heart Notes: *Jasmine, rose, fig leaf, carnation,*
                 ylang-ylang
   Base Notes: *Iris, plum, sandalwood, fig milk,*
                 date, vanilla

Davidoff enjoyed success with the men's version of Good Life. In 2000, Davidoff followed this success with Good Life for women, a sheer, floral Oriental fragrance blended to evoke feelings of happiness, contentment, and well-being. In short, of living the good life. Mirroring the simple serenity of the fragrance, the curved bottle is pure of line and easy to handle. Good Life is a versatile scent that is easy to wear from morning 'til night— ideal for the busy mother or career woman.

Introduced	*1999*
Price	*Mid-range*

GRACE DE MONACO

Scent Type   *Floral*
Composition
   Top Notes: *Mandarin, orange blossom,*
                 ylang-ylang
   Heart Notes: *Jasmine, May rose, tuberose*
   Base Notes: *Sandalwood, tonka bean,*
                 vanilla, ambrette, orris

Her Serene Highness Princess Grace of Monaco is lovingly remembered and honored with the creation of Grace de Monaco. HSH Princess Grace was known for her classic style, femininity and graciousness, as well as her devotion to the advancement of the performing arts and artists. An accomplished actress before marrying Prince Rainier III, and known as Grace Kelly, she received an Academy Award for the 1954 film *The Country Girl*. (We adored her in *High Society* and *Rear Window*, too.) A portion of the sales proceeds from the Fabergé Grace de Monaco fragrance line is donated to the Princess Grace Foundation. Founded in 1982, the foundation supports the education of young performing artists.

The fragrance, blended by Firmenich, is an elegant floral bouquet of warmth and glamour, of moonlit nights on Mediterranean shores. Gentle fruits and flowers are combined with sweet amber and sandalwood, while a touch of vanilla hints at luxury. Grace de Monaco is tastefully opulent, fit for a princess, or any sophisticated woman of the world.

Fabergé painstakingly created several limited-edition parfum bottles, based on original designs by Peter Carl Fabergé. Inspired by the Catherine Palace Egg and handcrafted in St. Petersburg, Russia, the crystal eggs are exquisite works of art, rendered in brilliant emerald green. A variety of atomizers, eggs, and flacons are available, each design as breathtaking as the next—definitely an heirloom presentation. We think HSH Princess Grace would have approved of this fabulous fragrance.

Introduced	*2000*
Price	*High range*

GRAIN DE FOLIE

Scent Type   Floral - Fruity
Composition
    Top Notes: *Lime, kumquat, rhubarb, clementine*
    Heart Notes: *Peony, jasmine, stephanotis, basil flower*
    Base Notes: *Tonka bean, acacia, musk, moss*

The legend of French couturier Alix Grès, born Germaine Krebs, lives on in a fragrance called Grain de Folie. Madame Grès, as she was professionally known, created such well-loved perfume classics as Cabochard and Cabotine and designed glorious, Grecian-draped gowns for Grace Kelly and Jacqueline Kennedy Onassis. Grain de Folie, French for "a little bit crazy," is a cheerful floral, enhanced with fruits such as kumquat and lime. The bottle sports the colors of a cockeyed optimist, in shades of lime green, blue, pink, and orange, with a carved bouquet cap of patchwork fruits and flowers. Engaging and fun, just right with a floppy straw hat and a cotton summer frock. Wear it and let yourself go just a little bit crazy.

Introduced	*2000*
Price	*High range*

GRAND AMOUR

Scent Type   Floral - Ambery
Composition
    Top Notes: *Honeysuckle*
    Heart Notes: *Hyacinth, lily*
    Base Notes: *Vanilla, myrrh, musk, balsam*

From Annick Goutal, the Parisian pianist-turned-perfumer, comes a rich, elegant fragrance. Goutal dedicated Grand Amour to her own great love, her husband, Alain Meunier.

Combined with the warmth of vanilla and myrrh in a sensual balsamic base, Grand Amour is an earthy melange of natural essences, including sweet honeysuckle and hyacinth. Expansive, exquisite, a fragrance for grand living, for the enjoyment of life at its fullest. Grand Amour is housed in Goutal's familiar gold and ivory packaging, topped with a golden butterfly to signify its creator's continual creative and personal metamorphosis.

Alas, Annick Goutal's untimely 1999 passing saddened many. The world weeps, for indeed, it has lost a grand lady.

Introduced	*1996*
Price	*Top range*

GREEN TEA

Scent Type   *Floral - Green*
Composition
    Top Notes: Lemon, peppermint, orange,
                 bergamot, rhubarb
    Heart Notes: Green tea, jasmine, celery seed,
                 carnation, caraway, fennel
    Base Notes: Oakmoss, amber, musk

Elizabeth Arden seeks to revive the inner spirit with Green Tea, a subtle, energizing blend with a dominant note of green tea and other natural ingredients. Hesperides, such as lemon and bergamot, provide a refreshing opening, followed by peppermint, which is a highly beneficial, energizing essential oil. Jasmine bestows a dual effect on the body's senses. Blended with spices and green tea, jasmine heightens sensuality while relaxing the nervous system—a state known as calm vitality. An excellent choice when a stressful day might otherwise leave you harried.

Aromas can pack a powerful psychological punch. Green tea, surging with renewed popularity, has long been recognized as an herbal healer for its immune system-enhancing, cholesterol-lowering abilities. It is even thought to slow the aging process with its cancer-fighting antioxidants. (Pardon me whilst I brew a "cuppa.")

Arden's Green Tea is presented in a simple, leaf-etched spray bottle. Well-priced line extensions include such restorative spa luxuries as oversized tea bags for the bath, and an exfoliating scrub. Cool and exhilarating. Mercy, I'm feeling younger already.

Introduced   *1999*
Price   *Mid-range*

GUÉPARD

Scent Type   *Chypre*
Composition
    Top Notes: Mandarin, geranium
    Heart Notes: Coriander, ginger, orange flower,
                 cinnamon
    Base Notes: Spices, woods, oakmoss

Guépard is the signature fragrance from the Swiss luxury purveyor known for its fine watches, jewelry, and accessories. The warm fragrance is mysterious and complex, a classic chypre composition of the highest order. Rich spices, including ginger, cinnamon, and coriander, are expertly blended in a smooth, sensual formula that envelops the wearer like a velvet cape. Guépard is long-lasting, rich enough for cool evenings, a subtly elegant statement that connotes class.

Presented in packaging of jade green and gold, Guépard is a work of art. Pale green frosted glass is encased in a gold-colored, basket-weave overlay, capped with an emerald orb. An imperial presentation.

Introduced   *1997*
Price   *High range*

HABANITA

Scent Type   Oriental - Ambery
Composition
    Top Notes: Bergamot, peach, orange blossom, raspberry
    Heart Notes: Rose, jasmine, ylang-ylang, orris, heliotrope, lilac
    Base Notes: Amber, oakmoss, leather, vanilla, musk, cedarwood, benzoin

Habanita is a warm Oriental blend from the Paris House of Molinard. Fruity top notes introduce the composition, which proceeds through rich florals to a final balsamic drydown of amber, leather, vanilla, and musk. Sweet and sensual, beautiful for evening and cool crisp days.

The original Molinard was established in Grasse in 1849 to supply wealthy vacationers and royalty, including Queen Victoria. A Paris presence was later established. The Grasse factory is now open for tours at certain times of the year. (60 blvd Victor-Hugo, telephone 93-36-01-62) Call ahead to the tourist office; this is a real treat!

Introduced   1921
Price   High range

HALSTON

Scent Type   Chypre - Floral
Composition
    Top Notes: Melon, greens, peach, bergamot, spearmint, tagetes
    Heart Notes: Jasmine, rose, cedarwood, orris, carnation, marigold, ylang-ylang
    Base Notes: Vetiver, amber, patchouli, musk, sandalwood, incense, moss

The signature fragrance from Halston is a distinctive fragrance that has been a bestseller for years. The chypre blend opens with energizing green notes supported by smooth fruity essences, followed by a classic French floral bouquet that rests on an amber base. Easy to wear, easy to enjoy.

Introduced   1975
Price   High range

HANAE MORI

Scent Type   Floral - Oriental
Composition
    Top Notes: Blackberry, strawberry, bilberry, black currant
    Heart Notes: Rose, jasmine
    Base Notes: Sandalwood, almond, rosewood

From the esteemed Japanese fashion designer Hanae Mori comes her signature floral fragrance of gracious elegance. Translated, her name means "flower of the forest." For inspiration, Mori sought out traditional Japanese aromas, such as cherry trees in bloom. A melange of berries opens the composition, which harmonizes with a classic floral heart. Accents of almond and rosewood add dimension to the sandalwood base.

The fragrance is delicately packaged in white cartons featuring Mori's beautiful butterfly motif; the various colors of butterflies indicate different fragrance strengths.

Elegant and refined—expect the Hanae Mori fragrance to flit and flutter into your heart.

Introduced   1996
Price   High range

HANAE MORI HAUTE COUTURE

Scent Type   *Floral - Aldehyde*
Composition
    Top Notes: *Bergamot, coriander, aldehydes*
    Heart Notes: *Jasmine, tuberose, gardenia,*
                     narcissus, lily of the valley
    Base Notes: *Iris, sandalwood*

Designer Hanae Mori regales us once again with an exquisite floral fragrance of impeccable pedigree. The scent is expansive and radiant, redolent of white flowers and warm woods. Suitable for a gala evening of grand proportions, or anytime you are comfortable in *haute couture*.

Pierre Dinand-designed bottles reside in a parade of ever-changing packages. Seasonal Hanae Mori *haute couture* designs grace the cartons, from red perfume cartons featuring wedding and ball gowns, to blue eau de parfum cartons with evening gowns, to pink eau de toilette boxes with casual wear. Hanae Mori Haute Couture is, indeed, a fragrance for the gracious life.

Introduced   1998
Price   *High range*

HAPPY

Scent Type   *Floral - Fruity*
Composition
    Top Notes: *Ruby red grapefruit, mandarin*
                     blossom, citrus, mountain laurel
    Heart Notes: *Boysenberry bush flower,*
                     morning dew orchid
    Base Notes: *Mimosa blossom, white lily,*
                     magnolia

Happy is a sparkling, effervescent fragrance from Clinique, a subsidiary of Estée Lauder. From fruity top notes and a heart of exotic flowers to the white floral base accord, Happy is a carefree composition. Packaged in an exuberant shade of lipstick red, Happy is an upbeat scent suitable for summertime daydreaming.

Introduced   1997
Price   *High range*

HEURE EXQUISE

Scent Type   *Floral - Aldehyde*
Composition
    Top and Heart Notes: Florentine iris, Turkish rose
    Base Notes: *Sandalwood*

Heure Exquise, which translates as "exquisite hour," is a romantically delicate scent. The refined essence of rose is combined with fragrant sandalwood. Creator Annick Goutal described it as a fragrance for the "sublimely feminine woman."

Introduced   1986
Price   *Top range*

HIRIS
♀♂

Scent Type   Floral - Semi - Oriental
Composition
    Top Notes: *Orange blossom, rose,*
                    coriander seed
    Heart Notes: *White iris, black iris, cedarwood*
    Base Notes: *Vanilla, ambrette seed,*
                    almond wood

Since 1837, the French house of Hermès has brought forth luxury goods of every description, from the finest leathers and silks to the most exquisite fragrances. Imagine classics such as Calèche and Amazone. Hiris, so named for liberal use of iris, combined with an "H" for Hermès, is an ethereal, yet warm, effusive scent of Old World sophistication.

The iris flower is named for the Greek goddess Iris, born of Electra and Thaumas, and the alter ego of Hermès. A messenger goddess, she is often depicted with a shimmering, rainbow scarf, leading souls to the great hereafter. Hence, the iris flower is often planted on gravesites to assist souls in their onward journey. The Florentine coat of arms also bears the iris, and every year in the Palazzo Vecchio the most brilliant irises are awarded recognition. Colors of every hue vie for attention, but the royal purple remains a perennial favorite.

Iris stands alone in the world of perfumery. It is the only flower whose scent is derived not from its velvety petals, but from the withered root, or rhizome. The root is then pulverized to a white powder from which the fragrance is extracted, as prized as platinum in the perfumer's palette. Perfumer Olivia Giacobetti states: "Hiris is born from a unique note, from an obsession with an exceptional material." Her passion for her craft is evident in Hiris; the scent unfolds with hints of rose and coriander and is warmed with cedarwood, vanilla, and a hint of almond wood.

Look for Hiris packaged in iris purple and Hermès' trademark orange. Hiris is a memorable scent of fine distinction for women and men, versatile and easy to enjoy.

Introduced   1999
Price   High range

HUGO WOMAN

Scent Type   Oriental - Fruity
Composition
    Top Notes: *Green apple, cantaloupe,*
                    water lily
    Heart Notes: *Florals, nectarine, peach, berry*
    Base Notes: *Siamwood, sandalwood, amber*

Following the success of Hugo for men, by Hugo Boss, Giorgio Beverly Hills rolls out Hugo Woman. Hip, young, and trendy, the scent targets the youth market. A sexy Oriental composition with fruity notes gives a provocative edge to the Givaudan Roure-designed scent.

The advertising tagline "Life is a journey, travel light" is in sync with the round, canteen-style flacon, which is topped with an aluminum cap attached by an orange strap. Presented in a Halloween-orange carton with blue lettering.

Introduced   1997
Price   Mid-range

HYPNOTIC POISON

Scent Type   *Oriental*

Composition

    Top Notes: *Bitter almond, caraway*

    Heart Notes: *Jasmine*

    Base Notes: *Vanilla, moss, jacaranda wood,*
                  musk

The original Poison formula was a shocking departure from the norm when it was introduced in 1986. Fourteen years later, the red hot Hypnotic Poison, from Christian Dior, replicates its predecessor's olfactory shock. Bitter almond and spice paves the way for an Oriental base of vanilla, musk, and woods. Dramatic and full-bodied, Hypnotic Poison is an ideal scent for Latin American holidays. Tango, anyone?

Packaging of sizzling red, black, and gold reflects the passionate nature of the fragrance. An opulent red resin coating lends a soft feel to the classic Poison bottle.

A rapturous scent—why not add a dash of spice to your life?

Introduced   *1999*

Price   *High range*

IL BACIO

Scent Type   *Floral - Fruity*

Composition

    Top Notes: *Honeysuckle, rose, jasmine,*
                  freesia, orchid, lily of the valley

    Heart Notes: *Peach, plum, melon, pear,*
                  passion fruit, osmanthus, iris

    Base Notes: *Amber, sandalwood, violet,*
                  musk, cedarwood

Il Bacio is an understated fruity floral melange from the Italian Princess Marcella di Borghese. Il Bacio, Italian for "the kiss," is an airy, feminine composition, created as a token of love. Il Bacio features floral top notes, animated by a well-rounded basket of succulent Mediterranean fruits. Il Bacio is a pretty springtime or light winter fragrance, easy to wear for daytime.

Il Bacio is encased in a fan-shaped bottle designed by Marc Rosen that the company says is "reminiscent of the palazzo arches seen in Venice." A knotted red cap, suggesting the "unbreakable bond of eternal love" adorns it.

Look for a Borghese lipstick in Il Bacio Red, said to be the perfect kissing lipstick. Venus would approve.

Introduced   *1993*

Price   *High range*

INDISCRET

Scent Type   *Floral - Fruity*
Composition
    Top Notes: *Mandarin, bergamot, galbanum,*
                  orange flower, tiger orchid,
                  white peach blossom,
                  orange blossom
    Heart Notes: *Jasmine, tuberose, rose, clove,*
                  rose geranium, basil, cypress,
                  ylang-ylang, iris, violet leaves
    Base Notes: *Sandalwood, amber, oakmoss,*
                  vetiver, patchouli, white musk,
                  guaiac wood

Famous Patrons
   Princess Nathalie Paley   *Marlene Dietrich*

Indiscret is one of the great classic fragrances of the twentieth century and the legacy of Lucien Lelong, renowned French couturier. Introduced in 1936, this magnificent perfume faded from the scene after Lelong's death, but was lovingly resurrected in 1997 by Lelong perfume and couture collectors Arnold Hayward Neis and his wife, Lucy de Puig Neis.

Rich and dramatic, Indiscret is a fragrance of impeccable pedigree. After being awarded the French *Croix de Guerre* for his efforts in World War I, Lucien Lelong opened his first *maison de couture* in 1919. By 1937, he was elected president of the French Fashion Syndicate, the *Chambre Syndicale de la Couture Française*. While Nazi troops occupied France from 1940 to 1945, Lelong toiled to keep the French fashion industry alive by foiling German attempts to move the industry to Berlin. He is widely credited with maintaining the fashion industry in Paris during World War II and, in the process, keeping some

three hundred thousand people employed. Among Lelong's staff were Hubert de Givenchy, Christian Dior, and Pierre Balmain, who later made their own marks in the world of fashion and fragrance.

In 1924, Lelong embarked upon his fragrant journey, establishing the *Societé des Parfums Lucien Lelong*. A prolific entrepreneur, he created more than twenty-five fragrances. Among them were lettered scents: N (for his wife, Princess Nathalie Paley), J, L, A, B, and C. Many of his fragrances masqueraded under different names in English-speaking markets: La Première (Opening Night), Orgueil (Pride), Joli Bouquet (Pretty Bouquet), Murmure (Whisper), and Mon Image (My Image). One of the most popular of these scents was Indiscret, the scent Arnold and Lucy Neis chose to commemorate the ideals of Lucien Lelong.

Indiscret, meaning "indiscreet," was reformulated with care by the French perfume house of Mane. The dramatic soul of the original formula prevails: sensual, captivating, expressive, sophisticated. Yesteryear's glamour is artfully blended with a new, modern attitude. Today's Indiscret features fresh top notes of mandarin, orange blossom and orange flower, with a green lift of galbanum. Following is an intensely feminine heart of jasmine, rose, and tuberose, with a twist of cypress and violet leaves, and finishing with a sultry, long-lasting base of sandalwood, amber, and vetiver. Indiscret is a fragrance for the art of grand living.

A sculptor and glass collector, Lelong favored glass for his bottle designs. Most of Lelong's many and varied bottles are priceless collectibles today. In designing the Indiscret bottle, Lelong draped a silk handkerchief and said, "That is how I want the Indiscret bottle to look—as if they were folds of classical drapery." Bottle designer Marc Rosen served as a consultant in the re-creation of the Indiscret bottle. Faithful to Lelong's original vision, Indiscret is captured in a frosted glass bottle, then nestled in brilliant fuschia satin, and boxed in shades of black and gold.

Finally, with deep admiration, this author bids a fond adieu to the man who left this world the day she entered it. Perhaps we passed in the corridor of life.

Introduced	1936
Reintroduced	1997
Price	High range

INFINI

Scent Type	Floral - Aldehyde
Composition	
Top Notes:	Aldehydes, peach, bergamot, neroli, coriander
Heart Notes:	Rose, jasmine, lily of the valley, carnation, ylang-ylang, orris
Base Notes:	Sandalwood, musk, vetiver, civet, tonka bean

From the House of Caron comes Infini, a floral with scintillating aldehydic top notes—a forever fragrance, in French, for the "infinite." The feminine bouquet is nestled in a soft wooded base, like a forest wood nymph in hiding. Its subtle, ethereal quality is fitting for casual or professional daytime wear.

Bottle designer Serge Mansau conceived the bottle. The clear glass flacon has a diamond-shaped cutout in the heart, matched by another diamond cutout in the angular crystal stopper. Crisp, asymmetrical lines complete the attractive object of art.

Introduced	1912
Reintroduced	1970
Price	High range

INITIAL

Scent Type	Oriental
Composition	
Top Notes:	Mandarin, black currant leaves
Heart Notes:	Jasmine, rose, almond, honey
Base Notes:	Pepper, patchouli

French jeweler Boucheron establishes a new tradition with Initial, a fresh Oriental composition from Firmenich perfumer Jacques Cavallier. Mandarin is blended with a classic accord of jasmine and rose, smoothed with almond and honey, and spiced with patchouli and black pepper. An easy-to-wear, full-bodied Oriental formula, it is ideal for the classic woman with a passionate nature.

After mining sapphires for the packaging of its Jaïpur line, Boucheron turned to the classic pearl for Initial. Designers at Desgrippes Gobé conceived the pearly white and gold presentation, selecting a feminine, teardrop-shaped bottled with a gold-colored cap, fashioned after a Boucheron pendant. Exquisite in presentation, rich in design, Initial is for new beginnings, for those all-important initial impressions.

Introduced	2000
Price	High range

INVITATION

Scent Type	Floral
Composition	
Top Notes:	Freesia, orange blossom, bergamot, frangipani, tangerine, lemon, tiare, greens
Heart Notes:	Rose, violet leaf, jasmine, violet, lily of the valley, ylang-ylang
Base Notes:	Amber, vanilla, sandalwood, cedarwood, musk, vetiver

Actress Susan Lucci, well known for her Emmy Award-winning role as Erica Kane on *All My Children*, threw her hat into the beauty ring with Invitation. Invitation is a two-in-one fragrance. The exotic floral scent infuses an eau de cologne version that is suitable for daytime, as well as a rich eau de parfum, an evening formulation. The two fragrance strengths are suspended in separate glass compartments, entwined like the fingers of a golden goddess.

Invitation is a unique concept and an entertaining fragrance. Lucci fans might also enjoy a visit to www.susanlucci.com.

Invitation: deserving of a speedy RSVP.

Introduced	*2000*
Price	*Mid-range*

IVOIRE

Scent Type	*Floral - Green*
Composition	
Top Notes:	*Jasmine, galbanum, bergamot, violet, mandarin, aldehydes*
Heart Notes:	*Turkish rose, lily of the valley, Tuscany ylang-ylang, carnation, pepper, nutmeg, cinnamon, berry pepper*
Base Notes:	*Vetiver, oakmoss, sandalwood, labdanum, amber, vanilla, patchouli, tonka bean*

From couturier Pierre Balmain, Ivoire is a green floral aroma, voluptuous and seductive, yet in an offhand, innocent manner. A woman at a gala who was dressed in creamy pale silk, stark among a sea of black tuxedos, supposedly inspired the name.

The sophisticated floral unravels with shimmering greens, flowing into a floral heart accented with spices and greens. The long-lasting base is composed of sweet amber and powdery woods.

After working with fashion legends—Christian Dior, Lucien Lelong, Robert Piguet, and Edward Molyneux—Pierre Balmain opened his boutique in Paris in 1946, where his designs were sought after by a privileged clientele. Before his death in 1982, he was honored as an Officer of the Legion of Honor, one of France's most esteemed positions.

Look for Ivoire products in creme and gold-colored packaging, as though dressed for a ball like the mysterious woman in pale silk.

Introduced	*1979*
Price	*High range*

J'ADORE

Scent Type	*Floral*
Composition	
Top Notes:	*Ivy leaves, champak flower, mandarin*
Heart Notes:	*White rose, orchid, violet*
Base Notes:	*Plum, blackberry, musk, woods*

A golden-haired model drenched in liquid gold is the advertising image put forth by Christian Dior for J'Adore, a recent addition to the house's legendary line of fine fragrances. J'Adore is an embraceable floral bouquet tempered with fruits and woods; it is a fragrance of adoration. A smoothly rounded, golden-hued bottle by Herve Van Der Straeten completes the tempting presentation.

Introduced	*1999*
Price	*High range*

JAÏPUR

Scent Type   *Floral - Fruity*
Composition
    Top Notes: *Plum, peach, freesia, apricot*
    Heart Notes: *Rose, iris, peony, acacia*
    Base Notes: *Sandalwood, amber, mush,*
        heliotrope

Jaïpur is an expansive floral fragrance from the venerable French jeweler Boucheron. A fruity opening accord lends lightness and gaiety to an otherwise sophisticated composition. A radiant springtime "let's do lunch" scent, equally appropriate for an evening at the theater.

Boucheron is well known for its exquisite packaging. For example, the signature Boucheron perfume is presented in a flacon styled to resemble a ring. Following tradition, Jaïpur is captured in a bracelet-style bottle of sapphire blue and gold. The inspiration for the design originated in 1928. Louis Boucheron received a commission from the Indian state of Punjab to set the gemstones of the Maharaja of Patiala in a bracelet. Tradition holds that the bracelet, or *nauratan*, was to be worn by brides for protection and good luck. The finest examples of these ornate, voluptuous designs are made in the Indian region of Jaïpur. Boucheron mined this memory for the Jaïpur flacon design. The result is simply sublime.

Introduced   *1994*
Price   *High range*

JAÏPUR SAPHIR

Scent Type   *Floral - Ambery*
Composition
    Top Notes: *Peach, cardamom, tangerine,*
        yuzu
    Heart Notes: *Magnolia, stephanotis jasmine,*
        heliotrope
    Base Notes: *Karmir wood, amber,*
        sandalwood, cinnamon wood,
        resin, vanilla

Prized for their clarity and radiance, the sapphires of Kashmir are legendary. French jeweler Boucheron drew inspiration from these miracles of nature to create Jaïpur Saphir, a tribute to one of the jeweler's most prized gemstones.

Jaïpur Saphir is a well-balanced floral with rich ambery tones. With a touch of green, a whisper of fruit, and a bouquet of flowers, the melange is warmed by a slightly spicy, ambery base of mystery and intrigue. Sensual and elegant, Jaïpur Saphir is a fragrance of classic proportion. Although it is versatile enough for day wear, we highly recommend wearing it for romantic evenings with your maharajah. The scent is beautifully clothed, of course, in sapphire blue and platinum-white hues. Clearly, Jaïpur Saphir is designed for the maharani in all of us.

Introduced   *1999*
Price   *High range*

JARDINS DE BAGATELLE

Scent Type *Floral*
Composition
  Top Notes: *Violet, aldehydes, lemon, bergamot*
  Heart Notes: *Orange blossom, tuberose, magnolia, gardenia, rose, jasmine, ylang-ylang, orchid, lily of the valley, narcissus*
  Base Notes: *Cedarwood, vetiver, patchouli, musk*

A classic floral garden fragrance from Jean-Paul Guerlain, Jardins de Bagatelle was created for the modern woman. Like most Guerlain fragrances, it carries with it an enchanting tale. It was inspired by and named after Queen Antoinette's gardens and château in the Bois de Boulogne, built for her in 1777. As in her gardens, spring florals blossom into a full-bodied white floral heart. The magic of white flowers is fragrant, long-lasting sweetness. Jardins de Bagatelle is a versatile, feminine fragrance that blooms from sunrise to sunset.

The romantic Bagatelle retreat was the result of a wager. Legend has it that one day the Queen and the Count of Artois, brother to Louis XVI, were enjoying a horseback ride through the French countryside. When they came upon a decrepit chalet, the Count bet the Queen that he would build a new château for amusement on the site in less than ten weeks. She took the bet, and in less than sixty-four days, Bagatelle was built. Though she lost the bet, she loved the new château and gardens.

As with most Guerlain fragrances, the scent was conceived as a reflection of its time. Jardins de Bagatelle was designed in the 1980s for the woman who is joyful and assertive, yet still feminine at heart.

Introduced *1983*
Price *Mid-range*

JE REVIENS

Scent Type *Floral - Aldehyde*
Composition
  Top Notes: *Orange blossom, aldehydes, bergamot, violet*
  Heart Notes: *Clove, rose, jasmine, hyacinth, lilac, orris, ylang-ylang*
  Base Notes: *Amber, incense, tonka bean, vetiver, musk, moss, sandalwood*

The couture House of Worth brings forth Je Reviens, a popular scent for more than sixty years. The fragrance opens with bright aldehydic top notes, then meanders along a floral path liberally doused with rare spices. Smoky incense and mellow amber linger long after the company has gone home.

Englishman Charles Frederick Worth established his fashion salon in Paris 1858, catering to a clientele of wealth and royalty, including the Empress Eugénie. From his shop on the chic rue de la Paix, he saw clients by personal referral only. Flowing, fluid garments became his trademark. His sons, Jean-Philippe and Gaston Worth, continued the business and created fragrances to give to clients, scents that proved so popular they were soon sold on a wider scale, an endeavor managed by great-grandson Roger Worth.

Je Reviens means "I will return." And it does, again and again. A perennial favorite. Look for Je Reviens in the blue aquamarine boxes.

Introduced *1932*
Price *Mid-range*

JE T'AIME

Scent Type   *Floral - Oriental*
Composition
    Top Notes: *Bergamot, mandarin, greens*
    Heart Notes: *Bulgarian rose, jasmine,*
                orange blossom
    Base Notes: *Sandalwood, patchouli, oakmoss*

Je T'Aime is a fine fragrance from Holzman & Stephanie Perfumes. Perfumer Esther Holzman and her daughter, Stephanie, who holds a master's degree in science, are the forces behind this family-owned business. Holzman dedicated Je T'Aime to her aunt, the Baroness Emmy de Hirzel.

Je T'Aime, meaning "I love you" in French, is a sensual floral Oriental arrangement. Using the richest of natural ingredients, Je T'Aime is a soaring sonata of rose and white flowers. Exotic touches of spicy patchouli and sweet sandalwood add depth and balance. Presented in Pochet bottles, Je T'Aime is housed in exquisite Holzman-designed cylinders and boxes of royal purple and gold. Je T'Aime is a romantic fragrance, perfect for a magical holiday.

Introduced   *1988*
Price   *High range*

JEAN PATOU COLLECTION
(See individual profiles on each fragrance)

ADIEU SAGESSE
Floral - Fruity
AMOUR AMOUR
Floral - Fresh
CÂLINE
Floral - Fresh
CHALDÉE
Oriental
COCKTAIL
Chypre - Fruity
COLONY
Chypre - Fruity
DIVINE FOLIE
Oriental - Ambery
L'HEURE ATTENDUE
Oriental - Spicy
MOMENT SUPRÊME
Floral - Ambery
NORMANDIE
Oriental - Ambery
QUE SAIS-JE?
Chypre - Fruity
VACANCES
Floral - Oriental

Famous Patrons
    Duchess of Windsor   *Josephine Baker*
    Mary Pickford   *Gloria Swanson*
    Barbara Hutton   *Elsa Maxwell*
    Constance Bennett   *Silvia de Castellane*
    Suzanne Lenglen   *Helen Wills*

In perfumery, French couturier Jean Patou is perhaps most remembered for his incomparable creations, Joy and 1000. Although Patou is no longer with us, the firm that bears his name continues to introduce fine fragrances such as Sublime and For Ever.

At the helm of the business Patou's great-nephews Guy and Jean de Moüy continue the family legacy, having re-created classic Patou perfumes. Jean de Moüy explains their impetus: "Our greatest desire was for these perfumes to be appreciated by the contemporary counterparts of those women who used to love wearing them; in other words, the most elegant, distinguished and also, more often than not, the most famous women in the world."

With their in-house perfumer Jean Kerléo, they re-created classic fragrances from formulas preserved by their great-uncle, the debonair Jean Patou. Jean de Moüy explains these classics "will give lovers of all things beautiful the opportunity of inhaling the scents of a glamorous and exciting era, famous for its seductive elegance…an era in which Jean Patou became a legend in his own lifetime."

In the 1930s, Patou provided a burl and glass cocktail bar in his salon to amuse the gentlemen while the women were being fitted. Along with the usual libations, an assortment of essential oils was also available to patrons so that they could create their own fragrances. The array of classic Patou fragrances takes us back to this ingenious cocktail bar tradition, reminding us of the excesses of the twenties, of the flamboyant jazz age, of aristocratic summers at the Riviera and Deauville, and of the racy Hispano Suiza automobile Patou motored throughout Europe.

Patou classic fragrances are available individually, as well as in a gift set of miniatures called *Ma Collection*.

See the individual fragrance profiles for fascinating history on each Patou classic fragrance.

| Introduced | 1925 to 1964 |
| Price | Mid-range |

JEAN-PAUL GAULTIER

Scent Type   Floral - Fruity
Composition
    Top Notes: Bulgarian rose, Chinese star anise, Tunisian orange blossom, Italian tangerine
    Heart Notes: Indian ginger, orchid, Florentine iris, ylang-ylang, rose, orange blossom
    Base Notes: Réunion Island vanilla, amber, musk

Famous Patrons
  Madonna

Flamboyant French designer Jean-Paul Gaultier offers a fragrance that's sure to raise a few eyebrows. Gaultier catapulted to international fame after Madonna displayed his conical corsets and fashions during her 1991 *Blond Ambition* tour.

The signature fragrance is a fruity floral, with a top note reminiscent of scented nail polish and face powder, scents Gaultier remembered from childhood and wanted to reproduce.

The packaging is equally outrageous; the glass is molded into the shape of a corseted bust. An earlier "torso" perfume bottle from Roman designer Elsa Schiaparelli, whose 1937 hyacinth and patchouli perfume was called Shocking, inspired the curvaceous flacon. Schiaparelli's Shocking was sold in a bottle modeled after a Venus de Milo bust that she received from her friend Mae West.

The Gaultier perfume bottle is adorned by a metal corset, while a soft drink tab forms the stopper. Look for it in the tin can package. Pure Gaultier, pure *avant-garde*.

| Introduced | 1993 |
| Price | High range |

JESSICA MCCLINTOCK

Scent Type   Floral - Green
Composition
    Top Notes: Black currant bud, bergamot,
                     basil, ylang-ylang
    Heart Notes: Rose, white jasmine,
                     lily of the valley
    Base Notes: Musk, woods

American designer Jessica McClintock is known for her delicate, flowing fantasy creations. To complement her designs, she created her signature fragrance, a scent as romantic and feminine as her fashions.

The fragrance owes its fruity green top notes to bergamot and basil, with a touch of cassis, the black currant fruit. The heart is a delicate, sparkling blend of classic florals, bolstered by musky background notes. The potion is packaged in clear glass bottles with lacy white and silver accents.

A sweet scent for daytime and soft evening wear; ideal for the incurable romantic in all of us.

Introduced   1989
Price   Mid-range

JICKY
♀♂

Scent Type   Fougère
Composition
    Top Notes: Bergamot, lemon, mandarin
    Heart Notes: Lavender, rosemary, basil, orris,
                     tonka bean
    Base Notes: Vanilla, amber, benzoin,
                     rosewood, spices, leather

Famous Patrons
     Jacqueline Kennedy Onassis
     Joan Collins   Brigitte Bardot
     Sean Connery   Roger Moore
     Kenneth Jay Lane

Jicky is a fresh fougère from Guerlain that has endured for more than a century. Citrus, lavender, vanilla, and amber form the dominant accords of the classic fragrance, a scent that is shared by men and women.

The Jicky story began in the 1850s when Aimé Guerlain was living in England, studying chemistry and medicine. He fell in love with a woman he nicknamed Jicky. All was bliss until his aging father, Pierre François Pascal, summoned him back to Paris to take over the family business. When he asked for Jicky's hand in marriage, her family would not allow it. He returned to Paris alone and brokenhearted.

More than thirty years later, Aimé Guerlain honored the great love of his life by creating a fragrance that bore her nickname. He was proud of the breakthrough modern blend that utilized revolutionary technology in the perfumer's palette.

For the floral notes, he discovered a new solvent technology that produced a potent pure flower essence. For the base accord, he employed another of his discoveries, synthesis, which came from a gum resin called benzoin. From this he extracted vanillin, a substance that shared the dominant theme of natural vanilla but lacked the background complexities. Guerlain found that when he blended vanilla and vanillin for the base note of Jicky, the result was a rounder, full-bodied fragrance. Jicky was a new breed of fragrance.

But the year was 1889, and respectable women wore light, single flower scents such as lavender, violet, or rose, or simple bouquets. With its notes of citrus, florals, woods, and spices,

Jicky was considered strong and scandalous among proper ladies. The only women who wore such distinctive fragrances were prostitutes, who presumably mixed strong fragrances so potential clients could identify them on the dark streets.

Indeed, men appreciated Jicky. Soon men who wanted to be slightly provocative began to wear it. By 1912 women's fashion magazines began to praise it and women embraced the complex fragrance once considered scandalous. Today, more than one hundred years later, the original formula Jicky remains popular with women and men, and Aimé Guerlain's great love is legend.

Introduced   1889
Price   High range

JIL

Scent Type   Oriental - Fruity
Composition
  Top Notes: Lavender, raspberry, herbs
  Heart Notes: Violet, iris, vetiver, cedarwood
  Base Notes: Amber, tonka bean, vanilla

German couturier Jil Sander's modern, minimalist style is reflected in Jil, an Oriental composition lightened by lavender and raspberry. A chic red and gray color combination underscores the sleek appearance of the packaging. Jil is rendered in brushed aluminum and opaque glass— a study in chic simplicity. For the self-assured, professional woman.

Introduced   1997
Price   High range

JIL SANDER NO. 4

Scent Type   Floral - Oriental
Composition
  Top Notes: Light rose, geranium, peach,
                plum, galbanum
  Heart Notes: Violets, jasmine, rose, tuberose,
                heliotrope, ylang-ylang,
                carnation, tarragon, myrrh
  Base Notes: Grey ambergris, moss, vanilla,
                sandalwood, patchouli, musk

Famous Patrons
  Kim Bassinger   Jacqueline Kennedy Onassis

Jil Sander is a German-born fashion design purist. Her No. 4 fragrance is introduced with a green fruity top note, followed by a delicate flowery heart enhanced with dry spices. The subtle Oriental background trails a sensual mix of woods, ambergris and vanilla. Her scent is the personification of today's woman—independent, successful, and charismatic. No. 4 is inherently seductive, like the Jil Sander fashions that have garnered international acclaim and industry awards.

Introduced   1992
Price   High range

JIVAGO 24K

Scent Type   *Floral*
Composition
    Top Notes: *Bulgarian rose*
    Heart Notes: *Asian jasmine, tuberose, orris*
    Base Notes: *Amber, woods*

Jivago 24K draws inspiration from the feminine and masculine ideals—the yin and yang of our spirits and souls. Jivago 24K is a sensual floral bouquet, redolent of jasmine-scented evening air and crystal bowls brimming with roses.

Israeli designer and entrepreneur Ilana Jivago envisioned the union of man and woman in the design of her first perfume, Jivago 24K. A carved-glass rock serves as the base for the diamond-faceted flacon, which slips snugly into a receptacle that holds it upright. Emerald green accents enhance the flacon, inside of which float flakes of 24-karat gold, symbolizing prosperity and the sun's energy. Her kissing J's logo further signifies the blending of two souls, the giving and receiving of love and devotion. Jivago 24K is a fragrance of infinite romance.

Introduced   *1994*
Price   *High range*

JIVAGO 7 NOTES

Scent Type   *Floral Semi - Oriental*
Composition
    Top Notes: *Orchid, pear*
    Heart Notes: *Jasmine, tuberose, lotus flower,*
                 cinnamon, peony,
                 lily of the valley
    Base Notes: *Vanilla, mango, amber,*
                 sandalwood, musk

"Alas! all music jars when the soul's out of tune," wrote Miguel de Cervantes, in *Don Quixote*. Fashion designer Ilana Jivago fine-tunes the soul with her musical scent, Jivago 7 Notes. Jivago's talents are wide-ranging; she wrote music to accompany her fragrance, and the jazzy, New-Age spiritual collection debuted with it.

The floral semi-Oriental composition is a smooth, lyrical blend of pear and orchid, white flowers and spicy cinnamon, vanilla, amber, and sandalwood. The result is a rich, diffusive melody. Jivago's fascination with the spiritual aspects of the number seven is reflected in the seven-planed diamond-faceted bottle.

A percentage of the proceeds from 7 Notes is donated to schools to aid young musicians—a generous gesture from a gracious lady.

Introduced   *1998*
Price   *Top range*

JO MALONE COLLECTION

AMBER & LAVENDER
Oriental
FLEURS DE LA FORÊT
Chypre
FRENCH LIME BLOSSOM
Floral
GARDENIA
Floral
GRAPEFRUIT
Citrus
HONEYSUCKLE & JASMINE
Floral
LIME, BASIL & MANDARIN
Citrus (♀♂)
NUTMEG & GINGER
Oriental - Spicy
RED ROSES
Floral

SANDALWOOD & CEDARWOOD
Chypre (♀♂)
TUBEROSE
Floral
VETYVER
Chypre (♀♂)
WHITE HYACINTH
Floral
WILD MUGUET
Floral

British perfumer and entrepreneur Jo Malone is taking the world by storm with her creative line of natural potions and lotions. Her first scent, Nutmeg & Ginger, was packaged in a plain wrapper. She says it was "Just a little something" she whipped up in her kitchen for friends and clients. Malone's best-selling scent is Lime, Basil & Mandarin, a unisex citrus scent she laughingly refers to as "the pension fund." Putting husband Gary to work, Malone has taken on the likes of New York City's venerable Bergdorf Goodman. Her glittering list of clients includes divas Barbra Streisand and Diana Ross, as well as royalty, such as the lovely, smart, and serene Queen Noor of Jordan.

Can't live with just one Jo Malone fragrance? Well, who could? Put several on your shopping list.

Introduced	*1991*
Price	*High range*

JONES NEW YORK

Scent Type   *Floral - Green*
Composition
   Top Notes: *Bergamot, mandarin, lime, jasmine, white rose, lily of the valley, ylang-ylang*
   Heart Notes: *Peach, plum, lavender, cypress, galbanum*
   Base Notes: *Sandalwood, amber, musk*

An understated classic floral, Jones New York is an ideal complement to the clothing line of the same name. The Dragoco-developed formula embraces florals and fruits, underscored with soft wooded notes. Easy to wear, soft and sparkling, the fragrance is packaged in Jones taupe and black with gold-colored accents.

Introduced	*1996*
Price	*Mid-range*

JOOP!

Scent Type   *Floral - Oriental*
Composition
   Top Notes: *Neroli, bergamot*
   Heart Notes: *Bulgarian rose, jasmine, orange blossom*
   Base Notes: *Vanilla, sandalwood, patchouli, coumarin*

From Parfums Joop!, German designer Wolfgang Joop introduces his version of a floral Oriental. Pronounce it "yope," to rhyme with "hope."

Beginning with a fresh citrus top note, Joop! dissolves into a rich heart note, then gives way to a sensual symphony of warm, exotic Oriental essences. Bursting with Joop! impact. Great for the trendy "let's do lunch" bunch.

Introduced	*1991*
Price	*Top range*

JOY

Scent Type   *Floral*
Composition
    Top Notes: *Aldehydes, peach, greens, calyx*
    Heart Notes: *Jasmine, Bulgarian rose,*
                    ylang-ylang, orchid,
                    lily of the valley, orris, tuberose
    Base Notes: *Sandalwood, musk, civet*

Famous Patrons
    Joan Rivers   *Mary Pickford*
    Gloria Swanson   *Barbara Hutton*
    Constance Bennett *Elsa Maxwell*

In 1930, the legendary Joy was introduced as the costliest perfume in the world. French couturier Jean Patou had set out to create a fragrance "free from all vulgarity" at any cost, as well as "impudent, crazy, and extravagant beyond reason." Indeed, the sumptuous scent quickly became revered as the world's most extravagant perfume and to this day remains one of the costliest perfume to produce, according to the Patou firm.

The dominant notes are absolute of jasmine and Bulgarian rose, two of the world's rarest and most expensive essences. Each ounce contains the essence from more than 10,000 jasmine flowers and twenty-eight dozen roses. Lavish quantities of the delicate jasmine and elegant rose are woven into a rich tapestry of more than a hundred essences, resulting in a scent that remains true to Jean Patou's vision. Each vessel of fragrance is still mixed and hand-sealed as it was at its inception in a process carefully overseen by Jean Kerléo, Patou's internationally recognized in-house perfumer, along with Patou's great nephews, who head the company.

Jean Patou launched his quest for Joy in 1926 when he took his assistant, cafe society woman Elsa Maxwell, with him to Grasse to work with perfumers on the new scent. Together they searched for a fragrance that would meet the exacting requirements of the best-dressed and most discriminating women of the world, the social leaders and accomplished women of their day. After exhaustive testing they were presented with the formula for Joy, a recipe that called for twice the amount of essential oils that other popular perfumes contained. But alas, the perfumer told them it was too expensive to be commercially viable. That cinched it. Hence was born the "costliest fragrance in the world," and women the world over had to have it.

Joy is timeless; as revered today as it was when it was introduced. It remains a strong, dynamic floral essence with an unmistakable stamp of wealth, breeding, and confidence.

Introduced   *1930*
Price   *Top range*

KISS & TELL

Scent Type   *Floral*
Composition
    Top Notes: *Orange blossom, ionicera,*
                    tangerine
    Heart Notes: *Tuberose, jasmine, narcissus,*
                    lily of the valley
    Base Notes: *Sandalwood, musk*

These days, everyone seems eager to kiss and tell, be it on a daytime talk show or in a celebrity "tell-all" autobiography. Capitalizing on this seemingly intrinsic human desire, Brad and Judy Levy, owners of Fragrance International, decided to do just that. But it was easier said than done.

The fragrance was more than three years in the making, and the bottle is an engineering triumph from master designer Robert du Grenier. The cleverly designed bottle is actually two bottles in one, with a spray cap on each end. The inner and outer chambers are filled with two versions of the same floral scent: Choose the lighter interpretation for daytime wear, or the opulent version for evening. Enjoy one scent at a time, or mix them in whatever ratio you deem fit. Then, kiss all you want—we'll never tell.

Introduced	*1999*
Price	*Top range*

KNOWING

Scent Type	*Chypre - Floral*
Composition	
Top Notes:	*Greens, coriander, orange, aldehydes*
Heart Notes:	*Rose, jasmine, lily of the valley, cedarwood, cardamom*
Base Notes:	*Amber, sandalwood, patchouli, spices, vetiver, orris, oakmoss*

Knowing is an understated composition, redolent of fragrant woods and soft spring flowers with a final aura of oakmoss and spice. Another fine fragrance from Estée Lauder.

Introduced	*1988*
Price	*Top range*

LA PARISIENNE

Scent Type	*Floral - Fresh*
Composition	
Top Notes:	*Linden, apple, greens*
Heart Notes:	*Bulgarian rose, violet, lily of the valley, jasmine, orris, hyacinth*
Base Notes:	*Amber, musk, vetiver*

Esther Holzman, of Holzman & Stephanie Perfumes, is the creative force behind the family-owned boutique firm that produces such classics as Misuki and Je T'Aime. La Parisienne is a sophisticated floral, developed with the Lake Forest woman in mind. Lake Forest is an exclusive area near Chicago, a village where Holzman and her family reside on a gracious estate. Inspired by the towering linden trees dotting their verdant grounds, Holzman developed La Parisienne—a light, all-natural, floral composition with a dominant note of white linden blossom.

La Parisienne is presented in graceful, clear Pochet bottles and wrapped in shades of Parisienne pink and gold. Feminine, delicate and endearing; La Parisienne is perfect for Paris in the spring.

Introduced	*1989*
Price	*High range*

LADY CARON

Scent Type   Floral - Fruity

Composition

     Top Notes: Neroli, jasmine, magnolia

     Heart Notes: Raspberry, rose, peach

     Base Notes: Sandalwood, oakmoss

From Parfums Caron comes a fragrance steeped in one man's dream of liberty and life. In 1939, when Nazi Germans threatened Europe, Parfums Caron founding father and master perfumer Ernest Daltroff fled Paris for the safety of the United States. Adrift and beleaguered, Daltroff felt his hope soar when his ship passed the Statue of Liberty—the gift from France, his homeland. Instantly, he pledged that someday he would create a fragrance to commemorate that moment, a scent that would convey his hopes, faith, and vision. And so, more than sixty years later, the fragrance, Lady Caron, debuts.

The lady in question is the Liberty Lady, whose embossed face shimmers on every bottle. Messages of hope adorn the cartons, as Daltroff's hopes surely nourished his hungry soul. Lady Caron is a classic, elegant, optimistic fragrance for the new millennium.

Introduced   2000

Price   Top range

LAGUNA

Scent Type   Floral - Fresh

Composition

     Top Notes: Moroccan lemon,
Calabrian tangerine,
Spanish verbena, pineapple,
Asian green galbanum, plum

     Heart Notes: Egyptian rose, Italian iris,
lily of the valley, jasmine

     Base Notes: Madagascar sandalwood,
Réunion Island vanilla, amber,
musk, coconut, cedarwood,
patchouli

Laguna is a shimmering floral from the fragrance line bearing the name of the late artist Salvador Dali. Packed with exotic fruits and spicy iris, Laguna is a modern eau de toilette with a youthful outlook. Refreshing, light, and "slightly impertinent," Laguna is said to have drawn its inspiration from the Pacific Ocean. Indeed, the fragrance is ideal for warm summer days or a plunge in a clear lagoon.

The fragrance flows in the trademark Salvador Dali flacon—a frosted glass rendering of voluptuous lips with a nose-shaped stopper. Outrageously fun! The outer package is colored in pale Caribbean Sea turquoise and embellished with Dali's signature. A 1981 Dali painting, *Apparition of the Face of Aphrodite of Knidos in a Landscape*, served as inspiration for the unusual packaging.

Introduced   1991

Price   Mid-range

LAILA

Scent Type *Floral - Fresh*
Composition
Notes:
Norwegian wild mountain flowers,
watermelon

Famous Patrons
Whitney Houston   Mariah Carey

Laila creator and entrepreneur Geir Ness cherishes his childhood memories of his native Norway. When he was a boy, his beautiful mother, Laila, introduced him to the many natural wonders of their homeland. Together they roamed the countryside, frolicked in pure mountain streams, and gathered bouquets of fragrant wildflowers. Years later, Ness drew upon these fond memories to create the first fragrance of Norway. With a flash of inspiration, he decided to use his mother's actual signature on the bottle. He silk-screened her name on the first one, and sent it to her for Mother's Day. Imagine her pride and delight upon opening it!

Brisk as a sparkling mountain stream, clean as a first snowfall, fragrant as a bouquet of wildflowers—these are the olfactory images of Laila. The sheer floral is rife with Norwegian wildflowers, while a hint of watermelon adds a watery freshness. Laila is ideal for daytime and warm weather wear, or anytime a sheer veil of scent is desired. Why not wear it high into the mountains for a special retreat, or for the season's first, pristine day of snow skiing?

Ness personally launched his line in Los Angeles, providing samples and gift baskets at the National Academy of Recording Arts and Science's Grammy nominations and awards parties. But you don't have to be a diva to enjoy Laila.

Introduced   1995
Price   *Mid-range*

L'AIR DU TEMPS

Scent Type   *Floral*
Composition
Top Notes: *Bergamot, peach, rosewood,*
neroli
Heart Notes: *Gardenia, carnation, jasmine,*
May rose, ylang-ylang, orchid,
lily, clove, orris
Base Notes: *Ambergris, musk, vetiver,*
benzoin, cedarwood, moss,
sandalwood, spices

Famous Patrons
Lana Turner

L'Air du Temps is a classic French fragrance from the Parisian firm of Nina Ricci. The fragrance is like a bouquet of spring flowers strewn in the sun across a bed of precious woods and subtle spices. L'Air du Temps is an easy-to-wear floral scent that floats effortlessly from day to evening. Graceful, feminine, innocent, and understated.

Italian-born Nina Ricci opened her couture boutique in 1932 amidst worldwide uncertainty. Closed in 1939 during World War II, the business reopened six years later under the direction of her son Robert. Before her death in 1970, Nina Ricci was awarded the French Legion of Honor for her collections and accomplishments.

Robert Ricci and Marc Lalique designed the lovely flacon. A pair of doves swoon atop the stopper, wings spread, beaks touching—a timeless image of love. As it was in 1948, the perfume is sold in crystal Lalique flacons of various hues.

L'Air du Temps remains a fragrance of infinite romance for lovers the world over.

Introduced   1948
Price   *High range*

LALIQUE

Scent Type	*Floral*
Composition	
Top Notes:	*Chinese gardenia, Sicilian mandarin, blackberry*
Heart Notes:	*Grasse magnolia, Tunisian orange blossom, peony, Bulgarian rose, ylang-ylang*
Base Notes:	*Réunion Island vanilla, Virginia cedarwood, East Indian sandalwood, Tibetan musk, Colombian amber, Yugoslavian oakmoss*

Famous Patrons
Alexandra (Mrs. Sidney) Sheldon

Lalique is a namesake fragrance from Lalique, maker of fine collectible glassware. The founder of the company, René Lalique, first collaborated with François Coty in 1906 to elevate the art form of the perfume bottle. Today, granddaughter Marie-Claude Lalique brings her vision of perfume and flacons full circle with a fragrance inspired by her gardens in Provence.

From her fragrant flowering oasis spills forth blossoms of magnolia and peony, her favorite flowers, and the main impression of the Lalique perfume. The challenge was to create these two essences by blending other essences from the perfumer's palette, for they do not exist as essential oils. This task accomplished, the blend was enlivened with touches of blackberry and mandarin, then softened with Colombian amber. Base notes of musk, vanilla, and woods create a long-lasting aura. The result is a subtle refined fragrance, remarkably like a Provençal spring garden in bloom.

The perfume resides in a package of vivid turquoise and understated terra cotta, and is draped with a gift: A crystal pendant suspended from a silk cord that can be worn as a necklace. Inside rests a flacon of clear and satin-finished mouth-blown crystal. Frosted trellises of sculpted leaves embrace the transparent center vial. The leafy vine motif is continued on the stopper and the crystal pendant.

Each year, Marie-Claude Lalique creates a new bottle collection. Her special collections are available in a limited number of stores, and are highly collectible.

Introduced	*1992*
Price	*Top range*

LAUREN

Scent Type	*Floral - Fruity*
Composition	
Top Notes:	*Wild marigold, greens, rosewood, pineapple*
Heart Notes:	*Bulgarian rose, lilac, violet, jasmine, lily of the valley, cyclamen*
Base Notes:	*Cedarwood, oakmoss, sandalwood, vetiver, carnation*

From American designer Ralph Lauren hails a light contemporary, feminine floral fragrance. Lauren opens with energizing greens and fruits, followed by a floral harmony with delicate undertones of spices and woods. As natural as the elegantly tailored, easy-to-wear Ralph Lauren designs—all timeless American classics.

Ralph Lauren explains: "My philosophy about fragrance, like fashion, is simple: Never accept substitutes for the best. And if the best doesn't exist, create it."

The understated fragrance is presented in ruby red flacons, accented with gold-colored caps. The clear lead crystal perfume flacon was inspired by antique regency inkwells and is now part of the permanent collection of the Cooper-Hewitt Museum in New York.

Introduced 1978
Price High range

LE DIX

Scent Type Floral - Aldehyde
Composition
Top Notes: Aldehydes, peach, lemon, bergamot, coriander
Heart Notes: Jasmine, rose, orris, lilac, lily of the valley
Base Notes: Vetiver, sandalwood, musk, amber, tonka bean, benzoin, Peru balsam

Le Dix is a classic fragrance from the celebrated Spanish couturier Cristobal Balenciaga. Le Dix debuted in Paris in 1947—the same year Christian Dior introduced his New Look collection of post-World War II fashion. Le Dix was one of the new postwar fragrances eagerly sought out by those who had denied themselves of luxuries for far too long during the war.

Balenciaga was born in northern Spain, but moved to Paris in 1937 during the Spanish Civil War. Creator of the pillbox hat, three-quarter sleeves, and flamenco dresses, he also trained other young designers, such as Ungaro and Courrèges. He designed for women of wealth and title, including those of the Spanish royal family. Today, his couture designs reside in the New York Metropolitan Museum collection.

Le Dix is French for "ten," named for his salon at No. 10, avenue Georges V, and indeed, it is a perfect ten with us.

Introduced 1947
Price High range

LE FEU D'ISSEY

Scent Type Oriental - Ambery
Composition
Top Notes: Rose, lily, coriander leaf, pepper
Heart Notes: Amber
Base Notes: Guaiac wood, benzoin, amber

Today, a fashion designer's rite of passage, commercially speaking, is the creation of a fragrance to call his or her own. However, Japanese designer Issey Miyake was initially hesitant when approached in the early 1990s about such an endeavor. Yet his concerns vanished when he met with Chantal Roos, who was president of Beauté Prestige. Their first successful collaboration was L'Eau d'Issey, a sheer, diaphanous marine fragrance launched in 1993. Le Feu d'Issey is the second act, a fiery, vibrant scent that reflects Miyake's evolving designs, trending toward a sizzling color range.

Amber is the dominant thread in this spicy yet understated tapestry of woods and florals from Firmenich perfumer Jacques Cavalier. The unusual bottle is a spherical design, made of synthetic material and shaded in crackling hot hues of golden red and sunset orange. Le Feu, which means "fire" in French, is one spicy scent; after all, some like it hot.

Introduced 1998
Price High range

LELONG

Scent Type Floral - Oriental
Composition
    Top Notes: *Bergamot, mandarin, magnolia, lilac, kadota fig*
    Heart Notes: *Jasmine, iris, ylang-ylang, tuberose, May rose, white and purple cattleya orchids, Sharry Baby orchid*
    Base Notes: *Oakmoss, sandalwood, vetiver, musk*

During the first half of the twentieth century, Parisian couturier Lucien Lelong was world-renowned, not only for his designs, but also for his fragrant creations. In 1997, Lelong perfume and couture collectors Arnold Hayward Neis and his wife, Lucy de Puig Neis, reacquainted the world with one of Lelong's most successful scents, Indiscret. Two years later, they introduced Lelong Pour Femme in honor of Lelong and his accomplishments.

An expansive, floral Oriental perfume in the French tradition, Lelong Pour Femme is warm and endearing, with a beautiful, lingering *sillage*. The glamour of the yesteryear is suspended on a silken veil of scent. Utterly exquisite.

The Neises engaged designer Marc Rosen to create the bottle as well as the presentation. It is the first fragrance bottle to incorporate a miniature working clock in its design. In fact, Lelong once designed gold wristwatches for the Elgin company; today these watches are prized collectibles. Inspired by the Paris Art Modern period, Rosen created the curved, arched crystal bottle, which is shouldered with *faux* tortoise shell. The execution is remarkable, and in time it is sure to become a collector's item. We love the beautiful double duty it serves on our desk.

Lucien Lelong believed that time was the ultimate luxury, and today, in our busy, interconnected world, that is certainly true. And so, through the mists of bygone years, Lelong is one way to have precious time on your hands.

Introduced   1999
Price   Top range

L'HEURE ATTENDUE
(See also Jean Patou Collection)

Scent Type Oriental - Spicy
Composition
    Top Notes: *Lily of the valley, geranium, lilac*
    Heart Notes: *Ylang-ylang, jasmine, rose, opopanax*
    Base Notes: *Mysore sandalwood, vanilla, patchouli*

Acclaimed French couturier Jean Patou crafted L'Heure Attendue to celebrate the liberation of Paris from the Nazi occupation during World War II. Formulated to reflect the happy peoples' *joie de vivre*, it is a spicy Oriental composition with an expansive, freewheeling personality.

L'Heure Attendue is a beautiful scent for evening and winter wear, a jubilant scent with the classic verve of yesteryear. Wear to express your own sense of freedom and exhilaration.

Introduced   1946
Price   Mid-range

L'HEURE BLEUE

Scent Type   *Floral - Ambery*
Composition
    Top Notes: *Bergamot, lemon, coriander, neroli*
    Heart Notes: *Bulgarian rose, iris, heliotrope, jasmine, ylang-ylang, orchid*
    Base Notes: *Vanilla, sandalwood, musk, vetiver, benzoin*

Famous Patrons
Julia Roberts	*Queen Elizabeth II*
Carolyn Roehm	*Catherine Deneuve*
Blaine Trump	*Teri Garr*
Liza Minelli	*Bianca Jagger*
Wendy Wasserstein	*Ursula Andress*
Pat Nixon	

L'Heure Bleue means "blue hour" in French, and it was reportedly inspired by the gentle blue-hued twilight of a pre-World War I Paris, a time of relative innocence.

Third-generation perfumer Jacques Guerlain conceived L'Heure Bleue for the sophisticated woman. He freely employed the latest synthetic ingredients to create a totally new scent, combined with passionate florals and dusky, exotic base notes including vanilla, musk, and aromatic woods. The resulting scent is tender yet penetrating, like a twilit evening in Paris, with undercurrents of bewitching sensuality, and a powdery *sillage*.

The perfume is captured in a heavy glass flacon adorned by scrollwork on the shoulders. The triangular stopper is shaped like a gentleman's hat, a *chapeau de gendarme*, from which a hand-tied silken tassel dangles.

L'Heure Bleue was a landmark scent of 1912 and remains an enchanting favorite. A classic French perfume, L'Heure Bleue is an elegant selection for the romantic at heart.

Introduced   *1912*
Price   *High range*

LIME, BASIL & MANDARIN
♀♂
(See Jo Malone Collection)

L'INTERDIT

Scent Type   *Floral - Aldehyde*
Composition
    Top Notes: *Aldehydes, mandarin, peach, bergamot, strawberry*
    Heart Notes: *Jasmine, rose, jonquil, narcissus, lily of the valley, orris, ylang-ylang*
    Base Notes: *Sandalwood, vetiver, musk, amber, cistus, benzoin, tonka bean*

Famous Patrons
    Audrey Hepburn

Renowned French couturier Hubert Givenchy created this aldehydic floral bouquet for actress Audrey Hepburn. It is said that for many years, Hepburn was the only woman allowed to wear the feminine fragrance. Givenchy was one of her favorite designers and created many of her clothes for films such as *Breakfast at Tiffany's*.

L'Interdit is a smooth blend of elegant floral notes in perfect harmony with bright aldehydes and succulent fruits. Balsamic base notes create an understated sensual aura. If fragrance were a movie scene, L'Interdit would be the opening sequence of *Breakfast at Tiffany's* with Hepburn draped in a black Givenchy evening dress gazing into the Tiffany window of sparkling jewels. Quietly alluring, L'Interdit is a fragrance of spare sophistication.

Introduced   1957
Price   High range

LIÙ

Scent Type   Floral - Aldehyde
Composition
    Top Notes: Bergamot, neroli, aldehydes
    Heart Notes: Jasmine, May rose, iris
    Base Notes: Amber, vanilla, woods

Famous Patrons
    Diana Ross   Ethel Kennedy
    Rose Kennedy

Every Guerlain fragrance begins with a story, before even the first drop of essential oil is selected. A character from Puccini's opera *Turandot* inspired the delicate Liù.

Liù is a charming romantic fragrance featuring a dominant bouquet of jasmine, rose, and iris. Exhilarating citrus top notes and powdery base notes round out the floral aldehyde composition. Inspired by a woman of tenderness and passion, whose love and generosity are boundless, Liù is understated and refined. A subtle fragrance, Liù is ideal for the professional woman with a multifaceted life.

Guerlain submitted this outline of *Turandot*:

> In the opera, the Princess Turandot dares any prince or nobleman who seeks her hand in marriage to successfully answer three riddles or be sentenced to death.
>
> One of her suitors, the Unknown Prince, accepts the challenge and proffers

triumphant responses to the riddles, thereby winning the Princess's hand. Sensitive to the Princess's opposition to the marriage, however, the Prince offers Turandot a challenge of his own: If she can guess his name, he will relinquish his right to her hand.

> The desperate princess kidnaps Timur, the Prince's father, and threatens to torture him until he reveals the guarded secret. To save Timur's life, Liù, the Prince's servant, acknowledges that she is the only one who knows the Prince's name. After admitting to Turandot that she is deeply in love with the Prince, Liù takes her own life, guarding the secret forever.

> The Prince grants Turandot one more chance at freedom by divulging his name: Calaf. Moved by Liù's amorous gesture, Turandot proclaims the Prince's true name to be Love.

A romantic story for a romantic fragrance.

Introduced   1929
Price   Mid-range

LIZ CLAIBORNE

Scent Type   Floral - Fruity
Composition
    Top Notes: Carnation, white lily, freesia, mandarin, marigold, greens, bergamot, peach
    Heart Notes: Jasmine, jonquil, rose, ylang-ylang, lilac, tuberose, lily of the valley
    Base Notes: Sandalwood, amber, oakmoss, musk

In 1976, American clothing designer Liz Claiborne introduced contemporary fashions to fit the way people lived. Ten years later, she created a signature fragrance that is just as comfortable and easy to wear.

A crisp, energetic blend of light florals, spirited greens, and sweet fruits, the eau de toilette essence is captured in bright lacquered triangles of primary red, blue and yellow. The perfume is housed in a playfully inverted triangle-on-triangle crystalline flacon.

Introduced	*1986*
Price	*Mid-range*

LIZSPORT

Scent Type   Floral - Green
Composition
    Top Notes: Bergamot, lemon, ivy, narcissus, grasses, mandarin
    Heart Notes: Rose, peony, phlox, mimosa, jasmine, lily, crocus
    Base Notes: Moss, musk, cedarwood

Liz Claiborne launches Lizsport, a casual fragrance for everyday living. A floral bouquet imbued with fresh–cut greens, the overall impression is crisp, clean, and carefree. From morning coffee through afternoon tea, from sports events to play dates, from luncheons to late night snacks, Lizsport glides effortlessly through a busy day.

Introduced	*1997*
Price	*Mid-range*

LOLITA LEMPICKA

Scent Type   Oriental - Fruity
Composition
    Top Notes: Ivy, anise seed
    Heart Notes: Iris, licorice, violet
    Base Notes: Vanilla, tonka bean, praline, vetiver, musk

Designer Lolita Lempicka's eponymous fragrance is an enchanting Oriental blend with fresh, fruity top notes. It is beautifully feminine, with a sensually sweet, powdery base. The fantasy–inspired fragrance is reminiscent of baroque designs of the early twentieth century. Indeed, many of Lempicka's fashion designs are fairy tale creations of luxurious fabrics.

The darling bottle is enough to make William Tell miss his mark. A hymn to romantic love, the lavender tinted, apple–shaped flacon is decorated with ivy leaves outlined in gold and white enamel. A brushed gold–colored cap and "stem" spray top the clever presentation. Finished with a playful chartreuse carton, the Lolita Lempicka presentation is absolutely stunning, reminiscent of the glamour and humor of early twentieth-century perfume bottles. Go ahead— take a bite out of this forbidden fruit.

Introduced	*1997*
Price	*High range*

LUCKY YOU

Scent Type   Floral - Fresh
Composition
    Top Notes: Ruby red grapefruit,
                        water hyacinth, freesia,
                        green leaves
    Heart Notes: Star jasmine, peony, blue poppy
    Base Notes: Sandalwood, amber, musk

Lucky in love, a lucky break, a lucky charm; Lucky You shares optimistic company in the lexicon of luck. From Lucky Jeans comes a duo of youth-oriented scents for women and men. Drawing on a 1950s Americana theme, Lucky You is packaged in apothecary-style bottles designed by Elizabeth Carlucci Cord. Firmenich perfumers blended the lighthearted scent. Spritz it on for lottery luck. Who knows? You might strike the mother lode.

Introduced   2000
Price   Mid-range

MA GRIFFE

Scent Type   Chypre - Floral
Composition
    Top Notes: Gardenia, greens, galbanum,
                        aldehydes, clary sage
    Heart Notes: Jasmine, rose, sandalwood,
                        vetiver, orris, ylang-ylang
    Base Notes: Styrax, oakmoss, cinnamon,
                        musk, benzoin, labdanum

Famous Patrons
    Barbara Walters

In French, *ma griffe* refers to a signature or personal stamp. Thus, couture designer Carven selected the name for her personal fragrance. Ma Griffe is a blend of earthy essences presented in brilliant green packaging. It is a timeless, easy-to-wear classic, steeped in mosses, flowers, and woody balsamics.

Carven made quite a splash with Ma Griffe. When she launched the fragrance, she hired a plane to drop thousands of tiny, parachuted perfume samples across Paris. The response was overwhelming.

Carven founded the House of Carven in 1944. From her Paris salon at the Rond Point des Champs-Élysées, she led the way in creating haute couture especially for petite women—she herself was just five feet tall. Along with her signature samba dresses, silk scarves, furs, and jewelry collections, she sold her fragrance creations. Though Ma Griffe was her personal scent, she also introduced other classics: Robe d'un Soir, Madame Carven, Vert et Blanc, and Variations.

Introduced   1946
Price   Mid-range

MA LIBERTÉ

Scent Type   Oriental - Spicy
Composition
    Top Notes: Heliotrope, citrus
    Heart Notes: Jasmine, rose, lavender, clove
    Base Notes: Sandalwood, vetiver, vanilla,
                        musk, cedarwood, patchouli,
                        nutmeg, cinnamon

From the House of Jean Patou comes a haunting ambrosial fragrance invented for the woman who is free with her emotions, the expressive woman with emotional liberty.

A subtle Oriental blend, Ma Liberté begins with saucy citrus top notes followed by a courtly floral heart enhanced with spicy clove. Fragrant woods are accented with cinnamon and nutmeg to produce a sweet sensual finish, fit for Aphrodite.

Declare your liberty with Ma Liberté.

Introduced	*1987*
Price	*Mid-range*

MACKIE

Scent Type	*Floral - Oriental*
Composition	
Top Notes:	*Peach, raspberry, pineapple*
Heart Notes:	*Jasmine, rose, jonquil, orange blossom, ylang-ylang, tuberose*
Base Notes:	*Sandalwood, vetiver, patchouli, amber, musk*

Mackie is the namesake fragrance from internationally renowned designer Bob Mackie. Fresh fruits introduce the scent, while rich white florals heighten the drama of the warm Oriental blend.

Mackie says, "A woman who wears my clothes is not afraid to be noticed." Ditto for his perfume. Mackie is the designer to the stars, the man behind some of Hollywood's most striking and alluring garments. Who can forget Cher's Academy Awards outfits? "Dare to be noticed—wear a Mackie Original," he says. Classic Mackie.

The sensual fragrance is captured in a multifaceted Pierre Dinand/Mackie–designed bottle, topped with a crystal stopper for added glamour and glitz. The ebony and ivory color theme reflects Mackie's love of piano. The dramatic outer package sports a brilliantly colored starburst prism.

Mackie...a glamorous fragrance for drop-dead drama.

Introduced	*1991*
Price	*High range*

MADAME ROCHAS

Scent Type	*Floral - Aldehyde*
Composition	
Top Notes:	*Hyacinth, neroli, aldehydes, greens, lemon*
Heart Notes:	*Bulgarian rose, jasmine, iris, lily of the valley, violet, orris, narcissus, tuberose*
Base Notes:	*Amber, cedarwood, sandalwood, moss, vetiver, musk, tonka bean*

Madame Rochas is a floral symphony of rich jasmine, rose, and iris. The full-bodied heart is embedded in warm exotic woods. The French approach is timeless and enduring, as fine today as it was upon introduction more than three decades ago. Its personality is spicy, delicate, and feminine.

Madame Rochas is presented in the signature Rochas color scheme of white, red, and gold. The octagonal cylinder is a copy of an eighteenth-century cut-crystal bottle Hélène Rochas unearthed in a Parisian antique shop. Classic design, classic fragrance, classic French.

Introduced	*1960*
Price	*Top range*

MAGIC

Scent Type   *Oriental - Fruity*
Composition
    Top Notes: *Cassis, bergamot, plum*
    Heart Notes: *Jasmine, almond oil,*
                      tuberose, geranium
    Base Notes: *Vanilla, clove*

Marilyn Miglin heads a beauty empire of fragrance, cosmetics and salons and is well known for her television appearances. Miglin's first fragrance success was Pheromone, which remains a favorite of many women.

Miglin's Magic is an intensely feminine, fruity Oriental composition with a spicy touch of almond oil and a hint of clove. A scent smoldering with sensuality—forbidden pleasures spring to mind. Miglin comments, "I have created classic fragrances for daytime and evening, but Magic is for midnight."

Introduced   *1999*
Price   *Mid-range*

MAGIE NOIRE

Scent Type   *Oriental - Ambery Spicy*
Composition
    Top Notes: *Hyacinth, cassie, bergamot,*
                    raspberry, galbanum
    Heart Notes: *Jasmine, ylang-ylang, Bulgarian*
                    rose, lily of the valley, narcissus,
                    honey, tuberose, orris
    Base Notes: *Spices, sandalwood, ambergris,*
                    cedarwood, patchouli, oakmoss,
                    musk, civet

Famous Patrons
    Isabella Rossellini

From Lancôme comes Magie Noire, or "black magic" in French. The spicy Oriental blend is as smooth as Far Eastern silk. Seductively understated, soothing and easy to wear, it is perfect for a little night magic.

The round bottle, designed by master bottle designer Pierre Dinand, sports a deeply indented V–shape, draped around the shoulders like a plunging neckline.

Introduced   *1981*
Price   *High range*

MANIA

Scent Type   *Oriental - Ambery*
Composition
    Top Notes: *Orange blossom, bergamot,*
                    greens, pittosporum
    Heart Notes: *Nutmeg, clove, amber, saffron*
    Base Notes: *Bourbon vanilla, white musk*

Giorgio Armani started a craze with Mania, a spicy fragrance of ambery incense. "The woman I had in mind when I created Mania is passionate, enthusiastic, full of desire," says Armani.

Mania opens with the freshness of bergamot combined with the lightness of sweet orange blossom; pittosporum, an evergreen shrub, contributes a herbaceous tone. Beneath a smoldering heart of nutmeg, clove, and amber lies a base of great refinement, a scent with the soul of Armani. The high-quality formula was blended by perfumer Jacques Cavallier, and the understated bottle was designed by Armani and Fabien Baron—a team of men who are clearly masters of their craft.

Introduced   *2000*
Price   *High range*

MANIFESTO

Scent Type	Green
Composition	
Notes:	Basil, bergamot, mandarin, white pepper, musk

Manifesto is actress and model Isabella Rossellini's first fragrance for Lancaster. Rossellini drew inspiration from her Swedish upbringing and from scents in her own back yard. Manifesto develops around a heart of basil, a green herb that Rossellini describes as humble and simple: "It doesn't make my mind wander." She also credits her mother, actress Ingrid Bergman, with inspiring her: "My mother revered practicality and down-to-earthness."

Manifesto is a comforting blend of fresh citrus, basil, and earthy musk. The scent is captured in a rounded, no-nonsense bottle of weighted glass designed by Alain de Mourgues.

Manifesto—wear it for casual days and carefree nights, wear it with ease and confidence.

Introduced	2000
Price	High range

MARIELLA BURANI

Scent Type	Floral - Fruity
Composition	
Top Notes:	Orange, lemon, bergamot, grapefruit, mandarin, aldehydes
Heart Notes:	Rose geranium, jasmine, peach, carnation, lily of the valley, iris, violet, coconut, ylang-ylang, cardamom
Base Notes:	Vanilla, sandalwood, vetiver, tonka bean, benzoin, tolu, musk, castoreum, cedarwood, oakmoss

Mariella Burani is the signature fragrance from the Cavriago-based Italian fashion designer. A fruity floral concoction, the scent is decidedly feminine. Fresh notes of delicate mandarin, blended with crisp grapefruit and bergamot, gracefully open the aromatic composition. Heart notes of jasmine, carnation, peach, and rose geranium add verve and depth, while base notes of vanilla and wood add strength and stability. A distinct aldehydic top note imbues the scent with a powdery impression, a nod to the charm of days gone by, when aldehydes were a new addition to popular scents of the nineteenth century. The overall effect is soft and subtle, yet the scent lingers like the memory of love's first foray. A beautiful choice for naturally feminine women, perfect for daytime, summer, and holiday wear.

The Mariella Burani packaging is delightfully reminiscent of the 1930s and 1940s—the era by which Burani is so greatly influenced. Her whimsical interpretation is depicted in the carved coral roses that adorn each bottle. To quote Burani, her fragrance and designs are for "women in bloom." The clear, rectangular, Pierre Dinand-designed bottles have a marvelously weighty feel.

Burani's combination of classic elegance and delicate femininity flows through the subtly hued packaging of peachy pink salmon.

For a change of pace, try Burani's Eau Rosée, a fruity floral fragrance with a distinct aldehydic, or powdery note.

| Introduced | 1992 |
| Price | High range |

MARINA DE BOURBON

Scent Type Floral - Fruity
Composition
  Top Notes: Lemon, watermelon, marigold, cistus, black currant leaves
  Heart Notes: Violet, orris, jasmine, rose, ylang-ylang, passion fruit
  Base Notes: Raspberry, peach, praline, tonka bean, vanilla, amber

Princess Marina de Bourbon is a descendant of the Bourbon dynasty—the family that ruled France from 1553 to 1848. Her forbear, King Louis XIV, arranged the construction of the palace of Versailles, leaving his mark upon the world of architecture.

Princess Marina's Paris showroom has featured the finest in leisure-oriented clothing and accessories since 1986. Recognized for her style, Princess Marina drew upon her taste and talent to create her signature scent, a composition she describes as being "clean, crisp, and elegant." The fragrance is a refined, fruity floral scent, with a hint of warm sensuality. A crystal stopper crowns the curved, elongated flacon; chic blue and white striped boxes encase the fragrance line. Truly elegant, a fragrance that is indeed fit for royalty.

| Introduced | 1996 |
| Price | High range |

MAROUSSIA

Scent Type Floral - Oriental
Composition
  Top Notes: Ylang-ylang, narcissus, black currant bud
  Heart Notes: Rose, jasmine, orange blossom, lily of the valley
  Base Notes: Amber, musk, vanilla, sandalwood

From Russia with love comes Maroussia, a warm ambery Oriental blend from native son and couturier Slava Zaitsev.

The sensual fragrance has mellow fruity top notes, quickly followed by a spicy floral heart that rests against a base accord of smoldering Oriental notes. The haunting melody creates a magnificent trail, or aura. Elegant and original.

Bottled in Moscow, Maroussia resides in ruby red and gold-colored flacons inspired by Russian Orthodox church domes. The fragrance is packaged in red boxes draped with an intricate print that is designed after Russian shawls and sensual Gustav Klimt paintings.

Close your eyes and imagine the snowy sleigh scenes from *Doctor Zhivago*. The romance of Russia…Maroussia.

| Introduced | 1992 |
| Price | Mid-range |

MASQUERADE

Scent Type	*Floral - Oriental*
Composition	
Top Notes:	*Freesia, mandarin, lily of the valley*
Heart Notes:	*Violet, passion flower, jasmine, osmanthus*
Base Notes:	*Sandalwood, musk, woods*

Fashion designer Bob Mackie hits his stride with Masquerade, an expansive floral Oriental. Masquerade is masked in black with a dazzling butterfly motif of yellow, blue, and violet; a full-bodied fragrance, perfect for the *bal masqué*, the traditional ball where ladies and gentlemen dance in disguise. "Oh, do be a dear and find my feathered mask, darling." We're already humming "Masquerade" from Andrew Lloyd Webber's *Phantom of the Opera*. Well, what better way to disguise and adorn yourself?

Introduced	*2000*
Price	*High range*

MICHAEL

Scent Type	*Floral*
Composition	
Top Notes:	*Moroccan incense, freesia*
Heart Notes:	*Tuberose, white peony, blue orris*
Base Notes:	*Vetiver, musk, cashmere woods*

Fashion designer Michael Kors celebrated the opening of his New York flagship store with his fragrance simply entitled Michael. "Glamorous but simple, indulgent but practical," Kors explains of the expansive floral scent. Feminine and chic, Michael is blended by Mane USA, and it features the dominant allure of tuberose, an extraordinarily fragrant white flower native to Mexico.

Look closely at the squared, architecturally rendered bottles, and a faceted "M" pops out; turn it sideways, and the "M" becomes a "K." For a real treat, try the Michael body products, which are named in a straightforward fashion—A Fabulous Body Lotion, A Sexy Body Shower, or our favorite, An Expensive Body Crème—at last, truth in advertising!

Introduced	*2000*
Price	*High range*

MILLENNIUM HOPE

Scent Type	*Floral - Fruity*
Composition	
Top Notes:	*Mandarin, strawberry, lily of the valley, black currant, tarragon*
Heart Notes:	*White tulip, jasmine, rose, violet, iris, osmanthus*
Base Notes:	*Musk, moss, vanilla, amber, tonka bean, sandalwood, vetiver, cedarwood*

Ilana Jivago greets the third millennium with Millennium Hope, a pair of women's and men's fragrances dedicated to universal love. Jivago comments, "By focusing our thoughts on unity and by taking positive actions coming from love, we become the hope and the promise of the new millennium."

The women's fragrance is an ethereal floral scent with a fruity opening accord that is sheer and sparkling. An ambery wooded base is blended with musk and vanilla to produce a warm, lingering effect on the skin. Jivago is known for her highly creative packaging designs, as evidenced in her previous fragrance, Jivago 24K. For Millennium Hope, a spherical, multifaceted bottle, representative of global unity, is carved from clear glass with a blue reflective base. Jivago enthusiastically calls Millennium Hope, "the scent for the next 1000 years."

Introduced   1999
Price   High range

MISS ARPELS

Scent Type   Floral - Fruity
Composition
    Top Notes: Freesia, basil, lemon,
                  watermelon, bay
    Heart Notes: Magnolia, jasmine, peony, lily
    Base Notes: Oak moss, sandalwood, vanilla

Fresh and invigorating, Miss Arpels is a light, fruity floral eau de toilette, developed for those with a youthful attitude. Sheer and summery, it is ideal for beach-bound days and languid evenings. Think balmy breezes and flowing white linen, endless white beaches and Mediterranean blue.

From jeweler Van Cleef & Arpels, Miss Arpels is a delightful scent with a well-bred background. Miss Arpels debuted in a multifaceted bottle designed by Serge Mansau, shaped to resemble a rough-cut diamond. Golden-hued four-leaf clovers adorn the bottle, as well as the debutante-white and gold-colored carton.

Introduced   1994
Price   High range

MISS DIOR

Scent Type   Chypre - Floral Animalic
Composition
    Top Notes: Bergamot, aldehydes, clary sage,
                  gardenia, galbanum
    Heart Notes: Rose, jasmine, lily of the valley,
                  carnation, orris
    Base Notes: Patchouli, oakmoss, amber,
                  vetiver, sandalwood, leather

A classic, impeccable floral fragrance, Miss Dior was created by French couturier Christian Dior.

Miss Dior was launched in 1947—the year Dior introduced his New Look. The New Look was actually a throwback to the pre-World War II years, full skirts, tiny waistlines, gloves, and bare shoulders, a far cry from the despondent styles of the war years. When consumers flocked to update their wardrobes with the New Look, they also snapped up his new fragrance, Miss Dior. The fragrance represented the re-emergence of the feminine, elegant style of the Belle Époque.

Today, the perennial French debutante Miss Dior is enjoying a resurgence, or second debut. She bows in a hound's tooth-embossed clear crystal flacon, with a pristine white satin bow at her neckline. Miss Dior is still lovely after all these years.

Introduced   1947
Price   High range

MISUKI

Scent Type   *Semi - Oriental*
Composition
     Top Notes: *Rosewood, bergamot, lemon*
     Heart Notes: *Orchid, jasmine, peach*
     Base Notes: *Amber, vanilla, sandalwood,*
                  patchouli

Misuki was the first fragrance from the exclusive Lake Forest, Illinois, firm of Holzman & Stephanie Perfumes. A family-owned, boutique perfumery steeped in European tradition, Holzman & Stephanie has since added other scents to its line, including La Parisienne and Fascination.

Founder Esther Holzman is a trained organic chemist. She also studied perfumery in Grasse, France, during her summer holidays on the French Riviera with her aunt, the Baroness Emmy de Hirzel, at the Baroness's Villa La Rato Penado, high above Grasse. Misuki is dedicated to another of Holzman's aunts, the Countess Evelyn de Prograny, who urged her niece to enter the fragrance business.

Misuki is a rich Oriental fragrance comprised entirely of natural essential oils, which linger superbly on the skin with a powdery whisper. A grand, entrance-making fragrance, Misuki enjoyed a Hollywood moment. It was featured in the Al Pacino film, *Scent of a Woman*. The Pochet bottle is swathed in a glorious red and gold Oriental print with gold-colored tassels and red satin ribbons. Elegant and alluring, Misuki is a classic town-and-country fragrance.

Introduced   *1987*
Price   *High range*

MITSOUKO

Scent Type   *Chypre - Fruity*
Composition
     Top Notes: *Peach, bergamot, hesperides*
     Heart Notes: *Lilac, rose, jasmine, ylang-ylang*
     Base Notes: *Vetiver, amber, oakmoss,*
                  cinnamon, spices

Third generation perfumer Jacques Guerlain developed Mitsouko for women of passion, intensity, strength, and introspection. Created on the eve of the Roaring Twenties, Mitsouko reflects the Far Eastern style that became the rage in the flamboyant years after World War I.

Mitsouko opens with fruity top notes of tangy bergamot and smooth, mellow peach. A lilac blend follows, dissolving into a woody chypre drydown, redolent of vetiver, oakmoss, and amber. Mitsouko is a sensual, voluptuous fragrance, like a dark, full-bodied Cabernet Sauvignon.

Mitsouko means "mystery" in Japanese and was inspired by a character in the Claude Farrère novel, *La Bataille*, or *The Battle*. The story revolved around the ill-fated love of an English officer and the wife of the ship's commander— a beautiful Japanese woman named Mitsouko. Farrère had mentioned another Guerlain fragrance, Jicky, in one of his novels, so Jacques Guerlain reciprocated the honor by naming his fragrance after a Farrère character. And so Mitsouko lives on, in print and in fragrance. It remains one of the great jewels of the House of Guerlain.

Introduced   *1919*
Price   *High range*

MOLINARD DE MOLINARD

Scent Type   *Floral - Fruity*
Composition
    Top Notes: *Fruits, citrus,*
                 black currant bud, greens
    Heart Notes: *Bulgarian rose, Grasse jasmine,*
                 narcissus, ylang-ylang
    Base Notes: *Amber, Réunion Island vetiver,*
                 incense

From the House of Molinard comes a classic floral bouquet, accented with sunny top notes of fruit and citrus.

In 1849 the House of Molinard opened a fragrance shop in Grasse, France, catering to the wealthy clientele that came to enjoy the French Riviera. To this day, the name of Molinard is associated with women of fine taste and privilege.

Molinard is known for its beautiful flacons, many created by Lalique and Baccarat. Today, the fragrance is presented in a rectangular Lalique bottle, festooned with a generous collar of frosted glass in which are sculpted graceful female forms. The bottle was originally designed in 1929 by Rene Lalique for the Molinard fragrance Les Iscles d'Or. Quite collectible.

Introduced   *1980*
Price   *High range*

MOMENT SUPRÊME
(See also Jean Patou Collection)

Scent Type   *Floral - Ambery*
Composition
    Top Notes: *Lavender, geranium, clove, bergamot*
    Heart Notes: *Jasmine, rose*
    Base Notes: *Amber, spices*

Moment Suprême is a classic Jean Patou concoction meant to capture the spirit of Paris at its most extravagant. Like the cultured city of light, the scent is enticing, sensual, and sophisticated. A high society fragrance, Moment Suprême is for the supreme moments of your life.

Introduced   *1929*
Price   *Mid-range*

MUST DE CARTIER

Scent Type   *Oriental - Ambery*
Composition
    Top Notes: *Bergamot, tangerine, lemon,*
                 aldehydes, peach, rosewood
    Heart Notes: *Jasmine, leather, carnation,*
                 ylang-ylang, orris, orchid
    Base Notes: *Musk, amber*

Famous Patrons
    Actress Josette Banzet, Marquise de Bruyenne

Extraordinarily rich and long-lasting, Must de Cartier is a dramatic Oriental fragrance from the world-renowned jeweler, Cartier. The perfume brims with exotic florals, spices, musk, and smoky amber. A splendid high-impact scent, ideal for luxurious days and opulent evening wear. The burnished topaz flacon is suspended in a gold-colored casing—a jewel in itself—and presented in a black carton.

For a translucent version of Cartier, try Must de Cartier II, a watery marine theme, packaged in a red carton. It's hard to go wrong when the label says Cartier.

Introduced   *1981*
Price   *High range*

MYSTIC

Scent Type   Floral
Composition
    Top Notes: Lily of the valley, cassis, narcissus
    Heart Notes: Marigold, apricot, heliotrope,
                      jonquil, wild rose, honeysuckle
    Base Notes: Vanilla, iris, patchouli

Mystic is an enchanting, expansive floral fragrance from Chicago-based entrepreneur Marilyn Miglin. It is tinged with the smooth suggestion of apricot and blended with vanilla; rich essences of jonquil, lily of the valley, and honeysuckle are particularly apparent. Feminine and intimate, Mystic is shrouded in a frosted bottle and encased in a transparent, lavender and amber tinted box. Miglin's tagline? "For the woman who transcends time."

Introduced   1998
Price   Mid-range

NAHÉMA

Scent Type   Floral - Aldehyde
Composition
    Top Notes: Peach, bergamot,
                      greens, aldehydes
    Heart Notes: Rose hyacinth, Bulgarian rose,
                      ylang-ylang, jasmine, lilac,
                      lily of the valley
    Base Notes: Passion fruit, Peru balsam,
                      benzoin, vanilla, vetiver,
                      sandalwood

Famous Patrons
    Natalie Cole   Madonna
    Sigourney Weaver   Joan Jett

Nahéma is a charming floral aldehyde with Oriental highlights. The Guerlain fragrance unfolds with the smooth freshness of fruit followed by a rich rose floral bouquet based on aromatic woods. An original, exotic blend, Nahéma is a fragrance for making grand entrances.

As with most Guerlain fragrances, Nahéma began with a story. A character in Scheherazade's *Thousand and One Nights* inspired the name. There were twin sisters, disparate in nature. Nahéma means "daughter of fire," bold and untamed. Passion and intensity governed one sister, while the other was tender and gentle. This duality of nature in the twins served as inspiration for Guerlain's fragrance, a scent that is powerful yet delicate, sensual yet innocent.

Nahéma is presented in a graceful, curvaceous bottle, a circular interplay of perfection. It is adorned with a single crystal drop—an elegant simplicity.

Introduced   1979
Price   High range

NAOMI CAMPBELL

Scent Type   Floral - Oriental
Composition
    Top Notes: Chinese star anise,
                      red pepper, bergamot
    Heart Notes: Queen of the Night cactus flower,
                      jasmine, magnolia,
                      cattleya orchid, fig
    Base Notes: Sandalwood, vanilla, cedarwood

Supermodel Naomi Campbell described her expectations of her ideal fragrance as "sensual, wild, mysterious, sexy, but always elegant."

Sleek, powerful, feline—these are the words often used to describe the doe-eyed Campbell, who was discovered at age fifteen in London's Covent Garden while wearing her simple school uniform. Campbell collaborated with perfumer Ursula Wandel of Givaudan Roure to create her own exotic signature scent. The resulting creation is feminine, warm, and tenacious. The model-thin bottle is long and lean, topped with a platinum-hued, conical cap.

Practice your catwalk moves while wearing this sensual scent.

Introduced   2000
Price   High range

NARCISSE NOIR

Scent Type   Floral - Oriental
Composition
    Top Notes: Orange blossom, bergamot,
                    petitgrain, lemon
    Heart Notes: Rose, jasmine, jonquil
    Base Notes: Persian black narcissus,
                    musk, civet, sandalwood

Famous Patrons
    Madonna

Created by the great perfumer Ernest Daltroff, founder of Caron, Narcisse Noir is based on the black narcissus, an exotic spring-blooming flower found in China and Persia. An Oriental blend of aromatic woods lends a sensual, lingering aura to the assertive floral arrangement.

Narcisse Noir was one of the most important fragrances brought forth in 1912, an industrious year in the history of perfumery. It remains a truly enduring, sophisticated classic. Although Daltroff died in the 1940s, his company and fragrances live on, a tribute to his remarkable talent.

Introduced   1912
Price   Mid-range

NAUTICA WOMAN

Scent Type   Floral - Fresh
Composition
    Top Notes: Grapefruit, bergamot, mandarin
    Heart Notes: Rose, lily of the valley
    Base Notes: Sandalwood, musk, amber

Sailing on the success of his men's Nautica scent, founder and fashion designer David Chu brings forth Nautica Woman. A fluid, fresh floral composition, the scent bursts open with a tangy fruit accord, then drops anchor with rose and sandalwood, forming a rounded heart and finish. *Très sportif!* A David Chu design, the simple, frosted bottle and sea-foam green packaging suggest fresh ocean breezes, and sunny skies above. Clear sailing ahead for David Chu.

Introduced   1997
Price   High range

NICOLE

Scent Type   *Floral*
Composition
    Top Notes: *Bergamot, peony, freesia, pepper*
    Heart Notes: *Rose, violet leaves*
    Base Notes: *Iris, musk, sandalwood, vetiver*

Nicole Miller's second women's fragrance is simply entitled Nicole. By comparison, it represents a mature evolvement from her first signature scent, Nicole Miller.

A study in classicism, of sense and sensibility, the fragrance is a well-mannered floral bouquet. Nicole is presented in graded rectangular bottles, sheathed in cartons of silver and copper hues. Wear it with a classy, Nicole Miller "LBD," or little black dress.

Introduced   1998
Price   *Mid-range*

NIKI DE SAINT PHALLE

Scent Type   *Chypre - Floral*
Composition
    Top Notes: *Greens, peach, bergamot, spearmint, artemisia*
    Heart Notes: *Jasmine, carnation, rose, ylang-ylang, cedarwood, orris, patchouli*
    Base Notes: *Oakmoss, sandalwood, leather, musk, amber*

Niki de Saint Phalle is a vivid chypre floral encased in an equally vivid bottle of deepest blue, featuring entwined multicolor snakes, slithering to the neck. Playful and dramatic.

Introduced   1982
Price   *High range*

NO REGRETS

Scent Type   *Floral*
Composition
    Top Notes: *Mandarin, ylang-ylang, galbanum, osmanthus*
    Heart Notes: *Lily, orange blossom, tuberose, gardenia, orris, night queen*
    Base Notes: *Oakmoss, tolu balsam, musk, sandalwood, vetiver*

No Regrets is an incandescent white floral fragrance from the Alexandra De Markoff cosmetic company. Brimming with attitude, No Regrets is designed for women who live life to the fullest, with no regrets. The charming bottles are simple, rectangular sprays, inscribed with scribbled notes on love and life: "Living well is the best revenge" and "Love is merely a madness." No Regrets is a fragrance for women who aren't afraid to speak their minds.

Introduced   1994
Price   *Mid-range*

NOA

Scent Type   *Floral - Fresh*
Composition
    Top Notes: *White peony, coriander, white musk, greens*
    Heart Notes: *White peony*
    Base Notes: *White musk, coffee, incense*

Parfums Cacharel, creator of the classic Anaïs Anaïs, introduces the youthful Noa for the new millennium. The fresh floral fragrance, created by Firmenich perfumer Olivier Cresp, is built around white notes of peony and musk. Ethereal and translucent, Noa is presented in a round flacon that signifies a new birth or reawakening—highly appropriate for a millennium scent. A *faux* pearl floats inside. The seed of new beginnings, perhaps?

Introduced	*2000*
Price	*Mid-range*

NOCTURNES

Scent Type	*Floral - Aldehyde*
Composition	
Top Notes:	*Aldehydes, bergamot, mandarin, greens*
Heart Notes:	*Rose, jasmine, ylang-ylang, tuberose, stephanotis, lily of the valley, orris, cyclamen*
Base Notes:	*Vanilla, amber, musk, sandalwood, vetiver, benzoin*

Famous Patrons
Madonna

Nocturnes hails from the esteemed Parisian firm of Caron. The ambrosial floral recipe is enhanced by stephanotis, a woody Greek vine that bears waxy white flowers with a full-bodied sweet scent. Sweet woods, vanilla, and amber create a lingering aura.

Ever curious, we researched the word "nocturnes" and discovered quite an artistic lineage. A nocturne may be a night scene painting. Or it may be a romantic musical composition, especially for the piano, evocative of dreamy night scenes. Think of it, Caron's Nocturnes could be the perfect fragrance for a dreamy evening with a handsome artist or pianist.

Introduced	*1981*
Price	*High range*

NORELL

Scent Type	*Floral*
Composition	
Top Notes:	*Greens, reseda, galbanum, bergamot, verbena*
Heart Notes:	*Carnation, hyacinth, rose, jasmine, ginger lily, calla lily, jonquil, ylang-ylang, heliotrope*
Base Notes:	*Musk, iris, sandalwood, myrrh, vanilla*

A classic floral fragrance, Norell zips open with snappy green notes, then does a slow dissolve to a rich, sophisticated floral heart. Spicy carnation and warm background essences create a luxurious ambiance, evocative of a Norell satin sheath.

In 1968, Revlon launched the fragrance with the endorsement of American designer Norman Norell, whose philosophy was that one should always buy the best one can afford. Norell was selected in part because he was a favorite designer of Lynn Revson, wife of Revlon founding partner Charles Revson.

The Norell name was subsequently sold and the formula was "updated." Later, in 1997, it was reformulated according to the original 1968 formula from International Flavors and Fragrances. Today, Norell is enjoying a revival, with Faye Dunaway serving as spokesmodel for the American classic. The glamour of Norell couture lives on in a courtly, refined fragrance that whispers of wealth.

Introduced	*1968*
Reintroduced	*1997*
Price	*Mid range*

NORMANDIE

(See also Jean Patou Collection)

Scent Type   *Oriental - Ambery*

Composition

    Top Notes: *Fruits*

    Heart Notes: *Carnation, jasmine, rose*

    Base Notes: *Vanilla, benzoin, oakmoss,*
                    cedarwood, woods

The year was 1935, and a swank new ocean liner called the *Normandie* carried the elite of business and society on its maiden voyage from Le Havre to New York. A new Atlantic crossing speed record was set, and each first-class passenger received Jean Patou's latest fragrance named in honor of the luxury liner. Patou described the fragrance as warm and determined, and packaged it in a miniature flacon surrounded by a replica of the ship. The passengers adored the spicy Oriental scent, and we do, too. But don't wait for your next Atlantic crossing to try it.

Introduced   *1935*

Price   *Mid-range*

NUIT DE NOËL

Scent Type   *Oriental*

Composition

    Top Notes: *Citrus*

    Heart Notes: *Rose, orris, jasmine, ylang-ylang*

    Base Notes: *Sandalwood, vanilla, oakmoss*

Famous Patrons

    Andrea Marcovicci

An exotic Oriental fragrance from the House of Caron, Nuit de Noël, French for "Christmas Eve," begins with exhilarating citrus top notes, followed by a heart of rare flowers. Orris adds a subtle violet-like note to the composition, while sweet vanilla, earthy oakmoss, and balsamic sandalwood are blended for a lasting aura. Nuit de Noël is a fitting fragrance for holiday galas or a romantic Christmas Eve.

Created in 1922, this classic is presented in a splendid black flacon, designed to accentuate the image of the dramatic scent. Wear it for memorable moments.

Introduced   *1922*

Price   *Mid-range*

Ô DE LANCÔME

Scent Type   *Citrus*

Composition

    Top Notes: *Mandarin, bergamot, lemon*

    Heart Notes: *Jasmine, rosemary, honeysuckle*

    Base Notes: *Sandalwood, vetiver, oakmoss*

The classic green citrus spritz from Lancôme is Ô de Lancôme, a refreshing scent for sultry days. Cool and chic, it's just the thing for the south of France, or any summery setting. Ô de Lancôme sparks a revitalizing lift—perfect for a spa visit, to keep you cool anytime, anywhere.

Introduced   *1994*

Price   *Mid-range*

Ô OUI

Scent Type   *Floral - Fruity*

Composition

    Top Notes: *Bergamot, clementine, freesia,*
                    hyacinth, nectarine

    Heart Notes: *Water lily, honeysuckle*

    Base Notes: *Musk, woods*

Ô Oui from Lancôme is an easy-to-wear scent with a carefree, youthful attitude. Perfumer Harry Freemont, of Firmenich, blended the sheer, sparkling floral fragrance. Ô Oui swirls around a fluid heart of honeysuckle and water lily, with fresh fruit accents. The summery scent is captured in a frosted flacon. Ideal for a Malibu summer, wear it with sarongs and sunglasses. Just say yes to Ô Oui.

Introduced	*1998*
Price	*Mid-range*

OBSESSION

Scent Type	*Oriental - Ambery*
Composition	
Top Notes:	*Mandarin, bergamot, peach, lemon, orange blossom, greens*
Heart Notes:	*Coriander, tagetes, armoise, jasmine, rose, cedarwood, sandalwood*
Base Notes:	*Vanilla, amber, oakmoss, musk, civet*

Famous Patrons
Rosie Perez

Obsession, the first fragrance from American designer Calvin Klein, quickly became a best-selling scent after its lavish debut. The passionate, long-lasting fragrance brims with exotic spices, vanilla, and amber. Heavy, provocative, compelling. It is a distinctive fragrance, formulated to last all night and into the morning. The cognac-colored liquid is a warm, wintry scent, perfect for cool days and cooler evenings.

The easy-traveling bottle is smooth and sparse, accented with amber hues tipped in gold-color, and presented in cartons of creme and navy.

For particular pampering, try the Obsession golden body glistener to enhance a summer tan, or slip into a scented bath to cast your petty cares aside…and let your mind wander to your own magnificent obsession.

Introduced	*1985*
Price	*Mid-range*

OH! DE MOSCHINO

Scent Type	*Floral - Marine*
Composition	
Top Notes:	*Tangerine, bergamot, rose*
Heart Notes:	*Pink lotus, orris, cyclamen, pink water lily, peony, lily of the valley, stephanotis*
Base Notes:	*May blossom, heliotrope, musk, sandalwood, orris*

Upon experiencing fashion designer Franco Moschino's fragrant creations, one is often moved with delight; indeed, an appropriate reaction is "Oh!" Thus, aptly christened Oh! de Moschino is a fashion-forward, sensually sheer floral fragrance developed around a watery marine accord. It's an ideal scent for daytime and warm weather wear, particularly for that long-overdue holiday to a chic Italian seaside resort—or the mountains, perhaps. Anyone for Lake Como? Quick, book us into the Villa d'Este.

Introduced	*1999*
Price	*High range*

OMBRE ROSE

Scent Type   Floral - Aldehyde
Composition
   Top Notes: Aldehydes, peach, rosewood, geranium
   Heart Notes: Lily of the valley, ylang-ylang, rose, orris, sandalwood, cedarwood, vetiver
   Base Notes: Vanilla, honey, iris, musk, cinnamon, tonka bean, heliotrope

Ombre Rose is from Jean-Charles Brousseau, a Parisian couturier known for his expertise in millinery and accessories. The rose floral bouquet is brightened with aldehydes, peach, and geranium, then warmed to a powdery finish by sweet vanilla, honey, and exotic woods. Vivid and long-lasting, Ombre Rose is an intense daytime or evening fragrance.

The perfume is presented in a burnished black hexagonal flacon, highlighted by a sculpted floral pattern. Other strengths are available in similar bottles of clear glass in bas relief. The bottle designs are based on an antique bottle from Brousseau's personal collection.

Introduced   1981
Price   Mid-range

OPIUM

Scent Type   Oriental - Spicy
Composition
   Top Notes: Plum, hesperides, clove, coriander, pepper, bay leaf
   Heart Notes: Jasmine, rose, carnation, lily of the valley, cinnamon, peach, orris
   Base Notes: Sandalwood, vetiver, myrrh, opopanax, labdanum, benzoin, benjamin, castoreum, amber, incense, musk, patchouli, tolu

Famous Patrons
   Tanya Tucker   *Jerry Hall*

Opium is an opulent Oriental blend from French designer Yves Saint Laurent. Smoldering and dramatic, the fragrance is unveiled with spicy, fruity notes that lead to a rich bouquet of heady florals. Underscoring the composition is an exotic melange of sweet aromatic woods and incense. Opium is a distinctive fragrance, made for grand entrances and seductive evenings. So potent you'll still detect it the next morning. Beautiful in cool weather, but spritz lightly in hot humid climates, when the body lotion and powder would probably suffice.

Opium caused quite a stir with its controversial name, but the exposure helped to make it a best-selling scent. For the extravagant launch party in 1977, a tall ship, the *Peking*, was rented from the South Street Seaport Museum in New York's East Harbor, with none other than Truman Capote at the helm. The ship was draped with banners of red, gold, and purple, and the Oriental theme was carried out with a thousand-pound bronze Buddha, laden with mounds of white cattleya orchids.

Yves Saint Laurent carried the Oriental theme into the packaging design. The perfume is held in a glass vial encased in a red plastic container, inspired by Japanese inros. Inros are small lacquered cases that were once worn under kimonos on silken cords and held aromatics, herbs, perfumes, and medicines. Look for Opium packaged in rich shades of scarlet and gold.

Introduced	*1977*
Price	*High range*

ORGANZA

Scent Type   *Floral - Oriental*
Composition
  Top Notes: *Honeysuckle, peony, rosewood*
  Heart Notes: *Tuberose, gardenia, ylang-ylang*
  Base Notes: *Amber, nutmeg, mace, vanilla,*
                    cedarwood

Givenchy brings forth a floral Oriental blend of exotic spices and fragrant white flowers, a well-mannered, pedigreed French fragrance of classic proportion. Refined and understated, Organza is an International Flavors and Fragrances composition for Givenchy.

The warm, expansive scent is displayed in a frosted hourglass silhouette, reminiscent of Givenchy house couturier John Galliano's creation of a fluidly draped, ice-white silk dress. The bottle, designed by Serge Mansau, is crowned with a cap fashioned after a stately Ionic Greek column. A tasteful combination of fragrance and presentation, Organza oozes style.

Introduced	*1996*
Price	*High range*

ORGANZA INDÉCENCE

Scent Type   *Oriental - Ambery Spicy*
Composition
  Top Notes: *Cinnamon, spices*
  Heart Notes: *Patchouli, jacaranda wood*
  Base Notes: *Amber, musk*

Givenchy's follow-up fragrance to Organza is Organza Indécence, a velvety Oriental composition. Using no floral essences, the formula was created entirely from fragrant woods, spices, and balsamics. Intoxicating and magnetic, Organza Indécence is a warm, full-bodied fragrance, suitable for cool weather wear and dramatic evening entrances.

The Serge Mansau-designed bottle is based on the original Organza pattern of a sleek female physique, with the same Ionic Greek column cap. The Organza Indécence bottle features rippling folds of sculpted glass partially enrobing the female silhouette. The overall effect is rich and regal, a sensual fragrance that whispers of passion and promise, of luxurious living at its best.

Introduced	*2000*
Price	*High range*

OSCAR DE LA RENTA

Scent Type   *Floral - Ambery*
Composition
   Top Notes: *Orange blossom, coriander,*
                     cascarilla, basil, peach, gardenia
   Heart Notes: *Jasmine, tuberose, ylang-ylang,*
                     May rose, lavender, orchid
   Base Notes: *Clove, sandalwood, amber,*
                     myrrh, lavender, patchouli,
                     opopanax

Famous Patrons
   Princess Margaret   Sharon Stone

In 1978, couturier Oscar de la Renta enchanted the world with his first fragrance foray. His signature scent is a delicate floral bouquet, intensely feminine, and reflective of his fashion designs. The formula includes rare florals set against a backdrop of powdery woods and soft spices. De la Renta took his inspiration from his mother's flower garden, in which grew the fragrant white flowers of his native country, the Dominican Republic. The result is a very wearable fragrance, excellent for daytime and warm weather, exquisite for evening. Soft, subtle, sweet, and sophisticated.

The best-selling fragrance is featured in a curved glass flacon from bottle designer Serge Mansau, and capped with a frosted glass flower with a dewdrop nestled among the petals. The fragrance garnered a pair of 1978 Fragrance Foundation FiFi Awards.

Oscar de la Renta's signature fragrance: A polished thoroughbred, romantically inclined.

Introduced   *1978*
Price   *High range*

PACO
♀♂

Scent Type   *Citrus*
Composition
   Notes: *Citrus, lavender, cola, vanilla*

From fashion designer Paco Rabanne comes Paco, a unisex scent that gets straight to the point. A simple, well-priced, fresh fragrance Rabanne says is designed to appeal to "everyone on the planet."

Rather than glass bottles, Paco is packaged in aluminum cans. In some locales, such as the Museum of Modern Art in New York, Paco is sold in sleek black and white Paco vending machines that accept credit cards only. The machines also house tester units, dispense shopping bags, and speak to shoppers. The epitome of hip—leave it to Paco!

Introduced   *1995*
Price   *Mid-range*

PALOMA PICASSO

Scent Type   *Chypre - Floral*
Composition
   Top Notes: *Bergamot, neroli,*
                     lemon, ambrette
   Heart Notes: *Jasmine, Bulgarian rose,*
                     ylang-ylang, coriander, clove
   Base Notes: *Patchouli, vetiver, sandalwood,*
                     oakmoss, moss, amber

From internationally acclaimed designer Paloma Picasso comes a signature fragrance as worldly, dramatic, and elegant as its creator. She states: "It is a fragrance for women, not girls. It is sophisticated, not naive or innocent." She calls it jewelry for the senses.

The lush chypre scent begins with brisk citrus top notes, dissolving into rich jeweled notes of jasmine and Bulgarian rose, poised against layers of spices and woods, warm ambers, earthy oakmoss, and exotic sandalwood. Presented in a flawless crystal ball, the perfume is wreathed by frosted French glass. It is packaged in Paloma's signature Florentine red, contrasted by matte black.

Paloma was born into a world of creativity, the daughter of artist Pablo Picasso and Francoise Gilot. She was christened Paloma, meaning "dove" in Spanish, after her father's dove, which was the symbol of the 1949 Peace Congress. She expresses her artistic genius in myriad ways, from her jewelry designs for Tiffany to her china and crystal creations for Villeroy & Boch.

She says: "As jewelry can please the eye and the hand, so fragrance can please the senses…revealing new sensory delights layer by layer. It is an intimate ornament that becomes part of your identity…a part of the mosaic of your life." Her philosophy is clearly evident in her signature fragrance, a jewel in itself.

Introduced   1984
Price   High range

PANTHÈRE

Scent Type   Floral - Ambery
Composition
  Top Notes: Ginger, pepper, black currant bud, peach, coriander, plum
  Heart Notes: Jasmine, narcissus, rose, tuberose, gardenia, heliotrope, carnation, ylang-ylang
  Base Notes: Musk, sandalwood, patchouli, amber, oakmoss, cedarwood, vanilla, tonka bean

The second women's fragrance from Cartier is a bewitching fragrance in a stunning package. Panthère is the fragrance counterpart to the sleek signature panther jewelry for which Cartier has been famous throughout the decades. For the Panthère perfume, lavish essences of florals, fruits, spices, and woods are blended to create an expressive, sensual scent. Panthère eau de toilette is a lighter, fresher version of the perfume, with additional top notes of lemon, mandarin, and grapefruit, while lily of the valley lightens the heart note.

The bottle, from Pochet et du Courval, is designed in the style of Cartier jewelry. Twin panthers perch on either side of the round flacon. An exquisite presentation, it is also one of the more affordable Cartier "jewels."

Introduced   1988
Price   High range

PARFUM D'ÉTÉ

Scent Type   Floral - Green
Composition
  Top Notes: Greens
  Heart Notes: Jasmine, rose, hyacinth, narcissus, peony
  Base Notes: Iris, oakmoss, sandalwood, musk

Created by fashion designer Kenzo, Parfum d'Été is a fresh tribute to summer. Lively greens and florals are combined with powdery iris, oakmoss, and woods. Initially invigorating and refreshing, the final mossy-woody impression is spirited and carefree, like the perfect summer holiday. Parfum d'Été is housed in a marvelously crafted, leaf-shaped bottle of frosted glass.

Introduced   1994
Price   High range

PARFUM D'HERMÈS

Scent Type   Semi - Oriental
Composition
    Top Notes: Aldehydes, bergamot,
                       galbanum, hyacinth
    Heart Notes: Egyptian jasmine, Florentine iris,
                       Nossi-bè ylang-ylang,
                       Bulgarian rose, labdanum
    Base Notes: Cedarwood, vetiver,
                       sandalwood, amber, spices,
                       incense, myrrh, vanilla

Parfum d'Hermès is a semi-Oriental fragrance from Hermès, rich, warm, and sensuous, with lush florals and exotic base notes, a refined day-to-evening fragrance with a proper pedigree.

Encased in a graceful oval bottle, the scent sports a delicate piece of metal reminiscent of a stirrup strap, a nod to the equestrian heritage of Hermès. Packaged in red, Parfum d'Hermès is a delightful addition to any fragrance wardrobe.

Introduced   1984
Price   Top range

PARFUM SACRÉ

Scent Type   Oriental - Spicy
Composition
    Top Notes: Pepper, cinnamon,
                       coriander, clove
    Heart Notes: Rose, jasmine, orange blossom,
                       mimosa
    Base Notes: Myrrh, musk, amber, vanilla

If the Parfum Sacré fragrance smells familiar, it is—Parfum Sacré is a classic scent that has been reintroduced by Caron. It is based on the original Caron Or et Noir fragrance, or "gold and black."

Parfum Sacré is composed of sacred essences, beginning with spicy top notes and giving way to a rich floral center, embedded in a precious blend of amber, musk, myrrh, and vanilla—a warm, long-lasting composition. Elegant and feminine, it is a timeless floral fragrance.

Introduced   1992
Price   High range

PARIS

Scent Type   Floral
Composition
    Top Notes: Rose petals, orange blossom,
                       mimosa, cassia, hawthorn,
                       nasturtium, bergamot,
                       greens, hyacinth
    Heart Notes: Rose, violet leaves, jasmine,
                       orris, ylang-ylang,
                       lily of the valley, lily,
                       linden blossom
    Base Notes: Sandalwood, amber, musk,
                       moss, iris, cedarwood, heliotrope

In this floral bouquet, Yves Saint Laurent has captured the very essence of the grand city of Paris.

Paris is a profuse bundle of flowers with rich sweet rose top notes and heady floral heart notes, set against warm woods and moss. An abundance of femininity sparkles in its spirit and soul. Paris is an extravagant, radiant fragrance, ideal for the romantic heart.

Think of Paris in the springtime, the Place Vendôme, the rue de Rivoli, the Louvre, the Musee D'Orsay…we love it. Look for Paris attired in—what else?—rose petal pink and chic jet black.

Introduced   1984
Price   Mid-range

PARURE

Scent Type   *Chypre - Floral Animalic*
Composition
  Top Notes: *Plum, bergamot, fruits,*
                    hesperides, greens
  Heart Notes: *Rose, lilac, jasmine,*
                    lily of the valley, jonquil,
                    narcissus, orris
  Base Notes: *Oakmoss, patchouli, spices,*
                    amber, leather

Famous Patrons
  Wendy Wasserstein

Parure is a sophisticated melange from fifth-generation Guerlain perfumer Jean-Paul Guerlain. An unaffected blend of chypre, fruit, and floral notes results in a lightly balanced, elegant scent. Distinctly feminine. Guerlain says it is "for an aesthetic, discerning woman, constantly in search of quality and truth."

Parure is French for "adornment," referring to precious luxuries. Where Guerlain created Chamade for the modern liberated woman, and Chant d'Arômes for youthful innocence, Parure was designed for the woman who is at ease with herself and appreciates the luxuries her life holds.

Introduced   *1975*
Price   *Mid-range*

PASSION
(See also Elizabeth Taylor's Passion)

PASSION

Scent Type   *Floral*
Composition
  Top and Heart Notes: Jasmine, tuberose
  Base Notes: *Vanilla*

Two years in the making, this warm, sensual fragrance was developed in Grasse, France, by Annick Goutal. Not to be confused with her own Gardénia Passion, nor with Elizabeth Taylor's Passion.

The heady combination of jasmine and tuberose is balanced by a tenacious drydown note of vanilla. A long-lasting, intensely feminine fragrance, Passion is appropriately named according to the Victorian language of flowers. White jasmine meant amiability, yellow jasmine conveyed grace and elegance, while Spanish jasmine denoted sensuality. And tuberose? Dangerous pleasures. Passion is a lively fragrance with a dangerous abundance of significant florals.

Introduced   *1986*
Price   *High range*

PAVLOVA

Scent Type   *Floral*
Composition
    Top Notes: *Hyacinth, bergamot, galbanum,*
                     black currant bud
    Heart Notes: *Rose, jasmine, tuberose, orchid,*
                     narcissus, orris
    Base Notes: *Sandalwood, musk, amber,*
                     cedarwood, benzoin, moss

Famous Patrons
    Ballerina Anna Pavlova

A tender, classic floral, Pavlova was created in honor of the glorious Russian ballerina Anna Pavlova, who lived from 1885 to 1931. Fragrance is a beautiful part of Russian ballet history. Legend has it that each ballerina was assigned a scent, a fragrance to be worn in extravagance all over the body and hair. Thus, the ballet was an experience not only in vision and sound, but also in smell. Patrons could close their eyes and imagine gliding through a flower garden, so sweet was the symphony of fragrance from the dancers. The Russian-born choreographer George Balanchine continued the tradition with the American Ballet Theater in New York City, which he founded in 1933.

    Pavlova is presented in dramatic black flacons, enhanced by delicate pink flowers that entwine the bottles. Others are of clear glass, featuring a graceful swan. Long after the fragrance is finished, the bottles will beautify any dressing table. They are as lovely as the fragrance, a delicate floral scent, fresh, soft, romantic, and understated.

Introduced   *1922*
Price   *Mid-range*

PENHALIGON'S COLLECTION

BLENHEIM BOUQUET
Citrus ($♀♂$)
BLUEBELL
Floral - Green
CORNUBIA
Floral - Oriental
ELIZABETHAN ROSE
Floral
ENGLISH FERN
Fougère ($♀♂$)
LILY OF THE VALLEY
Floral - Green
ORMOLU
Oriental
RACQUETS FORMULA
Chypre ($♀♂$)
VICTORIAN POSY
Floral
VIOLETTA
Floral

Established in 1870, Penhaligon's of London is an enchanting English perfumery that offers an extensive repertoire. Penhaligon's line resembles a page from storybook England, with its beribboned apothecary bottles. Bespoke grooming accoutrements include soaps, atomizers, shaving items, traveling sets, and silver toilette accessories. Penhaligon's also offers books, such as the ever popular *The Language of Flowers*, which was edited by managing director Sheila Pickles.

    In addition, the Language of Flowers collection features single-note scents for ladies. Penhaligon's is steeped in history. Take a tour back in time with the 1902 Blenheim Bouquet or the 1870 Eau de Verveine. Feel like a king with Esprit de

Roi, also from 1870, or revel in English Fern from 1911. Newer scents include the unisex Quercus from 1996, the rich, woody Ormolu from 1994, and the delicate Violetta, from 1996.

Journey to Penhaligon's and embark upon a fragrant treasure hunt through the pages of time.

Introduced   *Since 1870*
Price   *High range*

PERFUMES ISABELL COLLECTION

ATTAR
Floral - Oriental
CALLA
Floral - Oriental
CEYLON
Floral
MANDARIN
Floral - Fruity
PAPERWHITES
Floral
SAVANNA
Floral - Fresh

What do Caroline Kennedy, Madonna, and the fabulous Miller sisters have in common? Robert Isabell, florist extraordinaire, who specializes in weddings, parties, and gala events—he's on the speed dial of many a name in *Who's Who*. So popular were his fragrant bouquets that he decided to form Perfumes Isabell in order to bottle his most exquisite floral aromas. To date, he has offered six magnificent florals, with pastel sherbet-tinted formulas showcased in clear glass columns. Heavenly scents—simply close your eyes and imagine an atrium conservatory in luscious, aromatic bloom.

Introduced   *1996*
Price   *High range*

PERHAPS

Scent Type   *Floral - Oriental*
Composition
    Top Notes: *Mimosa, peach, orange*
    Heart Notes: *Jasmine, freesia, rose*
    Base Notes: *Sandalwood, amber*

Fashion designer Bob Mackie, often called the "Sultan of Sequins," makes an uncharacteristically quiet entrance with his latest fragrance foray, Perhaps. Coy and noncommittal, softer than his original namesake scent, Perhaps is a floral Oriental with fruity top notes, blended to suggest a champagne accord. Makes us quite giddy just thinking about it.

Perhaps is rendered in lady-like shades of peach and apricot. The peachy perfect springtime accoutrement.

Introduced   *1997*
Price   *Mid-range*

PETITE CHÉRIE

Scent Type   *Floral*
Composition
    Top Notes: *Peach, grasses*
    Heart Notes: *Musky rose*
    Base Notes: *Vanilla*

Famous Patrons
    Portia de Rossi

French fragrance creator Annick Goutal added another fine fragrance to her repertoire with Petite Chérie. Goutal envisioned Petite Chérie as part of a young woman's rite of passage, an innocent sexual awakening. Petite Chérie is a shimmering floral, presented in muted shades of soft green.

Introduced   *1998*
Price   *High range*

PHEROMONE

Scent Type   *Green*
Composition
    Top Notes: *Greens, spices*
    Heart Notes: *Florals, jasmine*
    Base Notes: *Exotic woods, bark, seeds,*
                   wine resins, wild grasses

Famous Patrons
    Cher
    Actress Josette Banzet, Marquise de Bruyenne

From Marilyn Miglin comes a precious fragrance called Pheromone. The company says the word "pheromone" means, "an organic scent signal used to communicate. From the Greek *pherein* (to carry) and *hormon* (to excite)."

When Marilyn Miglin decided to create a fragrance for her salon clientele, she searched the world for just the right formula. She journeyed to New York, Grasse, and finally Egypt, where she had ancient hieroglyphs translated to find recipes for perfume compounds. Says Miglin: "Ancient civilizations actually used fragrance to evoke behavioral responses." The ancient recipes were etched on stone temple walls, formulas for high priests and royalty. "The recipes we found contained ancient secrets that made perfume intriguing, long-lasting and communicative," reports Miglin. Thus, Pheromone was developed, a modern blend of 179 rare essences with a dominant green note.

Use the Pheromone Fluid Gold body moisturizer and Gold Dust body powder to achieve shimmering golden highlights on the skin. Perfect for a wintertime cruise, no?

Introduced   *1980*
Price   *Top range*

PLEASURES

Scent Type   *Floral - Green*
Composition
    Top Notes: *Lily, violet leaves, greens*
    Heart Notes: *White peony, rose, black lilac,*
                   karo karounde
    Base Notes: *Sandalwood, patchouli*

Danish philosopher Søren Kierkegaard once wrote, "Most men pursue pleasure with such breathless haste that they hurry past it." Let your senses revel in the moment; there is no need to hurry past Pleasures from Estée Lauder.

The simple pleasures of life take on an aromatic form in this easy-to-wear, joyful bouquet. Sprigs of meadow green and soft tendrils of sandalwood soothe the spirit and warm the heart, like a friend's gentle touch, a child's loving hug, or a partner's caress. Pleasures is a versatile, year-round scent suitable for those hectic times when you're juggling school, work, and family time. The scent is simply presented in a clear, smooth flacon. Real pleasures, like real happiness, need not be grand.

Introduced	*1995*
Price	*High range*

POÊME

Scent Type	*Floral*
Composition	
Notes:	*Blue poppy, datura candida, rose, freesia, narcissus, jonquil, mimosa, vanilla blossoms*

Lancôme's tribute to love and the written word is Poême, a lyrical fragrance styled for romance. Eschewing the traditional approach to fragrance architecture, second-generation perfumer Jacques Cavallier developed Poême by pairing Himalayan blue poppy with herbal datura candida. A bouquet of rich florals is interwoven, giving the fragrance an unusual, chameleon-like character.

Bottle designer Fabien Baron created the broad-shouldered, voluminous glass flacon. The packaging décor is bright and uplifting; Provençal shades of blue and canary yellow carry phrases of *amour* from French poet Paul Eluard. A fragrance of soulful poetic expression, Poême was introduced with scented bookmarks. In addition, Lancôme donated funds to benefit Reading Is Fundamental, a nonprofit children's literacy organization.

Introduced	*1996*
Price	*High range*

POISON

Scent Type	*Floral - Ambery*
Composition	
Top Notes:	*Coriander, plum, pimento, anise, rosewood*
Heart Notes:	*Rose, tuberose, orange blossom, honey, cinnamon, wild berries, cistus labdanum, carnation, jasmine*
Base Notes:	*Sandalwood, cedarwood, vetiver, musk, vanilla, heliotrope, opopanax*

Famous Patrons

Ms. Olympia bodybuilder Lenda Murray

The introduction of Poison rocked the fragrance world in 1986 with its controversial name and powerful aroma. Spicy, strong, and sensual, the long-lasting concoction from the House of Christian Dior is rife with the scent of exotic florals, fruits and woods. We detect a hint of raspberry, along with cassis, or black currant bud, with a distinct Oriental drydown.

The scent is passionately presented in a deep violet flacon and packaged in hues of emerald and royal purple. Poison is a rich, opulent scent, ideal for cold winters and hot, hot evenings.

Introduced	*1986*
Price	*High range*

POLO SPORT WOMAN

Scent Type   *Marine*
Composition
    Top Notes: *Citrus, water mint, melon*
    Heart Notes: *Freesia, ginger, water lily,*
                      mango, plum
    Base Notes: *Cedarwood, sandalwood, musk*

Ralph Lauren salutes the growing number of female athletes with Polo Sport Woman.

Polo Sport Woman is fresh and sheer, ideal after a brisk workout, competitive sport, or yoga and meditation. Soft floral notes are combined with sparkling citrus and marine notes—a refreshing experience, like an afternoon plunge into a shimmering lagoon. Polo Sport Woman is housed in an apothecary-style bottle with a barbell-inspired, silver-toned cap.

Introduced   *1995*
Price   *Mid-range*

PORTFOLIO

Scent Type   *Floral - Fresh*
Composition
    Top Notes: *Violet leaf, geranium, lemon,*
                      green grass, sea moss
    Heart Notes: *Rose, jasmine, hyacinth,*
                      clove bud
    Base Notes: *Vanilla orchid,*
                      sandalwood, musk

Portfolio, from Perry Ellis, is designed to fit the busy woman's lifestyle. A well-balanced floral bouquet, the scent opens with a fresh accord of greens, citrus, and soft florals. A classic floral heart of rose and jasmine is spiked with the exotic vanilla orchid flower which, when combined with sandalwood and musk, imparts a lingering, soft vanilla aroma. Portfolio is equally appropriate for private moments, career wear, or whenever an understated fragrance is desired. The scent is ideal for casual evenings, too, especially for a summery Sydney holiday.

Portfolio is presented in tall, frosted, opalescent white bottles. Delicate, salmon pink tints imbue the line with subtlety and taste.

Introduced   *2000*
Price   *High range*

PRIVATE COLLECTION

Scent Type   *Chypre - Green*
Composition
    Top Notes: *Greens, hyacinth, citrus*
    Heart Notes: *Jasmine, narcissus, rose,*
                      pine, reseda
    Base Notes: *Oakmoss, cedarwood,*
                      amber, musk

Famous Patrons
Princess Grace of Monaco

Private Collection is a fresh green chypre composition that was Estée Lauder's private perfume. As the story is told, Lauder often tried out a variety of scents while she was creating a new fragrance for her company. Naturally, she had a cache of personal favorites. When complimented on her scent one time, she was asked what it was; she replied that it was from her private collection.

Soon the word spread, and customers began asking for "private collection" at Lauder counters. Estée Lauder accommodated them, and thus was born Private Collection.

Introduced   1973
Price   Mid-range

PURE

Scent Type   Floral - Fruity
Composition
    Top Notes: *Topaz tangerine,*
                       to-yo-ran orchid, tagetes
    Heart Notes: *Gardenia, pineapple lily,*
                       osmanthus, peony, freesia
    Base Notes: *Incense, cinnamon, musk,*
                       amber, woods

Fashion designer Alfred Sung's Pure is a scent of surprising warmth, with a whisper of flowers, a hint of fruit, and a dusting of spice. A soothing blend the perfumer describes as an "inner sanctum lifescent" accord permeates the entire composition, so that the scent remains unchanged from the first whiff through the final phase. In simple, unadorned packaging of cream with black lettering, Pure evokes feelings of harmony and balance. Enter the Pure state of well-being.

Introduced   1997
Price   Mid-range

QUE SAIS-JE?
(See also Jean Patou Collection)

Scent Type   Chypre - Fruity
Composition
    Top Notes: *Peach, apricot, orange blossom*
    Heart Notes: *Jasmine, rose, carnation, iris*
    Base Notes: *Oakmoss, patchouli*

Que sais-je? is the second of Jean Patou's fragrant 1925 love trilogy, which also included Amour Amour and Adieu Sagesse. It was inspired by the moment when the will hesitates. Meaning "What do I know?" in English, Que sais-je? is a light, flowery chypre blend. Patou suggested this fragrance for fair-skinned blond women, but anyone can enjoy this fresh composition. We wouldn't hesitate for a moment.

Introduced   1925
Price   Mid-range

QUELQUES FLEURS

Scent Type   Floral
Composition
    Top Notes: *Greens, bergamot,*
                       orange blossom, lemon, tarragon
    Heart Notes: *Rose, jasmine, tuberose,*
                       lily of the valley, ylang-ylang,
                       carnation, heliotrope,
                       orchid, orris
    Base Notes: *Sandalwood, oakmoss, amber,*
                       musk, tonka bean, civet

Famous Patrons
    Sarah Bernhardt
    Actress Josette Banzet, Marquise de Bruyenne

One of the most important fragrances in history, Quelques Fleurs was the first true multi-floral composition, reportedly utilizing 313 different floral essences. Its development changed the approach to perfumery in the early 1900s, from subtle single florals to radiant multi-floral bouquets, and firmly established Paris as the foremost city of perfumery.

In 1987, Houbigant responded to consumer requests and reintroduced the fragrance—a devastatingly feminine scent, classic, and sophisticated, evocative of acres of intoxicating flowers. Beautiful for daytime into evening, with fresh green top notes amid expansive florals and ambery woods. A classic revisited.

Introduced	*1912*
Re-introduced	*1987*
Price	*Top range*

QUERCUS
♀♂

Scent Type	Citrus
Composition	
Top Notes:	Citrus
Heart Notes:	Jasmine
Base Notes:	Amber, sandalwood, guaiac wood

Established in 1870, the English house of Penhaligon's introduced Quercus, a bright, fresh scent that may be enjoyed by both sexes.

Quercus, Latin for "oak," opens with a bracing accord of hesperides, then moves gracefully into a warm heart of wooded amber. Sheer and clean, it is a fragrance of timeless appeal. Quercus is housed in classic Penhaligon's apothecary bottles.

Introduced	*1996*
Price	*High range*

RAFFINÉE

Scent Type	Floral - Oriental
Composition	
Top Notes:	Orange blossom, bergamot, plum, clary sage
Heart Notes:	Osmanthus, jasmine, tuberose, ylang-ylang, rose, carnation, orchid
Base Notes:	Sandalwood, spices, vetiver, cinnamon, vanilla, musk

Raffinée is a dramatic, opulent Oriental blend, rich and luxurious in the Houbigant tradition. In French the name refers to a refined elegance, an appropriate description.

A harmony of fruits and florals introduces the fragrance, followed by a full-bodied floral bouquet set against a warm backdrop of sweet spices, woods, and amber. Perfect for sophisticated day wear and black-tie evenings.

Continuing the top-drawer theme, Raffinée is presented in royal shades of lacquered red and gold.

Introduced	*1982*
Price	*High range*

RALPH

Scent Type	Floral - Fruity
Composition	
Top Notes:	Apple leaves, mandarin, freesia, loquat, osmanthus
Heart Notes:	Magnolia, linden blossom, boronia, orris
Base Notes:	Musk

Designed for the youth market, Ralph is a junior member of the Ralph Lauren world and was inspired by Lauren's daughter, Dylan. The color-coded fragrance develops around five colorful scent categories: green, orange, pink, purple, and blue. Go ahead, we'll let you match the notes, giving just one hint: freesia blooms in both purple and yellow.

The floral fragrance is packaged in cartons of the same array of bright colors. Unusual Ralph line extensions include a scented feather bracelet, and for fun in the tub, try the exploding It Rocks bath crystals. Ralph means to rock your world!

Introduced	*2000*
Price	*Mid-range*

REALITIES

Scent Type	Floral - Oriental
Composition	
Top Notes:	*Bergamot, chamomile, sage, osmanthus*
Heart Notes:	*Bulgarian rose, jasmine, white lily, carnation, freesia*
Base Notes:	*Vanilla, amber, sandalwood, peach*

Realities is the second fragrance launched by Liz Claiborne Cosmetics. Fresh top notes of herbs and bergamot are blended with a light floral accord, backed up by soft Oriental base notes blended with gentle peach. Realities is an easy-to-wear fragrance for daytime, office, and casual time; comfortable and relaxing.

A Claiborne spokesperson says that "Realities celebrates the intimacy and reality of a woman's life as she and her family truly live it," and that research showed that most women were "happy and content with their lives; fantasy escape was not for them." As the Claiborne ad says, "Reality is the best fantasy of all."

Realities comes in an artful flacon—a trio of stacked cubes, with the top cube as the cap, colored in teal. Very clean, very crisp—very Liz Claiborne.

Introduced	*1990*
Price	*Mid-range*

REALM

Scent Type	Oriental
Composition	
Top Notes:	*Sicilian mandarin, Italian cassia, Egyptian tagetes*
Heart Notes:	*Water lily, living peony*
Base Notes:	*Honey, vanilla*

Realm is a rich Oriental blend, and the first fragrance to include synthetic human pheromones.

Scientists have long acknowledged the existence of animal pheromones, the source of a kind of sixth sense in the animal world. Animals secrete a substance that affects the behavior of others of the same species. From the Greek *pherein* and *hormon*, pheromone literally means "to carry excitement." Animals use this silent language to send messages about danger, food sources, death, territorial boundaries, or sexual readiness.

Turning to the human species, neuroscientists found a small receptacle in the nose called the vomeronasal organ, or VNO. It seems that the VNO might be a human pheromone receiver independent of our sense of smell, a type of sixth sense. Erox Corporation scientists conducted tests with synthetic human pheromones and reported that test subjects experienced feelings of "warmth, comfort, happiness, and ease." As a result, these synthetic pheromones are placed at the heart of the Realm fragrance.

An Erox spokesperson comments: "We can create, for the first time, a whole new category of fragrance products with human pheromones. This marriage of technology with fine fragrances is a genuine breakthrough for the industry, because these perfumes can totally engage the senses."

Realm is packaged in a sleek modern flacon from Pierre Dinand.

While we can't vouch for the pheromonal effectiveness of Realm, it is a fine fragrance from an accomplished team of experts, and an exciting concept from the realm of science.

Introduced   1993
Price   Mid-range

RED

Scent Type   Floral - Aldehyde
Composition
    Top Notes: Osmanthus, ylang-ylang,
                  orange blossom, peach, bergamot,
                  spices, cassie, tagetes, hyacinth,
                  cardamom, aldehydes
    Heart Notes: Jasmine, carnation,
                  Bulgarian rose, marigold,
                  May rose, gardenia, tuberose,
                  orris, lily of the valley
    Base Notes: Amber, musk, patchouli,
                  sandalwood, oakmoss, vetiver,
                  tonka bean, cedarwood,
                  vanilla, labdanum

Red is a soft, sophisticated scent from Giorgio Beverly Hills. Each drop contains a blend of 692 ingredients—just a sampling is noted above. Red unfolds with green and fruity top notes that include peach and bergamot, aided by sweet orange blossom and ylang-ylang. A rich, yet subtle floral bouquet rests at the heart of the composition,

which dissolves into a lingering accord of fragrant woods. The fragrance is clothed in distinctive red and purple packaging.

Red is the sophisticated sister of Giorgio, quieter and more refined. Red is a fitting fragrance for career wear, from day into evening.

Introduced   1989
Price   Mid-range

RED DOOR

Scent Type   Floral - Amber
Composition
    Top Notes: Red roses, ylang-ylang,
                  peach, plum
    Heart Notes: Winter Oriental orchid,
                  jasmine, lily of the valley,
                  Moroccan orange blossom,
                  forest lilies, wild violets,
                  freesia, tuberose, rose
    Base Notes: Vetiver, honey, cedarwood,
                  sandalwood, amber, heliotrope,
                  musk, benzoin

Red Door takes its name from Elizabeth Arden's world-famous spas, the Red Doors. This lovely floral opens with an accord of fruits and red roses, followed by a floral bouquet featuring an Oriental orchid that blooms only in winter. Warm base notes of woods and amber round out the composition. Red Door is an enduring floral fragrance, suitable for high tea or career wear. Red Door is presented in an archway-shaped bottle topped with a cap of Red Door red.

It's like opening a door to a bouquet of heavenly red roses.

Introduced   1989
Price   Mid-range

RIVE GAUCHE

Scent Type   Floral - Aldehyde
Composition
    Top Notes: Aldehydes, bergamot,
                  greens, peach
    Heart Notes: Magnolia, jasmine, gardenia,
                  geranium, iris, ylang-ylang,
                  rose, lily of the valley
    Base Notes: Mysore sandalwood,
                  Haitian vetiver, tonka bean,
                  musk, moss, amber

Famous Patrons
    Woolworth heiress Barbara Hutton

From designer Yves Saint Laurent, Rive Gauche is a profusion of delicate, sweet white flowers, placed against a backdrop of woods and moss, all briskly introduced with ephemeral aldehydic notes. The result is a light, pleasing symphony. Look for Rive Gauche in the traditional midnight blue and black.

Introduced   1971
Price   High range

ROMA

Scent Type   Oriental - Ambery
Composition
    Top Notes: Sicilian bergamot,
                  black currant bud, mint
    Heart Notes: Rose, jasmine, lily of the valley,
                  carnation
    Base Notes: Civet, castor,
                  Singapore patchouli,
                  Yugoslavian oakmoss,
                  and balsamo, consisting of North
                  African myrrh,
                  Siamese ambergris, vanilla

Created by the renowned Italian fashion designer Laura Biagiotti, Roma is her love letter to her native city of Rome. Roma begins with the freshness of Sicilian bergamot, followed by an opulent floral bouquet. But Biagiotti's real secret behind this long-lasting fragrance lies in the discreet background notes of spicy balsamo, a blend that she says is based on a "seductive fragrance favored by women in ancient Rome." A chameleon-like spicy fragrance, Roma moves easily from casual daytime use to career and evening wear.

Subtle and complex, Roma was designed as a scent of eternal romance. Ancient Roman columns inspired the exquisite bottle, and the outer packaging is evocative of richly veined Italian marble. Roma is a fragrant tribute to a proud and ancient city.

Introduced   1987
Price   Mid-range

ROMANCE

Scent Type	*Floral*
Composition	
Top Notes:	*Tangerine, yellow freesia, ginger, marigold, chamomile, rose*
Heart Notes:	*Lotus flower, white violet, violet, night blooming day lily, paradisone*
Base Notes:	*Patchouli, oakmoss, musk*

Romance is a universal concept, as old as time itself. "Romances I ne'er read like those I have seen," wrote Lord Byron, in *Don Juan*. Romance is the language of the heart, except in Oscar Wilde's written opinion: "Romance should never begin with sentiment. It should begin with science and end with a settlement." We hope you'll discover your own version of romance.

American fashion designer Ralph Lauren traces this familiar path with his modern interpretation of Romance, a woody floral fragrance created by Firmenich. Classic florals are combined with warm, embraceable essences, stirring affections that will have you snuggling in no time. Packaging extends the modern theme: classic, rectangular bottles, silver-toned caps, and pretty-in-pink cartons. Romance is definitely a "date night" fragrance to dazzle the senses.

Introduced	*1998*
Price	*Mid-range*

ROSE ABSOLUE

Scent Type	*Floral*
Composition	
Notes:	*May rose, Turkish rose, Bulgarian rose, Damascus rose, Egyptian rose, Moroccan rose*

An international cornucopia of roses was gathered for this brilliant, fragrant exaltation from Annick Goutal. It is a superbly feminine fragrance celebrating the rose—the queen of flowers.

The scent of the rose is one of nature's most powerfully sensual aromas, and the rose is one of the most coveted flowers in history. In old Persia, the Sultan slept on a mattress filled with rose petals. Fountains of rose water adorned tables at feasts, and rose petals were often strewn among party guests. In the Victorian language of flowers, roses are the symbol of love. White roses represent purity and spiritual love; red roses mean true love; cabbage roses are ambassadors of love; a single rose denotes simplicity; burgundy roses mean unconscious beauty. But beware the yellow rose, for it represents decreasing love and infidelity.

Introduced	*1986*
Price	*Top range*

ROYAL SECRET

Scent Type	*Oriental*
Composition	
Top Notes:	*Citrus, African orange*
Heart Notes:	*Bulgarian rose, jasmine*
Base Notes:	*Sandalwood, musk, myrrh*

Germaine Monteil introduced Royal Secret in 1935, at a time when royal families still had secrets. The 1930s were the height of fascination with all things Oriental, and Royal Secret reflects this attitude with its eastern composition.

The fiery creation opens with fresh citrus notes, then combines a classic French heart of jasmine and rose with exotic base notes of sandalwood, musk, and myrrh. Royal Secret... as potent today as it was in 1935.

Introduced	*1935*
Price	*Mid-range*

RUSH

Scent Type	*Floral - Oriental*
Composition	
Top Notes:	*Freesia*
Heart Notes:	*Jasmine, gardenia*
Base Notes:	*Vanilla, patchouli*

Gucci pushes the avant-garde edge with Rush, a spicy floral Oriental fragrance with a sultry attitude. Classic florals are combined with sensual essences of patchouli and vanilla. Red and orange color the plastic-coated rectangular bottle, which is styled after a videocassette. Riveting and exhilarating, this rush of Gucci is the aromatic equivalent of a roller-coaster ride.

Introduced	*1999*
Price	*High range*

S.T. DuPont

Scent Type	*Floral*
Composition	
Top Notes:	*Mandarin, melon, black currant*
Heart Notes:	*Gardenia, ylang-ylang, cyclamen*
Base Notes:	*Patchouli, musk, amber, moss*

Since 1872, S.T. DuPont has been known the world over for luxury accessories, precision-crafted lighters, and fine menswear. Its sophisticated floral fragrance is equally well rendered, in a cylindrical bottle. The cap is fashioned after a cigarette lighter, and it snaps open and closed with the resounding click of quality. Look for the scent in a carton of muted sapphire. S.T. DuPont is a fitting fragrance of distinction for the elegant, understated woman.

Introduced	*1998*
Price	*Mid-range*

SABI

Scent Type	*Floral - Green*
Composition	
Top Notes:	*Orchid, galbanum, bergamot, hyacinth, rose*
Heart Notes:	*Rose, jasmine, orange flower, ylang-ylang, orris, narcissus*
Base Notes:	*Sandalwood, oakmoss, vetiver, patchouli*

Famous Patrons
Diane Sawyer

Henry Dunay, world-renowned jeweler known for his opulent designs, brings forth Sabi, a rich, full-bodied floral with a fresh green opening accord. The name, which means "simple elegance" in Japanese, also refers to a technique used to finish gold, a finish often employed on Dunay's highly collectible pieces—our own private passion!

The development of Sabi was a family effort; Dunay's perfumer brother, Richard Loniewski, had a hand in creating such classics as Saint Laurent's Opium and Giorgio's Red. Loniewski oversaw the fragrance development, while Dunay guided the flacon design. Dunay says the fragrance "will remind people what a rich, great fragrance should be." Indeed. The sensual, sophisticated floral is a romantic, refined scent, an obvious labor of love from two brothers at the height of their respective professions.

The limited-edition offering, sold in fine jewelry departments, was a $30,000 diamond-encrusted flacon that may be converted and worn around the neck suspended from a silken cord. The rest of the line, found in fragrance departments, is more reasonably priced, yet still remarkably beautiful. Ribbed glass is crowned with a gold-colored cap of deep "V" *faux pavé* diamonds. Overall, Sabi is a stunning achievement of both quality and presentation—a fragrance for the luxurious life.

Introduced	*1998*
Price	*Top range*

SAFARI

Scent Type	*Floral - Green*
Composition	
Top Notes:	*Tagetes, orange de Indes, hyacinth, black currant bud, jonquil, mandarin, galbanum*
Heart Notes:	*Italian jasmine, orange blossom, orris, genet, May rose, narcisse de Montagne*
Base Notes:	*Sandalwood, cedarwood, vetiver, patchouli, amber*

Famous Patrons
Actress Josette Banzet, Marquise de Bruyenne

Designed as part of the Ralph Lauren lifestyle, Safari is rich in attitude. Vigorous green notes accompany floral, citrus, and woody essences in the scent that was created for women of independent and adventurous spirit. Safari is an elegant selection for warm weather, career, and casually elegant evening wear.

The soft, sensual perfume is presented in curved flacons of hand-cut crystal, reminiscent of a gentle bygone era. Etched sterling silver hinged caps with tortoise shell accents complete the accoutrements a traveler might pack for an African safari. Imagine Meryl Streep in *Out of Africa*. Safari won two Fragrance Foundation FiFi Awards in 1990.

Lauren designed a whole world of products around the Safari theme: "A world without boundaries." He says: "I see the Safari woman as an expression of the dreams and yearnings that women have for adventure, romance, and intrigue. This elegant woman represents a state of mind in which she is surrounded by luxury, yet is always at ease and comfortable with where she is and who she is. She appreciates the finest in art, clothing, and her surroundings, and travels the world in search of experiences that interest and stimulate her." Oh, yes…that's us!

For a real Ralph Lauren immersion, visit his boutiques in New York and on Beverly Hills' Rodeo Drive—makes us want to start packing for a well-heeled safari.

Introduced   1990
Price   Top range

SALVADOR DALI

Scent Type   Floral - Aldehyde
Composition
  Top Notes: Aldehydes, mandarin, bergamot,
                  basil, greens
  Heart Notes: Jasmine, lily of the valley,
                  tuberose, rose, narcissus, orris
  Base Notes: Cedarwood, amber, vanilla,
                  sandalwood, musk, benzoin

Famous Patrons
  Princess Caroline of Monaco

Artist Salvador Dali lends his name to a fragrance as surreal as his paintings.

Bright aldehydic notes spill forth from the rich floral bouquet, while soft Oriental background notes add ambery verve. Splash it on for a busy day at the office or a slow stroll though your favorite museum.

The juice is poured into a signed flacon that mimics a partial visage. The humorous bottle is crafted in the shape of voluptuous lips, over which rests a nose-shaped stopper. We had to have this one just for the bottle.

Introduced   1983
Price   High range

SALVATORE FERRAGAMO

Scent Type   Floral
Composition
  Top Notes: Neroli, anise, cassis, green leaves
  Heart Notes: Florentine iris, rose,
                  lily of the valley, peony,
                  pepper, nutmeg
  Base Notes: Raspberry, musk, almond, woods

The Italian firm of Salvatore Ferragamo made its mark upon the world with a line of luxury footwear. Following in the footsteps of its founder, today's firm is dedicated to expanding the original vision. From shoes to accessories, clothing to home furnishings, the family-owned empire is on the rise under the watchful eye of Salvatore's successor, Ferruccio Ferragamo.

The women's Salvatore Ferragamo fragrance opens appropriately with neroli, distilled from the orange flower. The word "neroli" is from Italian, so named for Anna Maria de la Trémoille, a seventeenth century princess of Nerola. This intensely floral scent is built on a wooded raspberry foundation. Bolstered by rich florals of rose and iris with a dash of spice, the scent suggests the ultimate Italian holiday.

The sun-kissed formula is presented in twisted, cylindrical bottles of sleek, statuesque proportion. Designed by Thierry de Baschmakoff, the bottle visually portrays the personality of the scent. The presentation is complete—a sexy scent with a modern attitude.

Introduced   1998
Price   High range

SAMSARA

Scent Type   Floral - Oriental
Composition
    Top Notes: Bergamot, peach, lemon, greens
    Heart Notes: Jasmine, orris absolute,
                          ylang-ylang, rose,
                          narcissus, santal
    Base Notes: Amber, vanilla, sandalwood,
                          tonka bean, musk

Famous Patrons
    Cameron Diaz   Angela Lansbury
    Darryl Hannah   Brooke Shields
    Jaclyn Smith   Sally Jesse Raphael
    Sheena Easton

A 1989 addition to the Guerlain fragrance legend, Samsara is a tantalizing Oriental blend with exotic floral accents. The name is a Sanskrit word that signifies an infinite cycle of births and rebirths, repeated until perfection or nirvana is attained.

The rich fragrance is made using entirely natural ingredients. Dominant notes of jasmine, rose and ylang-ylang mingle with balsamic sandalwood and vanilla, while the seed of tonka bean adds a gingerbread-like aroma. Many of the ingredients used in Samsara are also used in aromatherapy to impart a sense of serenity. The result is a warm, beguiling fragrance, sensual and long-lasting.

Samsara was eleven years in the making. Perfection was essential for creator Jean-Paul Guerlain because the fragrance is a tribute to the woman he loves. Inspired by her grace and confidence, radiance, and generosity, he sought a feminine fragrance to honor her spiritual and physical beauty. "I was but the stonemason; she

was the architect," he says, and he still mixes a special version by hand just for her.

Jean-Paul Guerlain travels the Earth in search of the highest-quality ingredients for Guerlain perfumes. The company lists the sacred components they search out: "Jasmine, rose and tuberose from Mediterranean shores; sandalwood, cinnamon and bois de rose from Southeast Asia; geranium, verbena and palmarosa from Madagascar; bergamot from Calabria; vetiver from Réunion Island; and the essences of ylang-ylang and eucalyptus from the South Pacific." Indeed, Guerlain fragrances contain the essences of the world—or rather, the best of its essence.

Samsara comes in a perfume flacon inspired by ancient Asian artifacts. Colored deep red, the sacred color, it features lotus-like lines of elegant simplicity and is accented with a gold-colored sash and smooth cap. Graceful upturned edges remind us of pagodas that dot the verdant hills lining the shores of Taiwan, Korea, and Japan.

Introduced   1989
Price   High range

SÉXUAL

Scent Type   Floral - Oriental
Composition
    Top Notes: Japanese osmanthus, bergamot,
                          honeysuckle, freesia, clementine
    Heart Notes: Jasmine, gardenia,
                          red rose, neroli
    Base Notes: Cinnamon, myrrh,
                          vanilla, sandalwood

Canadian entrepreneur Michel Germain introduced a pair of sensual fragrances for women and men, entitled Séxual. Touted as an aphrodisiac, the women's floral blend is spiked with spicy highlights, including cinnamon, myrrh, and vanilla. Germain's wife, Norma, lent her long, lean back for the bare advertising photography. Voluptuous bottles by Pierre Dinand fill the hand with a smooth sensuality. Tastefully executed, Séxual is a fragrance for making love, and making love last.

Introduced	1997
Price	High range

SHALIMAR

Scent Type Oriental
Composition
    Top Notes: Bergamot, lemon, hesperides
    Heart Notes: Jasmine, iris, rose, patchouli, vetiver
    Base Notes: Vanilla, incense, opopanax, sandalwood, musk, civet, ambergris, leather

Famous Patrons

Meryl Streep	Dionne Warwick
Rita Hayworth	Lisa Hartman
Joan Collins	Britt Ekland
Shirley MacLaine	Gina Lollobrigida
Jeanne Hollenbeck	Josette Banzet

Shalimar is an intoxicating, yet subtly sensuous blend that has endured for more than sixty-five years. With a long-lasting base of spices and aromatic woods, it became the archetype for Oriental blends. A highly distinctive and dramatic fragrance, it was designed for the woman who is sensual, sophisticated and uninhibited...another grand entrance-making perfume from Guerlain.

A 1925 composition, Shalimar is reflective of its period, of a cosmopolitan Paris in the midst of celebration after World War I, of the Roaring Twenties, of exhilaration and new life. This attitude is mirrored in the zesty citrus top notes. Heady florals flow into a spicy base that is particularly rich in vanilla, incense, and sandalwood.

In creating Shalimar, Jacques Guerlain was inspired by a love story told to him by a Maharajah visiting Paris. The Guerlain company shared the story with us:

> More than 300 years ago, Shah Jahan succeeded to the throne of his father, Jahangir, and became the third Mogul Emperor of India.
>
> Jahan loved only one woman. Her name was Mumtaz Mahal.
>
> Some say he loved her unto madness, that she was not his wife but his fever. Victories, empires and riches were dust as compared to her...in his eyes, she alone was the balm that made life bearable.
>
> When she died, Jahan's hair turned white. He would burst into tears at the mention of her name. In her memory, he built one of the world's greatest wonders—the Taj Mahal at Agra.
>
> But the Taj Mahal is only an empty monument. While Mumtaz was alive, Jahan created a series of gardens for her at Lahore, gardens the like of which had never been seen before. He called them the gardens of Shalimar, the Sanskrit word meaning "abode of love."
>
> From every corner of the Earth, the most fragrant and delicate blossoms were brought. Deep pools were built with crystal fountains and terraces paved in marble. The rarest birds were summoned to sing here and lanterns were hung to rival the stars. In the gardens of Shalimar the lovers were truly happy, and Mumtaz bore fourteen children to her beloved Jahan.

Jacques Guerlain decided that the perfume should be called Shalimar, not Taj Mahal, because, you see, Taj Mahal marks the end of the story, and this love story can never end…

The flacon was designed by Raymond Guerlain and is also a reminder of the fountains in the gardens of Shalimar. The ornamental stopper in sapphire blue evokes the flow of the fountains' water.

Voluptuous and enveloping, Shalimar is a fragrance of eternal romance.

Introduced	1925
Price	*High range*

SIGNATURE

Scent Type	*Floral*
Composition	
Top Notes:	*White tulip, tangerine, nutmeg, Virginia creeper*
Heart Notes:	*Magnolia, rose, iris, gardenia, orchid, frangipani*
Base Notes:	*Sandalwood, amber, musk, rosewood, vanilla*

The second women's scent from S.T. Dupont is a tribute, the company explains, to "the poetry of writing." Established in 1872, the house of Dupont added fine writing instruments to its line in 1973. This heritage is reflected in the presentation of Signature; Dupont says the curved bottle is based on an inkwell, the "reservoir of our thoughts," and ensconced in a scarlet Ultrasuede box.

The floral fragrance develops around a rosy heart, while a powdery, ambery finish exudes warmth and charisma. Signature is aromatic poetry for the writer's soul; an upscale scent for women who have a way with words—or for those who would wish to.

Introduced	2000
Price	*High range*

SIRÈNE

Scent Type	*Floral - Oriental*
Composition	
Top Notes:	*Orange blossom*
Heart Notes:	*Lily, heliotrope, ylang-ylang*
Base Notes:	*Vanilla, sandalwood*

Paris-based couturier Vicky Tiel is renowned for exquisite draped and tailored designs. Sirène, an exquisite floral Oriental, reveals the same attention to detail that is required of a fine couture garment. The white flower bouquet is warmed with a classic vanilla and sandalwood base. Sirène is a romantic, elegant scent that hints of a mysterious past. The clear, classic perfume bottle is a work of art—the dip wand is a woman's sculpted silhouette.

In Greek mythology, sirens were sea nymphs who, with their enchanting songs, lured unsuspecting sailors to their demise. With Sirène, you can sing your own siren song and tempt your own sailor.

Introduced	1993
Price	*Top range*

SO DE LA RENTA

Scent Type	*Floral - Fresh*
Composition	
Top Notes:	Watermelon, gardenia, freesia, clementine
Heart Notes:	Tuberose, peony, narcissus, white lotus
Base Notes:	Vanilla, musk, woods

Dominican fashion designer, Oscar de la Renta, introduced So, commenting that the fragrance "personifies the spirit, energy and confidence of the twenty-first century."

So is a sheer floral composition of youthful exuberance, a feminine study of exotic white flowers and sensual musk—flirty and fun. So is pretty in pink, with a matte gold-colored cap and accents. It is an ideal scent for sheer summer wear, island hopping, and vacation flings.

Introduced	*1997*
Price	*Mid-range*

SO PRETTY

Scent Type	*Floral - Fresh*
Composition	
Top Notes:	Bergamot, dewberry, jasmine, orange blossom, mandarin
Heart Notes:	Rose, Florentine iris, diamond orchid, white peach, osmanthus
Base Notes:	Oakmoss, sandalwood, vetiver

So Pretty is soft and fresh, a jewel of a fragrance from Cartier. Built around an intensely feminine rose accord, So Pretty offers a bouquet of rich florals: the Centifolia rose from Grasse, the Damascena rose from Turkey, the Florentine iris, and the Diamond orchid from Brazil. The result is aptly named, for the youthful scent inspires the exclamation, "So pretty!" The fragrance is a fresh turn for Cartier, which serves as crown jeweler to nineteen royal houses.

A sensually curved flacon, trimmed with gold-colored fittings, houses the precious fragrance. Shades of gold and white suggest wedding day purity and innocence, with a refinement of regal proportion. So Pretty also received an industry award, the FiFi, presented by The Fragrance Foundation.

Introduced	*1995*
Price	*Top range*

SOLEIL

Scent Type	*Floral - Green*
Composition	
Top Notes:	Orange blossom, jasmine, ylang-ylang, freesia, mimosa, wisteria, seringa flower, black currant, marigold
Heart Notes:	Rose, iris, lilac, lily
Base Notes:	Sandalwood, musk, amber

From the legendary French firm of Fragonard comes Soleil, a delightful, spirited fragrance. The Grasse house of Fragonard is a family-owned business, operated by Jean François Costa and his two daughters, Françoise Costa-Fabre and Agnès Costa. Their great-grandfather, Jean Francois Costa, founded the firm and named it after a French painter from Grasse, Fragonard. The sisters developed the sunny floral scent with Givaudan-Roure perfumer, Jean Guichard. Evocative of pastoral Provence and the flowered fields of

Grasse, Soleil is a sun-drenched floral with fresh, meadow-green notes.

Soleil, French for "sun," is housed in a playful, baroque bottle designed by the Costa sisters with Joel Desgrippes. The rounded bottle features a spiked sun cap in golden tones. It's just the thing for a carefree summery frame of mind.

Introduced 1997
Price High range

SONIA RYKIEL

Scent Type Floral - Fruity
Composition
Top Notes: Mandarin, pineapple, passion fruit, black currant
Heart Notes: Lily of the valley, rose, violet, cyclamen
Base Notes: Sandalwood, caramel, cinnamon, vanilla, musk, patchouli, cedarwood

Before you slip into your Sonia Rykiel knitwear, spritz on her eponymous fragrance. It is designed to be just as comfortable and sensual as the easy, elegant fashions for which Rykiel is known. The fruity floral fragrance, blended by perfumer Jean-Louis Sreuzac, is a refined composition with a semi-Oriental base accord.

Complete with short sleeves and ribbing, the gleeful bottle is shaped like a Rykiel knit sweater. Emblazoned across the chest is the star-studded signature "Sonia Rykiel," spelled out with 149 dazzling rhinestones. The eau de toilette sports a similar signature in black. Eye-catching vermilion cartons complete the snazzy presentation of Sonia Rykiel.

Introduced 1998
Price High range

SPELLBOUND

Scent Type Floral - Ambery
Composition
Top Notes: Fruits, rosewood, coriander, orange blossom, pimento
Heart Notes: Rose, jasmine, tuberose, carnation, lily of the valley, carnation, heliotrope
Base Notes: Vanilla, amber, cedarwood, benzoin, musk, civet, opopanax

Estée Lauder brings us yet another fragrance destined to be a classic. Spellbound casts a potent spell with spices, rare flowers, and exotic woods woven into a sophisticated ambery blend with Oriental accents. A clove-like aroma adds impact to the dramatic, feminine statement.

The magical scent is encased in a classic glass bottle topped with a sleek brass ornament.

Introduced 1991
Price High range

SPLENDOR

Scent Type Floral
Composition
Top Notes: Sweet pea, wisteria, freesia, hyacinth, peony
Heart Notes: Water lily, magnolia, jasmine, poppy, rose
Base Notes: Satinwood, ebony wood, musk

The resurgence of old-style Hollywood glamour served as an inspiration for Elizabeth Arden's Splendor. A rich feminine floral, as warm as a tender embrace, Splendor is rife with the magical aroma of sweet pea. Expertly blended with ethereal freesia and wisteria, the classic floral heart develops into a musky, wooded base. The bottle is fashioned after a crystal decanter, dressed with a silver-colored collar and a crystal-ball stopper.

Classically inspired, Splendor is a scent that speaks of subtle enchantment, of refined luxury, of love, romance and indulgence—an ultra *femme* fragrance.

Introduced   *1998*
Price   *Mid-range*

ST. JOHN

Scent Type   *Floral - Oriental*
Composition
    Top Notes: *Freesia, mandarin, osmanthus,*
                   orange flower
    Heart Notes: *Jasmine, honeysuckle,*
                   moonflower, gardenia
    Base Notes: *Sandalwood, amber,*
                   apricot, musk

The eponymous scent from St. John founder and designer Marie Gray is an elegant floral Oriental blend—the ideal accompaniment to the timeless St. John suit. The fresh opening accord is rife with mandarin, freesia, and orange flower, while the jasmine heart and wooded floral base lend warmth, stability, and sophistication to this versatile, full-bodied scent. A touch of apricot in the base notes imparts a gentle trail, or *sillage*. St. John is sleekly attired in a black paillette-embossed carton with gold-colored accents. The ambery-apricot liquid is presented in a round flacon reminiscent of a bold St. John button, with the company's logo in the center.

For the confident woman of the world, St. John is a marvelous choice, a sensually elegant scent rich enough to linger through any dinner party or diplomatic reception.

Introduced   *1994*
Price   *High range*

STARDUST

Scent Type   *Oriental - Fruity*
Composition
    Top Notes: *Water hyacinth, tangerine,*
                   osmanthus, purple freesia
    Heart Notes: *Mimosa, jasmine, lily,*
                   carnation, peony
    Base Notes: *Plum, sandalwood, amber*

Stardust is the first fragrance from entrepreneurs Cynthia and Phillip L. Prime, founders of Parfums Llewelyn. The Oriental fragrance is an expansive blend of sweet fruits, rich florals, and lingering woods. Starburst is a sparkling scent of romance and intrigue. The heavenly diamond-faceted bottle, a Marc Rosen design and Brosse production, is crowned with a cap of sapphire blue and dusted with a sprinkling of stars. Stardust is a celestial scent, created to evoke a sense of new horizons as we forge ahead into the third millennium.

Stardust has a humanitarian heart and soul, too. Five percent of net sales is contributed to literacy programs, as well as to mentoring and job training programs for women and young girls. Bravo!

Introduced   *1999*
Price   *Top range*

STYLE

Scent Type   *Floral*
Composition
   Top Notes: *Mandarin, bergamot,*
                 apple blossom, chamomile
   Heart Notes: *Jasmine, lily of the valley,*
                 magnolia, geranium, carnation,
                 violet leaves
   Base Notes: *Sandalwood, amber, tonka bean,*
                 patchouli, musk

During the 1980s, the women of Beverly Hills and Hollywood turned to Gale Hayman for wardrobe advice, frequenting the Rodeo Drive boutique Giorgio Beverly Hills, which Hayman co-founded. Giorgio was headquarters for one-of-a-kind Academy Awards gowns and accessories, yet the shop's most successful offering turned out to be Giorgio, the blockbuster fragrance. Today, Hayman is still revered for her sense of style and glamour. Her best-selling book, *How Do I Look?* is a classic beauty guide, and her syndicated beauty column is a delight.

Hayman's love of fashion and fragrance began in her youth. Her unerring sense of style is evident in her 1999 introduction, a pair of scents called Style and Glamour, made to be worn separately or layered together. Style is intended for fresh daytime chic, while Glamour is the height of evening splendor.

Style is a casually sophisticated white floral perfume that can be worn, Hayman says, "from the boardroom to the bedroom." Style occupies a sleek bottle of frosted aqua, crowned with a sapphire-colored cap.

As Yves Saint Laurent once said, "Fashions fade, style is eternal."

Introduced   *1999*
Price   *Mid-range*

SUBLIME

Scent Type   *Floral*
Composition
   Top and Heart Notes: Jasmine, rose
   Base Notes: *Amber, musk*

Famous Patrons
   Actress Alessandra Martines

Sublime is a superb fragrance from the French firm of Jean Patou that brought the world the scent of Joy. The company says Sublime is "an instant of sheer happiness, of pure delight." It was designed for the modern woman, radiant and sensual, tender, and opulent, who is "equally at ease frolicking in a whimsical garden as she is basking in the Parisian sunlight on the banks of the Seine."

Famed French film maker Claude Lelouch provided the artistry evident in the photography of Italian actress Alessandra Martines, the sublime woman used in the print advertising. The flacon carries out the sublime vision—curved to fit a woman's hand, endowed with a gold-colored stopper in the shape of a flower bud...all in shades of brilliant amber and gold.

The scent is rife with pure floral essences, warmed by golden amber and sensual musk tones. Sublime is an opulent floral bouquet in the rich tradition of Jean Patou.

Introduced   *1993*
Price   *High range*

SUI DREAMS

Scent Type   *Floral - Oriental*
Composition
  Top Notes: *Tangerine, orange bitter, bergamot*
  Heart Notes: *Chinese peony, freesia*
  Base Notes: *Sandalwood, vanilla, anise, cedarwood*

Fashion designer Anna Sui targets a youthful audience with Sui Dreams, her second fragrance. The floral Oriental zings open with tangy citrus fruits, followed with white flowers and a wooded vanilla base that is sexy and smooth, funky and fresh—the fragrant equivalent of Sui's rococo-hippie clothing designs. Firmenich perfumer Phillipe Romano blended the blue-tinted scent. It is presented in a clever handbag-shaped bottle. Sui Dreams—sure to inspire sweet dreams.

Introduced   *2000*
Price   *High range*

SUN MOON STARS

Scent Type   *Oriental - Fruity*
Composition
  Top Notes: *Freesia, pear*
  Heart Notes: *Jasmine, heliotrope, narcissus, orange blossom*
  Base Notes: *Sandalwood, musk, amber, vanilla*

Famous Patrons
  Daryl Hannah

Recognizing a universal theme, Karl Lagerfeld brings us Sun Moon Stars—what more could we want? A lush, evocative floral Oriental composition, the scent begins with crisp fruity top notes, evolving into a delectable accord of florals, vanilla, and woods. The result is heavenly—a gustative celebration. Tenacious, warm, and expansive: A galaxy of possibilities emerge.

Sun Moon Stars is captured in a rounded flacon of the deepest celestial blue—a *boule bleu*—upon which are carved in relief the sun, the moon, and the stars.

Introduced   *1994*
Price   *Mid-range*

SUNFLOWERS

Scent Type   *Floral - Fruity*
Composition
  Top Notes: *Bergamot, melon, peach*
  Heart Notes: *Jasmine, cyclamen, tea rose, osmanthus*
  Base Notes: *Sandalwood, musk, moss*

Famous Patrons
  Model Vendela

Sunflowers is a brisk fruity floral from Elizabeth Arden, ideal for spa lovers. Arden calls it a "prestige fragrance without the prestige pricing." Created in response to all things natural, Sunflowers is light enough to be worn by women of any age, and is perfect for casual, outdoor, and warm weather use. We love it on the tennis court, or for a leisurely bicycle ride through the country.

Sunflowers is presented in a package with a sunflower cut-out, and the fragrance itself is in a simple clear glass bottle imprinted with the name in bright white and yellow.

A romantic note appears on the side of the box: "And the sun was shining when he held me and I felt a deep flowering of pleasure. All at once. Like a sunflower. Opening up." We just love the return to romance.

Introduced	*1993*
Price	*Mid-range*

SUNG

Scent Type Floral - Green
Composition
  Top Notes: *Orange, ylang-ylang, mandarin, bergamot, galbanum, lemon, hyacinth*
  Heart Notes: *Osmanthus, genet, jasmine, iris, lily of the valley*
  Base Notes: *Vanilla, orange blossom, sandalwood, ambrette, vetiver*

Sung is the first fragrance from international designer Alfred Sung. He states, "My perfume is an extension of my designs, an evolution, an intimate expression of a woman's wants and desires."

The signature white floral fragrance features sparkling fresh citrus blended with green notes and white flowers, set against a refined backdrop of woods and spices. Fresh and light, it is a classic fragrance that can be worn with equal ease on the shores of Palm Beach, to Manhattan galas or on Swiss ski slopes.

The feminine, sophisticated floral is encased in a classic Pierre Dinand bottle of clean, uncomplicated, symmetrical lines. Pure Sung.

Introduced	*1986*
Price	*High range*

SUNSET BOULEVARD

Scent Type Floral - Oriental
Composition
  Top Notes: *Green ivy, ylang-ylang, bergamot, water lily, lemon*
  Heart Notes: *Jasmine, orange blossom, lily of the valley, cyclamen*
  Base Notes: *Musk, mousse de Chine, amber, sandalwood, vetiver*

Gale Hayman has long been recognized for her sense of style. Co-founder of Giorgio Beverly Hills, founder of Gale Hayman Beverly Hills cosmetics, and beauty columnist and author (*How Do I Look?*), Hayman is well-versed in putting one's best foot forward.

Hayman captures the flair of Sunset Boulevard, the magic of Hollywood, and the style of Beverly Hills in this fragrance. A dramatic floral Oriental bursting with white flowers warmed with ambery woods, Sunset Boulevard is a sensually feminine scent. Hayman's signature leopard-patterned collar frames the neckline of the tall, chic bottle.

Discover the magic of Sunset Boulevard. And then, get ready for your close-up.

Introduced	*1998*
Price	*Mid-range*

SUSAN LUCCI INVITATION
(See Invitation)

SYLVIE CHANTECAILLE COLLECTION

DARBY ROSE
Floral
FRANGIPANE
Floral - Ambery
TIARE
Floral
WISTERIA
Floral - Fresh

Sylvie Chantecaille, a former cosmetics executive-turned-entrepreneur, boldly formed her own company and introduced three fragrances at once: Wisteria, Tiare, and Frangipane. Adventurous travels around the world served as her inspiration, including treks through India, Tibet, and Tahiti. The floral trio is redolent of exotic flowers she encountered on her journey. Frangipane, a jasmine found in Peru and the West Indies, embraces orange, jasmine, and vanilla. Tiare is rife with Tahitian white flower essences of gardenia, tuberose, and ylang-ylang. Wisteria, the sheerest of the family, also contains freesia, peony, and tarragon. A fourth fragrance was later added to the collection; Darby Rose is an expansive floral fragrance named for the roses that grow outside Chantecaille's New York residence.

The plain, rectangular bottles are topped with pewter-toned caps. Color is supplied by the fragrance tints: pink, green, and golden yellow. Chantecaille has since added a beauty division, featuring cosmetics in the same silvery-toned packaging.

Enjoy all four scents—simple, unfettered luxuries for everyday living.

Introduced   1997
Price   *High range*

TALISMAN

Scent Type	*Chypre - Fruity*
Composition	
Top Notes:	*Violet leaves, davana, litchi, rum, osmanthus*
Heart Notes:	*Hyacinth, rose, orchid, freesia, ylang-ylang, clove*
Base Notes:	*Amber, iris*

Talisman is the fifth fragrance from the house founded by Spanish couturier Cristobal Balenciaga, who created other classics such as Le Dix, Michelle, Quadrille, and Prélude. Although Balenciaga is no longer with us, his memory lives on under the stewardship of the new house designer, Josephus Melchior Thimister.

Talisman charms with a fruity opening accord that contains unusual notes, such as litchi, rum, and davana (a fruit progressed midway from plum to prune). The spicy floral heart holds hints of clove, while amber and iris render a final powdery impression. Perfumer Dominique Preyssas blended the fruity chypre scent.

A talisman is a touchstone, a good luck charm. Keep your horseshoes, rabbit's feet, and four-leaf clovers; if you want to be lucky in love, the magical Talisman may be just the thing.

Introduced   1994
Price   *High range*

TENDRE POISON

Scent Type   Floral - Fresh
Composition
    Top Notes: Galbanum, mandarin
    Heart Notes: Freesia, orange, honey
    Base Notes: Vanilla, sandalwood

Christian Dior's original Poison has gone green with its fresh counterpart, Tendre Poison. The fragrance is positioned to appeal to a younger market, or to those who want a change from the heady, erotic aroma of the original Poison.

Lightness is achieved with top notes of green galbanum and smooth fruity mandarin, before moving to an ethereal heart led by freesia. The base is soft yet tenacious, with the sweetness of sandalwood and vanilla.

Tendre Poison shares packaging and bottles with its mature sibling, though in green, of course. With Tendre Poison, Christian Dior proves the old adage false: The grass is not always greener on the other side.

Introduced   1994
Price   High range

TENTATIONS

Scent Type   Oriental
Composition
    Top Notes: Bergamot, pepper
    Heart Notes: Florals
    Base Notes: Myrrh, cedarwood

Tentations, meaning "temptations" in French, is a sizzling creation from Paloma Picasso. A fragrance designed for exotic living, Tentations is dramatic, passionate, and mysterious. Picasso,

daughter of artist Pablo Picasso, is an extraordinarily talented woman in her own right, as evidenced by her jewelry designs for Tiffany & Company, among other ventures.

Tentations is an expansive Oriental blend and is presented in hues of red and black, similar to Picasso's original signature fragrance. The bottle bears an intriguing filigree motif. Oh, so exquisite—why not yield to temptation?

Introduced   1996
Price   High range

THEOREMA

Scent Type   Oriental
Composition
    Top Notes: Tangelo, jasmine, Thia Shamouti
    Heart Notes: Osmanthus, spices
    Base Notes: Sandalwood, guaiac wood,
                    amber, macassar, sweet cream

The classically rendered Theorema is an Oriental blended addition to the House of Fendi fragrance line. A striking Italian style is evident throughout the seductive scent. To quote Lord Byron, "Italia! oh Italia! thou who hast the fatal gift of beauty."

Daring and defiant, Theorema is a vivacious blend of tangelo, spice, amber, and woods that conveys the romance of Rome and the verve of Venice. A warm, nuzzling scent, it is equally suitable for a cozy evening by the fireplace or a night on the town.

The classic Fendi leather handbag inspired the chic Theorema bottle. Stylish shades of black and gold add panache to the presentation.

Introduced   1998
Price   High range

TIEMPE PASSATE

Scent Type *Floral - Ambery*
Composition
 Top Notes: Bergamot, clementine
 Heart Notes: Montauk rose, ambrette
 Base Notes: Amber, cedarwood

Famous Patrons
 Jennifer Lopez

Inspired by a song of the same name, which was written by creator Antonia Bellanca's grandfather in the 1920s, Tiempe Passate, or "time past" in Italian, is a nostalgic floral harmony.

East Hampton-based florist-turned-perfumer Antonia Bellanca created her first fragrance, Antonia's Flowers, in 1985. In her quest to capture the fleeting aroma of flowers, Bellanca was attracted, quite naturally, to the art of perfumery. Today, Bellanca continues to slowly build her business in the traditional manner, by word of mouth. "Our customers spread the word for us," she says. Bellanca leads a balanced life, devoting time to being a wife and mother and to caring for a twenty-acre farm in East Hampton.

Radiant and diffusive, a classic bouquet warmed with sweet amber, Tiempe Passate is a fragrance of fairy tale legend. Montauk rose adds a dash of salty flavor; the effect is magical on the skin. Tiempe Passate is presented in a plum-papered box, which opens to reveal a graceful, petal-topped flacon mounted on a burgundy velvet pedestal. An atomizer is cleverly tucked to the side, giving women a choice of spray or splash. Well-designed, beautifully executed, an eau de parfum of great style and flair. Tiempe Passate is a touch of grace.

Introduced *1999*
Price   *High range*

TIFFANY

Scent Type *Floral - Ambery*
Composition
 Top Notes: Indian jasmine, Damascena rose,
       ylang-ylang, mandarin,
       orange blossom, Italian mandarin
 Heart Notes: Florentine iris, lily of the valley,
       black currant bud, violet leaves
 Base Notes: Sandalwood, amber,
       vanilla, vetiver

Famous Patrons
 Fashion designer Vera Wang

Tiffany is the signature fragrance from the world-renowned retailer of fine jewelry, timepieces, accessories, and tableware. An effusive bouquet of 150 floral notes, the Tiffany fragrance was created in 1987 in honor of the 150th anniversary of Tiffany & Company.

The fragrance begins with fruity top notes that give way to a refined semi-Oriental arrangement of florals, aromatic woods, and sweet vanilla. A sophisticated fragrance, Tiffany is equally suitable for the office and romantic dinners. A smidgen too rich? The Voile Parfume version is a lighter, alcohol-free formulation.

Tiffany Design Director John Loring and famed bottle designer Pierre Dinand created the elegant Art Deco bottle that houses the subtle, distinctive perfume. It is packaged, of course, in Tiffany's signature color of robin's-egg blue.

Introduced *1987*
Price   *High range*

TOCADE

Scent Type   *Floral - Oriental*
Composition
    Top Notes: *Magnolia, rose, mandarin,*
              bergamot
    Heart Notes: *Rose*
    Base Notes: *Vanilla, amber, cedarwood*

Tocade is a lighthearted offering from Rochas, the fragrance house that brought us Byzance and Femme. Tocade, in French, means an "impulsive infatuation." Tocade is a youthful, free-spirited fragrance created by Quest perfumer Maurice Rouchel. The playful composition unfolds with fruits and florals, then segues to a creamy finish of vanilla and amber.

Bottle designer Serge Mansau interpreted Tocade's spontaneity by applying bold primary colors of red, blue, and yellow; dashes of green and orange add spice to the whimsical, pointy-cap bottles. Vibrant and merry, Tocade is encased in bright Rochas-red cartons.

Introduced   *1994*
Price   *High range*

TOMMY GIRL

Scent Type   *Floral - Green*
Composition
    Top Notes: *Black currant bud, apple,*
              tangerine, mandarin, spearmint
    Heart Notes: *Heather, honeysuckle, violet, rose,*
              magnolia, jasmine, lily
    Base Notes: *Sandalwood, cedarwood*

Building on the success of his first fragrance, Tommy, fashion designer Tommy Hilfiger follows up with Tommy Girl, a veritable bouquet of wild flowers, as fresh as a sun-drenched meadow of springtime blossoms. A basket of fruits and a sprinkling of spearmint add character and clarity to this playful composition. Energetic and fun in a free-spirited, natural fashion, like a Hilfiger cotton pique shirt paired with casual chinos. In fact, Tommy Girl was launched in conjunction with Hilfiger's first women's clothing collection.

The container—designed to resemble a nineteenth-century apothecary bottle, shimmers in patriotic shades of red, white, and blue that reflect the spirit of the young American woman. Wear Tommy Girl and feel eighteen again.

Introduced   *1996*
Price   *Mid-range*

TOUCH

*(See Burberry Touch, or Fred Hayman's Touch
in Honorable Mentions.)*

TOVA

Scent Type   *Floral*
Composition
    Top Notes: *Bergamot*
    Heart Notes: *Jasmine, lavender*
    Base Notes: *Sandalwood*

Tova Borgnine began her beauty empire with just one product—a cactus root mask she created at home. From this, she built a cosmetic and fragrance firm that is frequently seen on the television shopping station QVC.

The Norwegian beauty immigrated to the United States with her mother, met and married actor Ernest Borgnine, then spread her entrepreneurial wings. In addition, she authored a book on style entitled *The Tova Difference*, and created a video, *Timeless Beauty*. Her signature fragrance is a floral harmony of fresh citrus, lavender, and jasmine, blended and balanced with sandalwood. Master designer Pierre Dinand created the classic curved bottle featuring sleek black accents. The final analysis: A study in chic, at an affordable price. Says Borgnine, "I am creating a little magic that will make people feel better about themselves."

Also try Borgnine's 1997 line addition, Tova Nights. A glamorous floral Oriental, Tova Nights is a bewitching blend of lily, rose, sandalwood, and patchouli. Another line addition, Tova.calm, includes soothing aromatherapy-inspired products.

Introduced	*1982*
Price	*Mid-range*

Très Chic

Scent Type	*Floral - Oriental*
Composition	
Top Notes:	*Bergamot, mandarin, lemon*
Heart Notes:	*Oriental rose, lily of the valley, jasmine, ylang-ylang, mimosa, orange blossom, tuberose, hyacinth*
Base Notes:	*Amber, sandalwood, orris, patchouli, vanilla, fruits*

A noble European heritage is evident in Très Chic, an expansive, floral Oriental perfume. Très Chic is blended from natural essential oils by French perfumer Michel Jarosz for the house of Holzman & Stephanie. Très Chic is the fifth fragrance from the talented mother-daughter team of Esther Holzman and her daughter, Stephanie.

European noblewomen by birth, they let their sense of style flow in the rich floral bouquet of jasmine and rose. A sparkling fruit accord adds lightness, while vanilla and fruited woods underscore the composition.

For Holzman & Stephanie's loyal clientele, the bottle carries yet another intriguing design. The hand-etched replica of the Eiffel Tower is a charming collectible, and indeed, it is a fitting choice for a fragrance entitled Très Chic.

Introduced	*2000*
Price	*High range*

Trésor

Scent Type	*Floral Semi - Oriental*
Composition	
Top Notes:	*Rose, apricot blossom, lilac, peach*
Heart Notes:	*Iris, heliotrope, lily of the valley, jasmine*
Base Notes:	*Amber, sandalwood, musk, vanilla*

From the French word for "treasure," Lancôme's Trésor is laden with fruits, florals, and long-lasting Oriental base notes. Blended by master perfumer Sophia Grojsman, Trésor is a saucy daytime fragrance, yet versatile enough to dress up for evening. Fresh, spirited, and innocent, we love it in warm weather, especially après spa.

The clear glass bottle is shaped like an inverted pyramid, designed by Areca to represent the glowing radiance of a woman in full bloom. Reflective of its fresh peach and apricot essences, the fragrance is presented in peach and salmon floral packaging. It is, indeed, a treasure.

Introduced	*1991*
Price	*High range*

TRIBÙ

Scent Type   *Floral - Fruity*
Composition
    Top Notes: *African tagetes,*
                   Italian violet leaves,
                   Belgian black currant bud,
                   Italian mandarin
    Heart Notes: *Bulgarian rose,*
                   Moroccan geranium,
                   Indonesian ylang-ylang,
                   Egyptian chamomile,
                   Moroccan jasmine
    Base Notes: *Indian sandalwood,*
                   Haitian vetiver,
                   Yugoslavian oakmoss,
                   Thai benzoin

Famous Patrons
    Sonia Braga   *Roberta Flack*

From the United Colors of Benetton comes Tribù, described by the company as a "fragrance and bath ritual collection that celebrates the tribal roots of all human beings, transcending time, cultures and ethnicity."

Sunny top notes register green apple, peach, and mandarin orange, followed by delicate flowers embedded in sweet lasting notes of sandalwood and ambery benzoin.

Made from healthy all-natural ingredients from around the world, Tribù is housed in an amber and red flacon designed by Tamotsu Yagi, and its packaging is made from recycled paper. The elongated bottle is part of the permanent collection at the San Francisco Museum of Modern Art. Yagi drew inspiration from an egg, one of the most primitive design forms, and a test tube, a symbol of the modern age. The ad campaign

from avant-garde award-winning photographer Oliviero Toscani depicted real people, not models, practicing ancient and modern tribal rituals, many culled from the archives of National Geographic.

Introduced   *1992*
Price   *Mid-range*

TRISH MCEVOY COLLECTION

NO. 1
Grapefruit & Yellow Freesia
NO. 2
Jasmine & Rose Honey
NO. 3
Snowdrop & Crystal Flowers
NO. 4
Gardenia Musk
NO. 6
Mandarin & Ginger Lily
NO. 7
(To Be Announced!)
NO. 8
Citrus Petals
NO. 9
Blackberry & Vanilla Musk
NO. 10
Lavender Spice (♀♂)

Makeup maven Trish McEvoy enters the perfume arena with a grand gesture. McEvoy tempts fragrance aficionados with a palate of nine scents, at last count, skipping No. 5 out of regard for Chanel No. 5. (At the time of printing, No. 7 had not been announced.)

The fragrances are composed of dominant single and double notes, exuding a certain nostalgia blended with modern-day charm. Clear glass bottles are a study in frank simplicity. Wear one number alone, or try your hand at combining scents for a new experience. Men—try the Lavender Spice.

Introduced 1998-2000
Price High range

TRUESTE

Scent Type Floral - Fruity
Composition
Top Notes: Peach, apricot, plum, black currant bud
Heart Notes: Tuberose, rose, orris
Base Notes: Sandalwood, oakmoss, cedarwood

Trueste is a spirited, youthful fragrance from Tiffany & Company. Created as a casual counterpart to the signature Tiffany fragrance, Trueste opens with soft fruits of apricot and peach, followed by a romantic rose and tuberose heart. Woods and oakmoss complete the fresh, easy-to-wear scent, which is blended by Chanel perfumer Jacques Polge.

Drawing inspiration from the jewels of Tiffany, Trueste is captured in clear, curved bottles designed by Pierre Dinand. The bottles are capped with cabochons of *faux* jewels: sapphire, citrine, ruby, emerald, and amethyst depending on the bottle size and formulation. Simply lovely— Trueste is a well-priced addition to the Tiffany fragrance line.

Introduced 1995
Price Mid-range

TRUSSARDI

Scent Type Chypre - Floral
Composition
Top Notes: Mandarin, violet
Heart Notes: Hyacinth, rose, ylang-ylang, iris
Base Notes: Juniper, coriander, oakmoss

The Italian firm of Trussardi has been at the forefront of classic fashion design for more than eighty years. A wide range of products, from accessories to clothing and leather goods, bear the Trussardi name and logo—the sleek greyhound.

Trussardi Donna is a classic floral chypre, blended with citrus and moss and a heart of rose with floral accompaniments. Sophisticated and well-mannered, Trussardi Donna is a full-bodied scent with a European pedigree. For summer days, try Trussardi Light, a watery sheer, fruity floral bouquet of water lily, wisteria, and rose.

Introduced 1982
Price High range

TRUTH CALVIN KLEIN

Scent Type Floral - Oriental
Composition
Top and Heart Notes: White peony, bamboo, white clover, sapling, patchouli, vetiver
Base Notes: Acacia flower, silk tree flower, white amber, vanilla, musk, woods

"Beauty is truth, truth beauty," wrote English poet, John Keats, in his work *Ode on a Grecian Urn*. Today, American designer Calvin Klein also takes aim at the heart of the matter with Truth, a multifaceted fragrance.

Truth Calvin Klein is a departure from Klein's previous fragrance ventures, in that Truth embraces two early Third Millennium trends: personalization and environmental scents. The Truth line contains items for body, bath, and bed, which are designed to be worn alone or mixed together to create a unique personal statement. For example, the Truth Bedtime fragrance may be mixed with the Truth eau de parfum. While their elements are similar, the scents differ. "We personalized and broke down the elements," explains Klein. Perfumers at Firmenich blended wooded notes with florals and musk to create a scent of lush sensuality, a Klein signature.

Truth body, bed, and bath products include such items as candles, incense, and bath grains. The body oil essences are offered in basic elements of the Truth formula: bamboo, vanilla, citrus, lilac, and sapling. Clear, rectangular bottles, designed by Fabien Baron, symbolize the naked truth.

Truth encourages experimentation and indulgence. Find your own version of the truth. For, as Pablo Picasso once said, "If there were only one truth, you couldn't paint a hundred canvases on the same theme." The same can certainly be said of perfumery.

Introduced	*2000*
Price	*Mid - to High range*

TUBÉREUSE

Scent Type	*Floral*
Composition	
Notes:	*Grasse tuberose*

Tuberose is an extraordinarily fragrant white flower, and perhaps the finest tuberose in the world is found in Grasse, France. Creator Annick Goutal described Tubéreuse as "a keynote of

irresistible fascination. A scent for the woman with mysterious powers of seduction." Tubéreuse is a heady, beguiling fragrance.

In the language of flowers, tuberose represents dangerous pleasures. Try this and report back to us—we have a steamy novel in the works and can use more material!

Introduced	*1986*
Price	*Top range*

TUSCANY

Scent Type	*Floral - Oriental*
Composition	
Top Notes:	*Mandarin, grapefruit, bergamot, rose, hyacinth, lily of the valley, herbs*
Heart Notes:	*Jasmine, honeysuckle, ylang-ylang, orange blossom, violet, carnation*
Base Notes:	*Sandalwood, vanilla, amber, musk*

Tuscany Per Donna is a fragrance from Aramis, an Estée Lauder company. It was introduced to complement Aramis' successful men's fragrance, Tuscany. The subtle scent takes its inspiration from the tranquillity of the Tuscan countryside and the Italian Renaissance woman.

Tuscany opens with a shimmering tumble of florals, citrus fruits, and herbs. The body unfolds with rich florals, then softens into a base accord of fragrant woods and sweet spices; like Italy in the spring.

Tuscany is housed in handsome copper and amber leaded glass flacons, and tapestry print packages.

Introduced	*1993*
Price	*Mid-range*

ULTRAVIOLET

Scent Type   *Oriental*
Composition
    Top Notes: *Pimento pepper*
    Heart Notes: *Japanese osmanthus*
    Base Notes: *Amber, vanilla*

Fashion designer Paco Rabanne, once known for his chain metal dresses, greets the third millennium, the Age of Aquarius, with Ultraviolet. A radiant Oriental blend, the scent is fresh and modern, with a sensual base of amber and vanilla.

Of course, packaging is futuristic, launching rounded, flying-saucer-shaped containers of vivid purple and silvered block letters. The elliptical bottle is a smooth creation of glass and metal, the modern material which for Rabanne has long held a fascination. Ultraviolet is held in a Space Age, sleeved container. Captain Kirk, Buck Rogers, and Judy Jetson must be green with envy. We've got Ultraviolet!

Introduced   2000
Price   *High range*

V/S VERSACE

Scent Type   *Floral - Fresh*
Composition
    Top Notes: *Orange blossom, ylang-ylang,*
                         lime, cinnamon
    Heart Notes: *Water lily, vanilla blossom,*
                         iris blossom
    Base Notes: *Cashmere musk, iris*

Introduced in tandem with the Versace ready-to-wear line, V/S Versace is a modern, sheer floral fragrance. The scent is captured in an upright, rounded bottle, crisp and clean of line, devoid of decoration. A bold fuschia VS logo is stamped on the bottle, which rolls onto its side as the fragrance is depleted. Simple and chic, V/S Versace is a study in the contrast of bright top and smooth base notes.

Introduced   1999
Price   *Mid-range*

VACANCES
(See also Jean Patou Collection)

Scent Type   *Floral - Oriental*
Composition
    Top Notes: *Hyacinth, hawthorn, galbanum*
    Heart Notes: *Lilac, mimosa*
    Base Notes: *Musk, woods*

Jean Patou's Vacances debuted in 1936—the year that paid vacations came into vogue for the French. Vacances opens with the fresh greens inherent in hyacinth and galbanum, followed by a floral heart and a soft Oriental base. Its elegance and versatility makes it an ideal accoutrement for a sunny vacation or a day at the horse races. If it's August, this must be Deauville....

Introduced   1936
Price   *Mid-range*

VAN CLEEF

Scent Type   Floral - Oriental
Composition
    Top Notes: Neroli, bergamot, raspberry,
                galbanum
    Heart Notes: Rose, jasmine, orange blossom
    Base Notes: Cedarwood, vanilla, musk,
                tonka bean

The signature fragrance from Van Cleef & Arpels jewelers is a feminine, refined fragrance with a superb pedigree. Breezy top notes of fruits and greens enliven a rich floral heart, while warm Oriental base notes linger with subtle opulence.

Look for the scent in an asymmetric gem-faceted flacon by designer Serge Mansau. Jewel tones of ivory, gold, and lapis blue clothe the precious fragrance.

Introduced   1993
Price   Mid-range

VANDERBILT

Scent Type   Floral - Oriental
Composition
    Top Notes: Orange blossom, apricot,
                bergamot, greens, mandarin,
                coriander, basil
    Heart Notes: Rose, jasmine, jonquil,
                mimosa absolute
    Base Notes: Musk, amber, moss, incense,
                vanilla

Vanderbilt was created in honor of Gloria Vanderbilt and her legendary family name, the very mention of which conjures up images of luxury and grandeur from a bygone era.

The romantic fragrance is a light floral Oriental. Herbs, fruits, and spices introduce the lush floral heart, where dominant essences of rose and jasmine reside. The background is a harmony of warm Oriental notes—powdery, rich, and sweet. Vanderbilt is a charming fragrance, fitting for women of any age.

The perfume is housed in a bottle designed by Bernard Kotyuk. It bears the Vanderbilt signature and is crowned with a Lalique-style stopper, in which a graceful swan is carved. The swan logo is carried throughout other packaging, symbolizing grace and elegance—Vanderbilt hallmarks.

Introduced   1982
Price   Mid-range

V'E VERSACE

Scent Type   Chypre - Floral
Composition
    Top Notes: Bergamot, lily of the valley,
                Bulgarian rose, jasmine,
                ylang-ylang, lily
    Heart Notes: Orange blossom, iris
    Base Notes: Balsamic wood, incense, amber,
                sandalwood, oakmoss

Famous Patrons
    Dame Elizabeth Taylor
    Cher   *Tina Turner*

Milano fashion daredevil Gianni Versace once said: "I don't care for half-measures. I believe in making clear-cut choices." Indeed. The late Versace is the designer who turned chain metal mail into evening wear. An extremist in his work, he was a risk taker who has ushered in striking styles for the young couture group.

V'E Versace derives its name from a shorthand, *simpatico* signature, with a Mediterranean slant.

A sensual fragrance, it resonates with vivid, white florals embedded in provocative base notes of incense and balsamic woods.

The bottle is described as "a cube which is not a cube," a modern, futuristic creation showcasing trademark Versace asymmetry. His own solid crystal inkwell served as inspiration. He also produced a limited-edition Baccarat crystal flacon.

Versace explained: "Human beings need room to express themselves, that is why we should have the courage to declare *Liberta de Profumo*! This expression allows us to break away from the roles and regulations that we often set for ourselves." An incredible legacy, indeed.

Introduced   *1993*
Price   *High range*

VENEZIA

Scent Type   *Floral - Oriental*
Composition
    Top Notes: *Wong-shi blossom,*
                 Indian mango, black currant bud,
                 rose, geranium, prune, osmanthus
    Heart Notes: *Jasmine, iris, ylang-ylang,*
                 cedarwood, ambergris
    Base Notes: *Vanilla, civet, sandalwood,*
                 musk, tonka bean

Famous Patrons
    Ann-Margret

For her second scent, Venezia, Italian fashion designer Laura Biagiotti took inspiration from the ancient city of canals, magical Venice. She describes Venezia as "Aromas from the Orient and the Occident merged into a perfume of infinite richness."

The initial prevailing notes of Venezia are the essence of fruits mingled with wong-shi blossom,

a rare gardenia-like flower that Marco Polo brought to Venice from the Orient. The flower was admired by Medieval Venetians. Italian poets called it "*l'eliser d'amore*," the elixir of love. Captivated by the rare essence, Laura Biagiotti based her fragrance upon it as a tribute to the irresistible city of Venice. As the fragrance develops on the skin, a bouquet of rich florals and woods emerges, giving way to a sensual balsamic Oriental base.

The spicy, seductive scent is encased in a Venetian-style glass bottle inspired by the Harlequin, the most important figure in Venetian carnivals. Fine gold shavings float in the perfume, while the cap is a recreation of the campanile of San Giorgio Maggiore. The gilded packaging features a winged lion, the symbol of Venice, in Harlequin colors of gold and red. The Venezia packaging and fragrance are splendid works of modern Italian art.

Introduced   *1992*
Price   *Top range*

VENT VERT

Scent Type   *Floral - Green*
Composition
    Top Notes: *Greens, orange blossom, lemon,*
                 lime, basil
    Heart Notes: *Rose, galbanum, lily of the valley,*
                 freesia, hyacinth, tagetes,
                 ylang-ylang, violet
    Base Notes: *Oakmoss, sandalwood, sage, iris,*
                 amber, musk

Vent Vert is a green floral from Paris couturier Pierre Balmain. The vibrant fragrance is fresh as spring, like a lush meadow blanketed with a rainbow of wildflowers and tender shoots of emerald grass.

Green and mossy notes are woven throughout the composition. In fact, Vent Vert is French for "green breeze."

The green theme is carried out in crisp mint green packaging. When you want a light, clean fragrance for daytime or professional wear, try Vent Vert, a fresh understated floral with a proven history.

Introduced   1947
Price   High range

VERSUS

Scent Type   Floral - Fruity
Composition
    Top Notes: Raspberry, black currant bud, plum
    Heart Notes: Tuberose, boronia, sandalwood
    Base Notes: Iris, amber, musk

Famous Patrons
    Model Carla Bruni

Maverick Gianni Versace formulated Versus to complement his expressive, avant-garde fashions. The family-run empire, now headed by his sister Donatella Versace, caters to dynamic youth, offering flamboyant body-hugging styles. The fruity floral fragrance is a youthful, defiant, sensual scent, positioned to appeal to the MTV generation.

Versace described the Versus woman as "electrifying, sensual and habitually unattainable." Supermodel Carla Bruni is the Versus woman, the woman who "creates her own rules and forges her own path."

The ruby red bottles and lipstick-red cap are accented by a gold-colored collar and deep sculpted "V." Defiant and dramatic…it's pure Versace.

Introduced   1992
Price   Mid-range

VERY VALENTINO

Scent Type   Floral
Composition
    Top Notes: Magnolia, lily of the valley, mandarin, bergamot
    Heart Notes: Jasmine, rose
    Base Notes: Sandalwood, vanilla

Italian couturier Valentino first imprinted his vision of style on the fragrance world with the introduction of Valentino in 1978. Twenty years later, Very Valentino Pour Femme made headlines in Europe, and in 2000, the United States embraced the fragrance. And for men, there is Very Valentino Pour Homme.

Of his fragrant endeavor for women, Valentino says: "Very Valentino is a highly seductive fragrance. Subtle, yet romantic, its essence lingers on your skin, and in your mind." Modern, feminine, self-assured, Very Valentino opens with a fresh accord, followed by a robust heart of rose and jasmine, and ends with a sensual melange of sandalwood and vanilla. The essence of Valentino couture, Very Valentino is a scent of smooth sophistication. Classic rectangular bottles complete the elegant theme; less is most definitely more. *Bravissimo!*

Introduced   1998
Price   High range

VOL DE NUIT

Scent Type   *Oriental - Ambery Spicy*
Composition
  Top Notes: *Orange, mandarin, lemon,*
                bergamot, orange blossom
  Heart Notes: *Jonquil, aldehydes, galbanum*
  Base Notes: *Vanilla, spices, oakmoss,*
                sandalwood, orris, musk

Famous Patrons
  Claudette Colbert   *Barbra Streisand*
  Michelle Pfeiffer   *Diana Rigg*

Another timeless classic from Jacques Guerlain, Vol de Nuit is a spicy Oriental scent designed for the elusive, assertive woman, and is one of the most sophisticated scents from the House of Guerlain.

Vol de Nuit, French for "night flight," is presented in one of our favorite Guerlain flacons. The dramatic gold-colored amber bottle is molded with the shape of French Air Force wings. Indeed, Vol de Nuit was created in homage to the daring aviators of the 1920s, and was named after the Antoine de Saint-Exupéry novel of the same name. Saint-Exupéry, also an avid aviator, was the author of many works, including *Le Petit Prince*.

The fragrance captures the essence of adventure, the spirit of exploration, the radiance of independence. It is an assertive scent of the 1930s; ideal for the woman of today.

Introduced   *1933*
Price   *High range*

WEEK END

Scent Type   *Floral - Fresh*
Composition
  Top Notes: *Citrus, greens*
  Heart Notes: *Hyacinth, cyclamen, nectarine,*
                iris, rose
  Base Notes: *Cedarwood, musk, sandalwood*

Burberry's Week End for women is the casual companion to the signature Burberry of London fragrance. Fresh top notes of citrus and greens provide a sparkling lift to the relaxed floral heart. A smooth, easy drydown imbues the scent with an enticing air of unhurried bliss. Toss a Burberry trench coat over your shoulders and head for the English country estate for a long, leisurely weekend.

Introduced   *1998*
Price   *High range*

WEIL DE WEIL

Scent Type   *Floral - Green*
Composition
  Top Notes: *Tangerine, neroli, greens,*
                galbanum, hyacinth
  Heart Notes: *Lily of the valley, honeysuckle,*
                ylang-ylang, acacia farnesiana,
                May rose, narcissus
  Base Notes: *Sandalwood, vetiver, civet,*
                musk, oakmoss

The classic Weil de Weil begins with saucy citrus and lively green notes, blended with a symphony of fragrant white flowers, and couched in a bed of sandalwood warmed by woody vetiver and soft, erotic musk. Fresh and spirited, with a hint of a mysterious past.

Weil de Weil…a green floral bouquet well worth the experiment.

Introduced   1971
Price   Mid-range

WHITE CAMELLIA

Scent Type   Floral
Composition
    Top Notes: Mandarin, aldehydes, jasmine,
                    rose, cassia
    Heart Notes: Geranium, peony, rose
    Base Notes: Sandalwood, amber, musk

Following the success of St. John's classic signature scent is White Camellia, a lighter, more modern floral fragrance. The scent's ethereal femininity is achieved through the use of white flowers and aldehydes.

The white camellia is frequently used to adorn St. John designs, hence the name. Company president Kelly Gray, daughter of founder Marie Gray, states, "It's feminine and light and clean." Recommended for daytime divas or a summery sail, preferably in St. John sportswear.

White Camellia is captured in a leaf-shaped, inner container, suspended in a clear rectangular, Brosse-designed bottle with silver-colored accents. It's a delightful scent that is bright and breezy, light and lovely.

Introduced   1998
Price   High range

WHITE DIAMONDS

Scent Type   Floral
Composition
    Top Notes: Italian neroli,
                    living Amazon lily, aldehydes
    Heart Notes: Egyptian tuberose, Turkish rose,
                    Italian orris, living narcissus,
                    living jasmine
    Base Notes: Italian sandalwood, patchouli,
                    amber, oakmoss

As with her first fragrance, Passion, Dame Elizabeth Taylor again proves able to blend her extraordinary sense of style with her innate sense of scent. She calls White Diamonds "the fragrance that dreams are made of."

A dazzling combination of floral essences and sparkling aldehydes are blended to create a floral fragrance that is delicate yet tenacious, with a subtle Oriental base. White Diamonds is a sophisticated floral bouquet—versatile enough to be worn for casually elegant days and lavish evenings…anytime you'd wear diamonds.

White Diamonds inhabits a brilliant bottle. The White Diamonds eau de parfum columnar spray bottles are adorned with a generous band of shimmering *faux* and *pavé* crystal stones, while the oval-shaped perfume bottle is dressed with a glittering rhinestone bow. We love it; diamonds may be a woman's best friend, but *faux* diamonds cost much less to insure.

The packaging has received numerous accolades from industry peers, notably a 1992 FiFi Award from The Fragrance Foundation, the fragrance industry equivalent of an Oscar. Taylor was graciously on hand to accept the honor.

Introduced   1991
Price   High range

WHITE LINEN

Scent Type   *Floral - Aldehyde*
Composition
    Top Notes: *Aldehydes, peach, citrus oils*
    Heart Notes: *Jasmine, lilac, rose, hyacinth,*
        lily of the valley, orchid,
        ylang-ylang
    Base Notes: *Amber, cedarwood, sandalwood,*
        honey, benzoin, tonka bean

Estée Lauder was searching for the fragrance embodiment of white linen, the look and the meaning—clean, crisp, and classic. Always right. She achieved this in the development of White Linen, the fragrance.

Airy top notes of shimmering aldehydes introduce the delicate floral bouquet. The scent lingers on background notes of warm woods and spices to create an aura of understated elegance. Romantic and gentle, White Linen is a feminine scent with a polished demeanor. It is ideal for warm weather and subtle daytime wear...anytime you'd slip into pressed white linen.

Introduced   *1978*
Price   *High range*

WHITE SHOULDERS

Scent Type   *Floral*
Composition
    Top Notes: *Neroli, tuberose, aldehydes*
    Heart Notes: *Gardenia, jasmine, orris,*
        lily of the valley, rose, lilac
    Base Notes: *Sandalwood, amber,*
        musk, oakmoss

Famous Patrons
    Barbara Bush

White Shoulders is an enduring floral, as charming today as when it was introduced. The predominant note is tuberose, sweet, delicate, and feminine, with a powdery soft finish. It is a timeless, tenacious fragrance, and attractively priced.

Legend has it that White Shoulders was inspired by a baron's love for a woman with exquisite porcelain shoulders, the woman whose cameo still embellishes each pink package.

White Shoulders whispers of a bygone era, of daring low-cut ball gowns, billowing satin, and rustling taffeta. An intoxicating scent, it enchants each new generation.

Introduced   *1935*
Price   *Mid-range*

WILLIAM OWEN COLLECTION

ADORATION
Floral
(See Adoration)

CELIA'S ULTIMATE GARDENIA
Floral

COQUETTE
Oriental

DESIRE
Floral - Fruity

ISIS
Floral

L'AMOUR
Floral

REVERIE
Green

Fourth generation-British perfumer William Owen took the creative reins of his family's London-based business at the tender age of twenty-five. His legion of admirers grew to include royalty, such as the late Diana, Princess of Wales, as well as celebrities and other women of refined taste. Now residing in Palm Beach, Owen continues to create fine specialty perfumes.

The flirtatious Coquette is a warm Oriental scent, while Celia's Ultimate Gardenia is an expansive floral fragrance, created for Owen's sister. Isis is feminine and delicate, a blend of white rose and violet. As with Owen's fragrance Adoration, Isis was created for Princess Diana. The natural fragrance is derived from the type of flowers grown at Owen's family estate on the coast of Wales.

All Owen fragrances can be worn alone, or layered and mixed with others in the collection. Owen encourages experimentation and often refers to his scents as "moods." All scents are hand-assembled, which sets them apart from mass-produced competitors. A multitalented artist, Owen's fine sketches also grace the cartons of several scents in the line.

Owen fragrances are available in a variety of plain or jewel-encrusted flacons. Swarovski Austrian crystals of various colors adorn the bejeweled selections, such as green for Reverie, and golden yellow for Isis. In fact, Owen was kind enough to send us our very own Isis to try, in a gold-colored moiré box tucked inside an elaborate outer box of champagne silk brocade. The French crystal flacon is wrapped with a delicate gold-colored cord—a magnificent presentation from a talented man with an eye for exquisite detail.

Owen's fragrances make us feel as though we were back in Britain, punting along the River Cam through Cambridge, in a narrow wooden boat with an Oxford man at the helm, an English spring breeze rustling our lace petticoats....

Price   *Mid- to high range*

WINGS

Scent Type   *Floral - Oriental*
Composition
   Top Notes: *Ginger lily, green osmanthus,*
                      passion flower, gardenia,
                      marigold, blue rose
   Heart Notes: *Cattleya orchid,*
                      shaffali jasmine, heliotrope
   Base Notes: *Woods, amber, musk*

This free-spirited composition from the Giorgio stable was inspired by the "Winged Victory" sculpture at the Louvre museum in Paris. Wings consists of 621 ingredients, blended to evoke spontaneity, positiveness, and exhilaration. The result is a delicate balance of sprightly top notes and warm base notes. Wings is presented in a graceful glass bottle topped with a blue stopper to represent clear blue sky.

A crisp, invigorating fragrance with a soothing melody, ideal for career days and casual evenings, for the woman who knows no boundaries.

Introduced   *1992*
Price   *Mid-range*

WISH

Scent Type   *Oriental - Fruity*
Composition
   Notes: *Fruits, florals, woods, spices*

From Chopard, the Swiss watch and luxury goods maker established in 1860, comes Wish, which follows on the heels of the firm's previous success, Casmir. Nathalie Lorson of International Flavors and Fragrances created the crisp Oriental composition, which is enhanced by fruity top notes and rich wooded notes. Wish is a sensual fragrance, suitable for cool weather and wishful evenings. The fresh formula is designed to appeal to the youthful consumer, or at least, those with a youthful outlook. Mightn't we all qualify on that count?

Wish is cleverly packaged in a faceted, diamond-shaped flacon that lies at an angle like a giant gemstone—calling to mind the Hope Diamond, surely the secret desire of many wishful women.

Introduced *1998*
Price   *High range*

Y

Scent Type *Chypre - Fruity*
Composition
 Top Notes: *Greens, aldehydes, peach,*
    gardenia, mirabelle, honeysuckle
 Heart Notes: *Bulgarian rose, jasmine,*
    tuberose, ylang-ylang, orris,
    hyacinth
 Base Notes: *Oakmoss, amber, patchouli,*
    sandalwood, vetiver, civet,
    benzoin, styrax

Y was the first fragrance introduced by couturier Yves Saint Laurent. Completely different from his later flamboyant creations, Opium and Paris, Y is a light fragrance, delicate, feminine, and subtle. A fruity chypre with greens and woods, it is perfect for warm days and active wear. Well, Y not?

Introduced *1964*
Price   *High range*

YOHJI

Scent Type *Oriental - Fruity*
Composition
 Top Notes: *Bergamot, galbanum, linalol*
 Heart Notes: *Florals, praline, fruits*
 Base Notes: *Vanilla, vanillin, musk,*
    sandalwood, coumarin

From Japanese fashion designer Yohji Yamamoto comes a signature scent of spare sophistication. The Oriental composition from master perfumer Jean Kerléo consists of two major movements. The opening is rife with greens and citrus, while a floral-praline impression sets the stage for a wooded, ambery finish. Mysterious and intriguing, the scent is multilayered like a woman's personality, or like a Yamamoto design.

The Yohji bottle sports minimalist elements. The reclining clear glass vial bears Yamamoto's signature in navy blue. With a nod to his clothing designs, the vial is wrapped from view and presented in a clear, plexiglass box. *très avant-garde.*

Introduced *1996*
Price   *High range*

YOUTH DEW

Scent Type *Oriental - Ambery Spicy*
Composition
 Top Notes: *Orange, bergamot, peach, spices*
 Heart Notes: *Clove, cinnamon, cassie, rose,*
    ylang-ylang, orchid, jasmine
 Base Notes: *Frankincense, amber, vanilla,*
    oakmoss, clove, musk, patchouli,
    vetiver, spices

Famous Patrons

Madonna	*Duchess of Windsor*
Gloria Swanson	*Dolores Del Rio*
Joan Crawford	

Youth Dew was the first fragrance produced by Estée Lauder and became the first sensational American fragrance hit when it was introduced as a bath oil for everyday use. During World War II, perfume had been difficult to obtain, and American women were not accustomed to using fragrance every day. They did use bath oils, however, and Lauder seized upon this, marketing her new scent as a bath oil and perfume. She often hinted that Youth Dew was based on a formula her uncle had created for a Russian princess. Women were swept away by the mystery and the spicy, heady fragrance.

The opulent scent has endured as one of Estée Lauder's most popular fragrances. Youth Dew is a strong, long-lasting scent, perfect for cool weather and dramatic evenings…or anytime you want to be noticed.

Introduced	*1953*
Price	*Mid-range*

YSATIS

Scent Type	*Chypre - Floral Animalic*
Composition	
Top Notes:	*Mandarin, bergamot, ylang-ylang, galbanum, orange blossom, coconut, rosewood, greens, aldehydes*
Heart Notes:	*Rose, jasmine, polianthes, iris, tuberose, ylang-ylang, carnation, narcissus*
Base Notes:	*Bay rum, vetiver, patchouli, oakmoss, sandalwood, clove, vanilla, amber, musk, honey, civet, castoreum*

Ysatis is another best-selling fragrance from the House of Givenchy. Pronounce the name "ee-sah-tees." The chypre floral composition unfolds with fruity top notes, followed by an exotic floral accord and warm base notes. Givenchy once described the fragrance as having a "seductive charm." Easy to wear, sophisticated, not over-powering. Ysatis is versatile enough to follow a woman through a busy day from morning meetings to evening interludes. Look for it in a columnar Art Deco-inspired flacon designed by Pierre Dinand.

Introduced	*1985*
Price	*High range*

YVRESSE
(See Champagne)

ZAHAROFF

Scent Type	*Floral - Oriental*
Composition	
Top Notes:	*Lily of the valley*
Heart Notes:	*Rose, water lily, jasmine*
Base Notes:	*Amber, iris*

A family affair, Zaharoff was originally created for Mariana Zaharoff, a fashion designer whose credits include the television series *Dynasty* and *Dallas*. But it is her son, the movie-star-handsome George, who has taken the reins of Parfums Zaharoff. The women's version of Zaharoff is a rich floral Oriental, blended by Quest. Zaharoff is a worldly fragrance of sophistication for the chic professional woman, or the woman who has it all. And for her man? The Zaharoff men's version, of course.

Introduced	*1997*
Price	*High range*

MEN'S FRAGRANCES

212

Scent Type Green
Composition
    Top Notes: Grapefruit, mandarin, ginger, green leaves
    Heart Notes: Aquatic molecules, iron woods, guaiac wood, sandalwood
    Base Notes: Musk

Carolina Herrera, the Venezuelan-born fashion designer, partnered with Antonio Puig Perfumes and Firmenich to produce 212 Men. Now based in New York, Herrera sought to capture the essence of the New York City man. The fragrance name refers to the Manhattan area code.

The 212 Men fragrance opens with citrus and greens, then evolves into an aquatic heart and a sensual, musky base. The scent is designed for the man who is suave and debonair—a man about town. Confident, elegant, and dashing, the subtle, sophisticated scent has a charming personality. A versatile, understated fragrance with a clean finish, 212 Men is appropriate anywhere the well-traveled man might venture.

Bottle designer Fabien Baron created a modern, cylindrical bottle of aluminum to house the blue-tinted scent.

For another Carolina Herrera creation, try Herrera for Men, an elegant, fresh Oriental fragrance that debuted in 1991.

Introduced 1999
Price High range

ALLURE

Scent Type Oriental - Woody
Composition
    Top Notes: Bergamot, mandarin, citron
    Heart Notes: Jamaican pepper, labdanum
    Base Notes: Sandalwood, patchouli, cedarwood, tonka bean

Chanel master perfumer Jacques Polge sought to bottle a man's charisma and character in Allure Homme, the male counterpart to Chanel's successful Allure for women. Polge designed Allure with four facets: fresh, woody, sensual, and spicy. Allure opens with a zesty citrus accord, then dissolves into a warm, vibrant heart of spices and woods.

Packaging is classic Chanel. A chic rectangular bottle is topped with a champagne-colored cap and nestled in a tobacco-brown carton. Simple and masculine, Allure is an appealing fragrance of quality. It is attractively priced and is also offered in a variety of grooming products.

Introduced 1998
Price Mid-range

ARAMIS

Scent Type Chypre
Composition
    Top Notes: Citrus, green leaves, sage, thyme
    Heart Notes: Clove, cardamom
    Base Notes: Oakmoss, patchouli, vetiver, sandalwood

Introduced in 1965, Aramis from Estée Lauder remains a favorite among men's fragrances.

Aramis is a classic chypre composition, a category characterized by the marriage of citrus and oakmoss, with the addition of spicy patchouli. Green leaves, thyme, and sage form a fresh herbal accord, and spices of clove and cardamom create a warm heart. A superb lingering base is blended from vetiver and sandalwood, and a distinct leathery impression adds fullness.

A perennial favorite that is versatile and easy to wear, Aramis is a classic choice.

Introduced   1965
Price   Mid-range

BIJAN FRAGRANCE FOR MEN

Scent Type   Oriental - Woody
Composition
   Top Notes: Bergamot, mandarin, lavender, rosemary, orris
   Heart Notes: Nutmeg, cinnamon, clove, sandalwood, vetiver, patchouli
   Base Notes: Amber, oakmoss, musk

Famous Patrons
Ricky Martin   Luis Miguel
Sylvester Stallone   George Lucas
Steven Spielberg   Adnan Kashoggi
George Benson   Julio Iglesias
Jack Nicholson   Jack Lemmon
Charles Bronson   Chevy Chase
Arnold Schwarzenegger
President Bill Clinton

Since 1976, Beverly Hills-based menswear couturier Bijan has dressed the most powerful men in the world. For clients ranging from kings and presidents to captains of industry, he designs entire wardrobes from head to toe. Malcolm Forbes once referred to Bijan as "the first miracle in men's fashion." But the final touch, Bijan's namesake fragrance, is his *pièce de résistance*.

An award-winning scent, Bijan Fragrance for Men is an enticing blend of crisp citrus and rich spice, smoothed with a wooded Oriental base. Rich and full-bodied, the scent exudes wealth, power, and style. An erotic enigma, Bijan Fragrance for Men lingers superbly on the skin.

The trademark Bijan bottle is an amazing artistry in glass. The rounded flacon has a hole in the center, around which the fragrance swirls to delight the eye. From formula to presentation, Bijan Fragrance for Men is an opulent work of art for the worldly, sophisticated man.

For an even more indulgent experience, look to Bijan's Perfume for Men, a rich Oriental perfume of a different formulation than Bijan's Fragrance for Men. It is presented in an exquisite Baccarat collector's bottle, and is available from Bijan's "by appointment only" shop in Beverly Hills. Furthermore, it is one of only ten American fragrance bottles on permanent display at the Smithsonian Institute.

Bijan's fragrance collection mirrors his design ethos: "Quality, elegance and simplicity—the essence of great style."

Introduced   1987
Price   Top range

BOUCHERON

Scent Type   *Citrus*
Composition
    Top Notes: *Verbena, bergamot, orange, basil*
    Heart Notes: *Basil, coriander, juniper, rose,*
                 iris, geranium, ylang-ylang, clary
    Base Notes: *Sandalwood, vetiver, patchouli*

In 1858, Frédéric Boucheron opened his first jewelry shop in the exclusive Palais Royal section of Paris. Only nine years later, he garnered a gold medal for his designs at the Paris Universal Exhibition of 1867. This was a clear sign of the road ahead for the Boucheron family. Today, descendent Alain Boucheron heads the family empire, which expanded into fragrance in 1988.

Boucheron Pour Homme is the first Boucheron fragrance for men. Fresh citrus is blended with aromatic and wooded essences; the result is refined and sophisticated. Boucheron offers a concentrated eau de parfum version, along with the classic eau de toilette formulation. A full complement of grooming products offers the elegant gentleman an array of choices for layering and extending the fragrance.

The Boucheron bottle is strong and sturdy in the hand. Crafted from fine materials of clear and frosted glass, a *faux* sapphire cap, gold-colored gadroons (or rings), and a Boucheron signature, the overall effect is one of European classicism at its finest.

Introduced   *1991*
Price   *High range*

CASSINI

Scent Type   *Fougère*
Composition
    Top Notes: *Mandarin, sweet basil,*
                 chamomile, rosewood, guava,
                 osmanthus
    Heart Notes: *Lavender, oregano, geranium,*
                 verbena, jasmine
    Base Notes: *Vetiver, musk, vanilla,*
                 tonka bean, sandalwood, amber,
                 incense, benzoin

Cassini for Men is a dashing fragrance from the European couturier Oleg Cassini. He calls it a "gutsy fragrance," saying: "In the men's arena I am respected as an athlete. My direction is appealing to the man who is free in his thinking, who is motivated by the outdoors and sports. You have to respect the body, improve the body and mind." A ten-handicap golfer and accomplished equestrian, Cassini cuts a trim figure in the worlds of sports, society, and fashion.

Cassini was born a count in Paris, to the Italian Count and Countess Cassini. His grandfather served as Russia's ambassador to the United States. After apprenticing for Jean Patou in Paris, Cassini operated his own boutique, then headed to Hollywood where he designed for the studios. Exuding a unique charm, he wooed and won the hearts of many lovely women, including actresses Grace Kelley and Gene Tierney. His designs have graced many a well-dressed man: President John F. Kennedy, Michael Jordan, George Hamilton, Anthony Quinn, Ted Turner, Charlton Heston, and Burt Reynolds.

Cassini for Men is a fresh fougère, supported by a warm, wooded base. Cassini calls it an "erotic fragrance." He explains: "I am producing the invisible, the extra dimension, that makes a man attractive. There is nothing in the world more attractive to the other sex than a great fragrance." Clean, wholesome, fresh, and well-balanced, Cassini is a fine, versatile fragrance with an aristocratic heritage.

| Introduced | 1994 |
| Price | High range |

CERRUTI 1881

Scent Type	Citrus
Composition	
Top Notes:	Bergamot, lemon, basil, lavender, rosemary, juniper berry, cumin, clove, tarragon, artemisia, cypress
Heart Notes:	Ylang-ylang, rose, lily of the valley
Base Notes:	Sandalwood, amber, patchouli, wood musk, balsam fir

From Italian designer Nino Cerruti comes Cerruti 1881. Understated, citrusy, and naturally fresh, the scent evokes the breezy Mediterranean outdoor lifestyle. A sunny opening accord bursts with sparkling citrus and subtle spicy accents. The lingering wooded base imparts a smooth civility for any gentleman. Versatile and well-mannered, Cerruti 1881 moves with ease from sunny shores to city doors.

An herbal green carton reflects the herbaceous spices in the heart of Cerruti 1881. We love the frosted bottle, which is embossed with raised numerals—1881. European casual and Cerruti chic. For more Cerruti, try Cerruti Image, a fresh, aromatic fougère designed to appeal to the youthful man.

| Introduced | 1990 |
| Price | High range |

CREED COLLECTION
(See women's section for Creed Collection unisex scents)

BOIS DU PORTUGAL
Oriental

EROLFA
Marine

GREEN IRISH TWEED
Green
(see Green Irish Tweed)

GREEN VALLEY
Chypre

RUSSIAN LEATHER
Chypre

Since 1760, Creed fragrances have been recognized for their quality. At last count, Creed was offering thirty-two specialty scents to the public, many of them originally created for royalty, dignitaries, and celebrities.

Many Creed fragrances are designed to be worn by both men and women, but some are strictly for the male club. Bois du Portugal is a rich woody Oriental, while Erolfa is a fresh marine composition. Green Valley is a fresh chypre, or woody-mossy blend, and Russian Leather contains richer chypre elements. Creed offers a wide range of fragrance wardrobe possibilities for the well-dressed man.

Look for the classic Creed cartons with the Prince of Wales crest. Whichever scent you choose, you'll find quality and taste in abundance.

| Introduced | Since 1760 |
| Price | Top range |

DÉCLARATION

Scent Type　　　　*Chypre*
Composition
　Top Notes:　　*Bergamot, bitter orange, birchwood*
　Heart Notes:　*Cardamom, wormwood*
　Base Notes:　　*Vetiver, oakmoss, cedarwood*

French jeweler Cartier entered the fragrance arena in 1981 with a pair of fragrances for men and women, named Santos de Cartier and Must de Cartier. Sultry, spicy, and seductive, both remain popular. In 1992, Pasha, a complex fougère for men, was introduced.

Déclaration represents a new generation of Cartier fragrances. The contemporary chypre is a blend of citrus and oakmoss. A dash of spice and a wooded base add depth and balance to the composition. Housed in a tall, clear bottle and wrapped in a sleek package of blue and silver-toned shades, Déclaration is well-presented line. Dare to declare your mark, your independence, your love.

Introduced　　　　*1998*
Price　　　　　　*High range*

DRAKKAR NOIR

Scent Type　　　　*Fougère*
Composition
　Top Notes:　　*Verbena, lemon rind*
　Heart Notes:　*Lavender, coriander,*
　　　　　　　juniper berry
　Base Notes:　　*Sandalwood, patchouli,*
　　　　　　　fir balsam

French designer Guy Laroche launched Drakkar Noir in 1982, and it remains a favorite.

Named for a Viking ship, Drakkar Noir conveys a sense of power, adventure, and charisma. A dynamic formula, Drakkar Noir opens with a burst of citrus, then segues into a lavender heart with spicy accents. Sandalwood, patchouli, and fir balsam form a lingering impression that is sensual and magnetic. Rich and diffusive, Drakkar Noir is the choice for the self-assured man.

A brooding, black bottle captures the essence of Drakkar Noir. A full line of grooming products allows a man to coordinate his dressing ritual. In addition to the classic eau de toilette, the After Shave Balm is a nice selection for those with sensitive skin. Low in alcohol, the balm is designed to soothe and heal.

Drakkar Noir is a classic scent for the active, accomplished man who conquers the world—or at least his corner of it!

Introduced　　　　*1982*
Price　　　　　　*Mid-range*

EMPORIO ARMANI HE

Scent Type　　　　*Chypre*
Composition
　Top Notes:　　*Cardamom, sage, yuzu*
　Heart Notes:　*Vetiver*
　Base Notes:　　*Sandalwood, cedarwood,*
　　　　　　　musk, guaiac wood

Italian fashion designer Giorgio Armani takes a distinctly modern approach for Emporio Armani He, called "Lui" in Europe. The crisp chypre opens with spicy cardamom, green sage, and yuzu fruit; it develops around an earthy heart of vetiver, then evolves into a wooded base. The use of guaiac wood, also known as guaiacum, adds a resinous quality to the woody-mossy composition. The scent is a refined, contemporary blend that is versatile to wear.

Emporio Armani He is contained in a sleek, soft-touch spray sheath, called a "flowpack." The espresso-colored unit is the size of a cell phone and is wrapped in a foil packet. Uniquely modern, spare, and elegant, Emporio Armani He is a fragrance for the fashion-forward man who appreciates quality and understated style.

Introduced   1998
Price   High range

ESCADA

Scent Type   Oriental - Woody
Composition
    Top Notes: Bergamot, mandarin, lemon
    Heart Notes: Clary sage, cognac
    Base Notes: Sandalwood, vanilla

Escada developed an elegant escort for its signature women's fragrance in Escada Pour Homme. The company introduced Escada Pour Homme with a quote from Aeschylus in *Prometheus Bound*: "When we match partners, then I fear not."

The sophisticated scent opens with a fresh accord of citrus fruits. Sandalwood and vanilla combine to create a smooth, long-lasting impression of spice and wood. Like the women's signature fragrance, Escada Pour Homme is easy to wear from day through evening. A midnight-blue fluted flask with gold-colored accents continues the masculine theme.

An elegant fragrance of power and prestige, Escada is ideal for gentlemen of distinction. For a casual Escada fragrance, try Escada's Casual Friday, a khaki-clothed, fresh fragrance with a sweet, subtle tinge of vanilla.

Introduced   1993
Price   High range

GREEN IRISH TWEED

Scent Type   Green
Composition
    Top Notes: Violet leaves, verbena
    Heart Notes: Iris
    Base Notes: Sandalwood, ambergris

Famous Patrons
    Cary Grant   Prince Charles of Wales
    Robert Redford   Richard Gere
    Quincy Jones   Clint Eastwood
    Naomi Campbell

Green Irish Tweed was created for Cary Grant, which speaks volumes for the fragrance, its attitude, and its character. Casually elegant, fresh and sporty, Green Irish Tweed moves with ease through the vagaries of life. The House of Creed blends the green freshness of violet leaves with the powdery root of iris, sandalwood, and ambergris. Harmonious and genial, Green Irish Tweed develops on the skin as comfortably as a favorite tweed jacket.

Introduced   1985
Price   High range

HABIT ROUGE

Scent Type *Oriental*
Composition
 Top Notes: *Bergamot, orange*
 Heart Notes: *Spices, patchouli*
 Base Notes: *Vanilla, leather*

Famous Patrons
 Robert Redford *Alec Baldwin*
 Richard Gere

 Guerlain's Habit Rouge, translated from French as "red hunting coat," was inspired by a rider's red habit. Blended by perfumer Jean-Paul Guerlain, the fragrance has attained classic status. An Oriental blend of verve and vitality, Habit Rouge opens with fresh citrus top notes, then meanders along a spicy path to a base of vanilla and patchouli, finally leaving a leathery, individualistic impression.

 A weighty rectangular bottle captures the intoxicating essence. Habit Rouge is a fine selection for gentlemen of taste and refinement who appreciate the sensuality and subtlety of Guerlain formulations. And, quite naturally, it's the ideal fragrance for a rousing morning of horseback riding.

Introduced *1965*
Price *High range*

HALSTON Z-14

Scent Type *Chypre - Spicy*
Composition
 Top Notes: *Bergamot, citrus*
 Heart Notes: *Herbs*
 Base Notes: *Amber, patchouli, musk,*
     cedarwood, oakmoss

Famous Patrons
 Soccer star Laszlo Marton

 Nearly three decades ago, American fashion designer Halston enjoyed smashing success with Halston Z-14. An intoxicating aroma, it remains a favorite. The magical scent opens with a crisp, citrusy accord that evolves into a chypre base of moss and woods. Amber, patchouli, and musk form a rich, velvety tapestry that lingers magnificently on the skin, while the spicy herbal accents warm the depths of one's soul. Halston Z-14 is a handsome choice for wintry days and elegant evenings.

 A masculine scent of power and privilege, Halston Z-14 is an exotic, charismatic fragrance. A rich, coffee-colored flacon is smoothed and rounded to further enhance the scent's smoldering sensuality. Halston Z-14 is expansive—a fragrance for the accomplished man who lives life to its fullest.

Introduced *1976*
Price *Mid-range*

HÉRITAGE

Scent Type   Oriental - Woody
Composition
    Top Notes: Citrus
    Heart Notes: Coriander, pepper
    Base Notes: Vanilla, tonka bean, patchouli,
                 cedar, leather

Drawing upon its rich heritage, Guerlain sought to create a fragrance of heirloom quality—a scent to last through the ages. Many Guerlain fragrances have attained heirloom status, such as the unisex Eau de Cologne du Coq, from 1894, and Eau de Cologne Impériale, from 1853. (*See the women's fragrance section for these profiles.*)

Héritage contains hesperides, or fresh citrus notes, in the opening movement. As the scent progresses, spices and woods become increasingly apparent. The final touch is the "Guerlinade," a secret, enchanting blend of vanilla and tonka bean that is the imprint of Guerlain and underscores many Guerlain compositions. The faceted bottle, designed by Guerlain glass sculptor Robert Granai, has architectural roots. Packaging is rendered in an understated red with gold-toned accents. Refined and confident, Héritage is an elegant statement for the self-assured man.

Another Guerlain fragrance of note is Coriolan, named for the noble warrior immortalized in music and literature by Beethoven and Shakespeare. Introduced in 1998, Coriolan is a crisp chypre fragrance of freshness and vitality.

Introduced   1992
Price   High range

HUGO

Scent Type   Fougère
Composition
    Top Notes: Green apple, cedar leaves,
                 spearmint, pine needles
    Heart Notes: Lavender, jasmine,
                 geranium leaves, sage, clove
    Base Notes: Oakmoss, woods, leather

Youthful, adventurous and charismatic, Hugo, from Hugo Boss, cops a distinct attitude. It is an unconventional scent geared toward the rugged individualist, whereas the designer's first fragrance, Boss, is tailored to the casually elegant man.

Possessing an "outdoorsy" personality, Hugo is inspired by aromas of Acadia National Park in Maine. Foresty fresh notes of pine and cedar are blended with spicy geranium leaves, lavender, and sage. Earthy oakmoss is rounded with a wooded finish and a leathery impression.

When the mood strikes, strap on a backpack and hike the Himalayas—don't forget to take Hugo, already dressed for the occasion in a canteen-style bottle with decoy-green canvas accents.

Introduced   1995
Price   Mid-range

JAÏPUR

Scent Type	Oriental - Woody
Composition	
Top Notes:	Heliotrope, bergamot, lemon
Heart Notes:	Cinnamon, nutmeg, clove
Base Notes:	Amber, tonka bean, vanilla

In the 1920s, French jeweler Louis Boucheron traveled to India. While visiting Jaïpur, Boucheron became intrigued by the "astronomical garden" developed by Maharaja Jai Singh II, the Jantar Mantar. Boucheron, an engineer by training, made many sketches of the garden and its instruments and stone structures.

Years later, these sketches served as inspiration for the architecturally styled bottle of Jaïpur Homme. Silver- and gold-toned metals are crowned with a Boucheron signature, a *faux* sapphire. The golden-hued liquid is a spicy Oriental blend—a vibrant, sensual composition that recalls Boucheron's adventurous journey to the legendary city of Jaïpur. We found the subtle heart note of cinnamon particularly intriguing, and truly reminiscent of our own Orient travels.

A polished balance of elegance and sensuality, Jaïpur Homme is a compelling blend of warmth and charisma, of power and attraction.

Introduced	1997
Price	Top range

JORDAN

Scent Type	Oriental - Woody
Composition	
Top Notes:	Mandarin, bergamot, bitter orange, sage, greens, white ivy, cypress
Heart Notes:	White nutmeg, black pepper, cardamom, jasmine
Base Notes:	Sandalwood, cashmere musk, oak, blond woods, amber

Famous Patrons	
Jay Leno	Tom Brokaw

When sports superstar Michael Jordan partnered with Bijan, the Beverly Hills menswear couture designer, for the original Michael Jordan cologne, they far surpassed the traditional expectations for fragrance launches. The mega-hit fragrance, sold in department stores and sporting goods chains, is joined by the Jordan-Bijan team's second scent, Jordan by Michael.

Since his basketball retirement, Jordan has stepped into the business arena. He is often recognized for his superb sense of style, which Jordan displayed in designing the scent with Bijan. Blended by perfumers at Givaudan-Roure, the Jordan fragrance is described as a fresh fougère and Oriental combination. A spirited citrus beginning gives way to a fresh green accord, which dissolves into an aromatic heart of North Carolina woods, chosen for the memory of Jordan's Carolina childhood. A white amber note evokes subtle style and worldly elegance. At the base is the warmth of musk, a masculine accord that is at once comforting and sensual. The Jordan fragrance is a superbly rendered composition of elegance and refinement, suitable for the well-dressed executive.

Jordan's beautiful wife, Juanita, shares the spotlight with her husband in the advertising campaign. Jordan's familiar silhouette graces the blue and silver-toned cartons. The sleek bottle sports shades of pale, Mediterranean-blue (or perhaps, Caroline blue, for his alma mater, UNC at Chapel Hill). The bottle is crowned with a modern, silver-toned spray mechanism—a design that rests comfortably in the hand.

Even off the basketball court, Jordan continues his winning streak, with Bijan as a teammate. Now, there's a dynamic duo!

Introduced	*1999*
Price	*Mid-range*

KOUROS

Scent Type	*Fougère*
Composition	
Top Notes:	*Lavender, artemisia, coriander, clove*
Heart Notes:	*Honey, jasmine, rose*
Base Notes:	*Incense, patchouli, oakmoss, vanilla, galbanum, vetiver, sandalwood*

French couturier Yves Saint Laurent once remarked to Andy Warhol, "Fashions fade, style is eternal." Saint Laurent's Kouros proves this adage, with two decades of popularity behind it.

Kouros is a rich fougère blend, balanced with an opening accord of green herbs and spices. The honeyed heart leads to a mossy, wooded base, which lingers on the skin with a hint of green galbanum and incense.

Saint Laurent once stated: "We must never confuse elegance with snobbery." Kouros is undeniably elegant, an impeccable choice for the sophisticated man, a classic scent of depth and magnetism.

Introduced	*1981*
Price	*High range*

LAGERFELD

Scent Type	*Oriental - Spicy*
Composition	
Top Notes:	*Bergamot, coriander, basil*
Heart Notes:	*Lavender, rose, clove*
Base Notes:	*Tabac, tonka bean, patchouli, oakmoss, musk*

Famous Patrons
Sir James Halper

Couturier Karl Lagerfeld made fragrance history with his signature Lagerfeld, a rich, sensual, Oriental fragrance that remains a favorite. Lagerfeld opens with a fresh herbal accord that is smooth and sophisticated, setting the stage for a lavender heart underscored with spicy clove. The dominant theme is one of spice and woods, as the artful blend of patchouli, tonka bean, and musk develops and becomes one with the skin. The lingering accord contains a touch of tabac, or tobacco, that conjures images of silk smoking robes and wood-paneled gentlemen's clubs.

Presented in understated shades of taupe, gray, and silver, Lagerfeld is a classic fragrance, known to inspire nuzzles and more.

For a fresh view of Lagerfeld, try Lagerfeld Photo, a clean, crisp scent ideal for summer wear.

Introduced	*1978*
Price	*High range*

LALIQUE

Scent Type   *Floral - Oriental*
Composition
   Top Notes: *Mandarin, blackberry, gardenia*
   Heart Notes: *Orange blossom, rose, peony,*
      ylang-ylang, magnolia
   Base Notes: *Musk, sandalwood, vanilla,*
      cedarwood, oakmoss

Lalique Pour Homme is the first men's fragrance from Lalique, the French luxury goods firm that specializes in crystal. The fragrance, a wooded floral with fresh, fruity accents, was blended by Dragoco and inspired by the company's past. Company founder René Lalique created exquisite hood ornaments for luxury cars from 1925 to 1932. Referred to as "car mascots," these were frequently fashioned after animals. Suitably, for the initial collector's edition, a crystal lion's head was featured atop a substantial crystal flacon. Remove the ornament and it becomes a paperweight. Of course, every year a different animal is featured. Why not collect them all?

The Lalique fragrance is also reminiscent of the Roaring Twenties. A refined floral with an ambery wooded base, Lalique is a scent of immense elegance and class. It is a versatile, *recherché* fragrance that reverberates with style—ideal for the well-dressed man of the world.

Introduced   *1997*
Price   *High range*

LANVIN

Scent Type   *Fougère*
Composition
   Top Notes: *Mandarin, neroli, bergamot*
   Heart Notes: *Lavender, sage, mint,*
      coriander, cardamom
   Base Notes: *Amber, musk, vanilla,*
      sandalwood, violet wood

French couturier Jeanne Lanvin opened her first shop for ladies in 1885, and in 1926 she became the first French designer to create a couture line for men. The company that bears her name continues her legacy today, emphasizing luxurious fabrics, attention to detail, and timeless classics.

Lanvin's 1927 fragrance creation, Arpège for women, remains popular. Lanvin L'Homme, an elegant composition, has the potential to rise to such legacy status. Blending fresh, spicy, aromatic, and wooded essences, Lanvin is relaxed and easy to wear. After a fresh burst of citrus, the scent dries down to a well-balanced fougère base of woods and musk. Mediterranean blue and chrome accents convey the contemporary feeling of the fragrance, which was created by Firmenich perfumer Alberto Morillas. The pale blue liquid is suspended in a smooth, rounded bottle, which fits easily in the hand.

Lanvin is available in an eau de toilette, as well as in grooming products. A popular product is the non-oily, alcohol-free After Shave Balm—a soft touch to ease a strong man.

Introduced   *1998*
Price   *High range*

MICHAEL JORDAN

Scent Type   *Fougère*
Composition
   Top Notes: *Grapefruit, lemon,*
                       cedar leaf, cypress
   Heart Notes: *Lavender, fir balsam, geranium,*
                       clary sage, juniper berry, nutmeg,
                       coriander, cardamom, green tea,
                       clove leaf, incense, suede
   Base Notes: *Sandalwood, patchouli,*
                       rosewood, cognac, musk

Famous Patrons

   The Chicago Bulls   *Dustin Hoffman*
   Mel Gibson   *Spike Lee*
   David Letterman   *Jack Nicholson*

Basketball great Michael Jordan joined a new dream team to bring his eponymous cologne to market. Along with Jordan, Beverly Hills menswear designer and fragrance tycoon Bijan, perfumer Givaudan-Roure, and Bijan fragrance division president Sally Yeh won over fragrance fans with a real slam-dunk!

"The scent isn't serious or contrived," says Jordan. "It's relaxed and really makes you feel good. For me, that's a winning formula." Bijan adds: "Michael Jordan represents the best of the best—in every respect. I admire and respect him for his great talents and for his integrity, enthusiasm, and spirit."

Jordan, often referred to as "His Airness," drew upon memory during the creative development stage. The cologne develops around five accords, or aroma blends, captured through new fragrance technology. The first, called "rare air," evokes the tropical air of a Costa Rican beach, with grapefruit, lemon, and cedar leaf. The second accord is "cool," reminiscent of the fresh Appalachian air near Jordan's North Carolina childhood home. A green note, "Pebble Beach," was inspired by golf, one of Jordan's favorite pastimes. "Home run" is a hit—an accord of green tea, clove leaf, incense, and suede, that brings back memories of Jordan's favorite leather baseball glove. Finally, a "sensual" accord combines woods and musk, creating a long-lasting base. The overall effect is fresh and lively; the Michael Jordan fragrance is a bright scent with an optimistic attitude.

Gold Medal Olympian, Chicago Bulls guard, four-time NBA Most Valuable Player: Jordan is a modern-day hero and role model. He lends his distinct "headshot" to the black and red carton. A basketball motif is debossed into the clear glass bottle, a presentation sure to be a hit with sports fans. Jordan comments on his fragrant venture, as well as life in general, "It's all about having fun and feeling good."

Introduced   *1996*
Price   *Mid-range*

OLD SPICE

Scent Type   *Fougère - Spicy*
Composition
   Top Notes: *Bergamot, lemon, carnation,*
                       anise, orange
   Heart Notes: *Lavender, ylang-ylang,*
                       cinnamon, jasmine
   Base Notes: *Amber, incense, vanilla, nutmeg,*
                       musk, patchouli, sandalwood,
                       oakmoss, vetiver, tonka bean

Since 1937, Old Spice has graced many a man's dressing table; the scent is a beloved classic. The spicy fougère blend combines classic fougère elements of citrus, lavender, and oakmoss. Delicious culinary spices set it apart in the fougère category. Nutmeg, vanilla, and incense are supported by velvety amber, while sandalwood, patchouli, and vetiver provide an earthy, wooded base that launches memories of exotic ports of call.

A mass-market fragrance, Old Spice is well-priced and simply packaged in a creamy porcelain-style bottle with a sketch of a tall-masted sailing ship. Wear it in memory of the good old days.

Introduced   1937
Price   *Mid-range*

PENHALIGON'S COLLECTION

HAMMAM BOUQUET
Oriental - Woody
LORD'S
Citrus

Established in 1870, Penhaligon's of London is an English perfumery that offers an extensive repertoire. The woody Oriental, Hammam Bouquet, dates from 1872, and the citrusy Lord's was created in 1911. See the women's section for a variety of unisex scents, including Racquets Formula, English Fern, Quercus, and Blenheim Bouquet. Penhaligon's English Classics is a collection of eaux de cologne for gentlemen.

The classics according to Penhaligon's: Worth studying.

Introduced   *Since 1870*
Price   *High range*

PLEASURES

Scent Type   *Fougère*
Composition
   Top Notes: *Nectarines, green leaves*
   Heart Notes: *Coriander, pimento, ginger*
   Base Notes: *Sandalwood flowers, forest moss*

Casual, clean, and comfortable—that's the personality of Estée Lauder's Pleasures for Men. Fresh greens and nectarine are blended with culinary spices, and a mossy base creates an ambiance of ease and tranquility.

The versatile scent is presented in subtle shades of gray and silver, and the simple, understated bottle is topped with a man-size pewter-colored cap. Pleasures is ideal for those who cherish the simple pleasures in life—for weekend warriors, soccer dads, and gentlemen farmers.

Introduced   1997
Price   *Mid-range*

POLO

Scent Type	*Chypre*
Composition	
Top Notes:	*Basil, chamomile*
Heart Notes:	*Leather, tobacco*
Base Notes:	*Oakmoss, patchouli*

Upon its debut, Ralph Lauren's Polo quickly achieved superstar status. Packaged in the familiar hunter green and gold bottle, Polo is a crisp chypre formula that zips open on a green herbal note. The heart holds masculine impressions of leather and tobacco, while the oakmoss and patchouli blend results in a classic chypre combination. A well-balanced composition, Polo is at ease in a variety of settings, from the classroom to the boardroom—not to mention the polo club, of course.

A fresh addition to the Ralph Lauren fragrance line is Polo Sport. It's ideal for summer and sporting events—take it to the gym.

Introduced	1978
Price	Mid-range

ROCABAR

Scent Type	*Chypre*
Composition	
Top Notes:	*Juniper berries, cypress, lavender, walnut, cinnamon, nutmeg*
Heart Notes:	*Cypress, atlas cedar*
Base Notes:	*Balsam, vanilla*

Founded in 1837, French luxury goods purveyor Hermès is known for its high quality leather goods, scarves, accessories, clothing, and housewares. Hermès debuted on the fragrance scene with an invigorating unisex scent, Eau d'Hermès, in 1951. The fresh Eau d'Orange

Verte, introduced in 1979, was the firm's second unisex scent. Exclusively for men are the spicy and aromatic Équipage and the leathery chypre, Bel Ami. Both are scents of true distinction.

The firm's third fragrance just for men is Rocabar. Its name is derived from the phrase "*rug a barres,*" which describes a striped horse blanket, usually placed under a well-made Hermès saddle. Perfumers Bernard Bourgeois, of Hermès, and Gilles Romey, of Quest, collaborated on the Rocabar formula. They sought to capture the aromatic sensation of fresh wind on the face during an exhilarating horse ride. An ambery wooded accord is combined with balsam and spice, and the final effect is warm, rich, and lingering.

Serge Mansau designed the smooth, clear bottle. Rocabar is wrapped with a miniature rocabar blanket and presented in a box of Hermès orange, gold, and navy. Equine inspired, Rocabar is a thoughtful gift for any member of the horse-lovers set.

Introduced	1998
Price	Top range

SALVATORE FERRAGAMO

Scent Type	*Chypre*
Composition	
Top Notes:	*Grapefruit, fig leaves, geranium, cyclamen*
Heart Notes:	*Clove bud, cardamom*
Base Notes:	*Vetiver, sandalwood, cedarwood, "bio" musk*

From the partnership of Ferragamo and Bulgari, called Ferragamo Parfums, comes Salvatore Ferragamo Pour Homme. The modern chypre scent opens with the sharpness of grapefruit. Spicy cardamom and clove warm the heart, while the fragrance develops around a traditional note of vetiver. Contemporary and versatile, the scent exudes Italian chic.

Burgundy packaging sets the masculine theme; the handsome glass bottle is collared and capped with silver-colored metal. Salvatore Ferragamo is available in eau de toilette and after shave formulas. Bath and body products are also available, for head-to-toe grooming, Italian style.

Introduced　　　*1999*
Price　　　*High range*

TOMMY
♀♂

Scent Type　　　*Fougère*
Composition
　　Top Notes:　　*Cape Cod cranberry,*
　　　　　　　　New England apple pie
　　Heart Notes:　*Texas yellow rose,*
　　　　　　　　Kentucky blue grass
　　Base Notes:　*Mid-Atlantic driftwood*

In creating his first fragrance, Tommy, designer Tommy Hilfiger chose a theme and ingredients as American as apple pie.

A light scent with a wooded base, Tommy develops around regional North American fragrance accords. The apothecary-style bottle is topped with a silver-colored cap inspired by a Tommy Hilfiger button. Packaging in patriotic red, white, and blue completes the theme.

Envisioned as a unisex scent, Tommy is casual, youthful, and easy to wear—ideal for the blue-jean lifestyle.

For a slightly richer Hilfiger experience, try Freedom for Him, a citrusy-spicy 1999 introduction that is imbued with a casual elegance for the modern man.

Introduced　　　*1995*
Price　　　*Mid-range*

VERY VALENTINO

Scent Type　　　*Oriental - Woody*
Composition
　　Top Notes:　　*Anise, sage, nutmeg*
　　Heart Notes:　*Pipe tobacco, coriander, thyme*
　　Base Notes:　*Amber, sandalwood, musk*

Valentino, the Italian couturier known only by his first name, interprets a man's desire for luxury with Very Valentino Pour Homme.

The fragrance is an Oriental blend that unites a crisp opening accord with the rich impression of pipe tobacco. Anise contributes a minty accent; imagine the aroma and flavor of anisette liqueur. The dominant accords of Very Valentino are nutmeg, tobacco, and sandalwood. A base of musk, amber, and sandalwood warms to the skin, as a hint of pipe tobacco imparts a refined, aromatic sweetness that is just right, never overwhelming.

Very Valentino is a superbly executed fragrance of quiet elegance and discreet sensuality. Packaged in a rectangular bottle of chic gray and black, the scent receives high marks for its well-executed appearance.

Very Valentino is a versatile, understated fragrance that may be worn for a variety of occasions and seasons. Destined to become a classic.

Introduced　　　*1999*
Price　　　*High range*

VETIVER
♀♂

Scent Type	Chypre
Composition	
Top Notes:	Citrus
Heart Notes:	Vetiver, spices
Base Notes:	Tobacco, sandalwood, tonka bean

Famous Patrons

Andy Garcia	Harrison Ford
Paul McCartney	Arnold Schwarzenegger
John Fairchild	Michael Caine
Peter Sellers	Anne Bass
Jodi Foster	Naomi Campbell

The venerable House of Guerlain is well known for its wide array of fine fragrances for women and men. From the unisex fougère Jicky to the memorable Mitsouko and Shalimar for women, Guerlain has proved its mastery of the art of perfume.

Vetiver, like most Guerlain fragrances, began with an inspiration. The story is told of Jean-Paul Guerlain, then a young perfumer, who happened upon a country squire who had just left his estate. A woody green aroma clung to his clothes, mingled with the smoky sweetness of tobacco. Guerlain's nose surely tingled with excitement. The result is a woody green blend, freshened with citrus, spiked with tobacco and spice, smoothed and rounded with tonka bean. Derived from a woody root, vetiver is a tenacious essential oil. Although Vetiver was made for men, women gravitate toward it, too, and their skin chemistry evokes a subtle difference. Vetiver is classic formula, understated and refined, a scent of casual ease.

Introduced	1959
Price	High range

XERYUS ROUGE

Scent Type	Oriental
Composition	
Top Notes:	Green cactus, tarragon, kumquat
Heart Notes:	Red pepper, geranium, cedar leaves
Base Notes:	Sandalwood, cedarwood, ambergris

Givenchy warms the cockles of the heart with Xeryus Rouge, a spicy Oriental fragrance with a passionate nature. The name is reminiscent of Xerxes the Great, the fearless King of Persia in the fifth century B.C.

Xeryus Rouge opens with zesty notes of cactus and kumquat. A spicy heart and a woody, balsamic base create an impression of rich complexity, of smoldering sensuality, of power and prestige. An opulent French fragrance of distinction, Xeryus Rouge is a fine choice for romantic evenings, formal occasions, and cool weather wear. Reflecting its hot-blooded nature, the fragrance is captured in a bold, blood-red bottle. Enigmatic and superbly lingering, Xeryus Rouge is a refined fragrance, fit for a king.

Introduced	1996
Price	High range

PART 3

CROSS REFERENCE BY SCENT TYPE

WOMEN'S AND UNISEX FRAGRANCES BY SCENT TYPE

FLORAL

1000
24, Faubourg
273
360 Perry Ellis
Acte 2
Adoration
Amazing
Anne Klein (HM)
Antonia's Flowers
Arôme 3 (♀♂) (HM)
Baby Doll (HM)
Beautiful
Believe (HM)
Bellodgia
Bill Blass (HM)
Black Tie (HM)
Blonde
Bobbi
Bulgari
Bulgari Eau Parfumée
Burberry Touch
Capricci (HM)
Carolina Herrera
Catalyst
Ce Soir ou Jamais
Celia's Ultimate Gardenia
Cerruti 1881
C'est Si Bon
Ceylon
Channel No. 22
Charlie (HM)
Chloé
Christian Lacroix
Coeur-Joie (HM)
Courrèges in Blue (HM)
Darby Rose
Delicious
Demi-Jour *(HM)
Diamonds & Emeralds *(HM)
Dilys *(HM)
DKNY
Donna Karan
Duende
E by HRH Princess
Elizabeth
Eau du Ciel
Ecco *(HM)
Elizabethan Rose
Enjoli (HM)
Estée
Evelyn
Evening in Paris (HM)

Extravagance
Fabergé
Fantasia (HM)
Fantasia de Fleurs
Fascination
Ferentina
Fidji
Fleur d'Interdit
Fleurissimo
Fleurs de Bulgarie
Fleurs de Rocaille
Forever (HM)
Fracas
Fragile
Fred Hayman's Touch (HM)
French Lime Blossom
Gabriela Sabatini (HM)
Gardenia
Gardénia
Gardénia Passion
Gianfranco Ferré
Giorgio
Golconda
Grace de Monaco
Heure Exquise
Honeysuckle & Jasmine
Ice Water (HM)
Impératrice Eugénie
In Love Again *(HM)
Invitation
Isis
Ivana (HM)
J'Adore
Jardins de Bagatelle
Jivago 24K
Joy
K de Krizia (HM)
Kenzo (HM)
Kiss & Tell
L'Effleur (HM)
L'Air du Temps
Lalique
L'Amour
Lavande Velours (♀♂)
L'Eau de Monteil (HM)
Lumière (HM)
Mad Moments (HM)
Madeleine de Madeleine (HM)
Mea Culpa (HM)
Michael
Michelle (HM)
Mon Ange (HM)
Muguet Millésime *(HM)

Mystic
Nicole
Nina (HM)
No Regrets
Norell
Ocean Dream *(HM)
Paperwhites
Paris
Passion
Pavlova
Petite Chérie
Poême
Quadrille (HM)
Quelques Fleurs
Quelques Violettes (HM)
Red Door
Red Roses
Romance
Rosa Magnifica
Rose Absolue
S.T. DuPont
Salvatore Ferragamo
Scaasi (HM)
Signature
Soir de Paris (HM)
Sparkling White
    Diamonds *(HM)
Splendor
Spring Flower
Stiletto (HM)
Style
Tatiana (HM)
Tiare
Tova
Tubéreuse
Tubereuse Indiana
Tuberose
Tweed (HM)
Very Valentino
Vice Versa *(HM)
Vicky Tiel (HM)
Victorian Posy
Violetta
Vivid (HM)
White Camellia
White Diamonds
White Hyacinth
White Shoulders
Wild Muguet
Wind Song (HM)
Womenswear (HM)
Ylang & Vanille

FLORAL - GREEN

Andiamo *(HM)
Bluebell
Cabotine
Chanel No. 19
Dazzling Silver
Eau de Camille
Energizing Fragrance (HM)
Envy
Fleurs d'Elle (HM)
Flirt
Green Tea
Ivoire
Jessica McClintock
Jones New York
Léonard de Léonard (HM)
Lily of the Valley
Lizsport
Parfum d'Été
Pleasures
Sabi
Safari
Soleil
Sung
Tommy Girl
Vent Vert
Weil de Weil

Laguna
Laila
Le Muguet de Rosine (HM)
Loving Bouquet *(HM)
Lucky You
Moods (HM)
Nautica Woman
Noa
Portfolio
Rare Orchid (HM)
Relaxing Fragrance (HM)
Savanna
So de la Renta
So Pretty
Tendre Poison
Tilleul (HM) (♀♂)
V/S Versace
Week End
Wisteria

FLORAL - FRUITY

Adieu Sagesse
Amarige
Amazone
America
Basic Black (HM)
Birmane
Byblos
Calyx (HM)
Champagne
Cherry Blossom *(HM)
Claire de Nilang
Dazzling Gold
Deci Delà
Design
Desire
Diamonds & Sapphires *(HM)
Eau de Charlotte
Eau de Givenchy
Eau d'Hermès (♀♂)
Elysium (HM)
Exclamation (HM)
Ferré
Flora Nerolia
Folavril
For Ever
G
Gènèration *(HM)
GFF
Gieffeffe (HM)
Giò (HM)
Grain de Folie
Happy

FLORAL - FRESH

212
Acqua di Giò
Acte 2 En Fleurs
Amour Amour
Anaïs Anaïs
April Fields (HM)
AV (HM)
Bouquet de Provence
Câline
Cashmere Mist
Champs-Élysées
Curve
Destiny
Diorissimo
Dolce Vita
Eau d'Ivoire
Eternity
Eternity
Face à Face
Flore
Floret
Frangipani
Freedom
La Parisienne

Il Bacio
Indiscret
Jaïpur
Jean-Paul Gaultier
Josie (HM)
La Prairie (HM)
Lady Caron
Laura Ashley No.1 (HM)
Lauren
Lily Chic *(HM)
Listen *(HM)
Liz Claiborne
Magnetic (HM)
Mandarin
Mariella Burani
Marina de Bourbon
Millennium Hope
Miss Arpels
Molinard de Molinard
Ô Oui
Petit Guerlain (HM)
Pure
Quartz (HM)
Que Viva *(HM)
Ralph
Romeo Gigli (HM)
Senso (HM)
Sonia Rykiel
Sunflowers
Sweet Courrèges (HM)
Tribù
Trueste
Versus
XS (HM)

FLORAL - MARINE
Cool Water Woman
Dune
Fleur de Diva
Oh! de Moschino

FLORAL - ALDEHYDE
Anna Sui
Antilope (HM)
Arpège
Bois des Îles
Calandre
Calèche
Channel No. 5
D & G (HM)
Farouche (HM)
First
Fleur de Fleurs (HM)
Fleurage (HM)
Gucci No. 1 (HM)
Hanae Mori Haute Couture
Infini
Je Reviens
Lady Stetson (HM)
Le Dix
L'Interdit
Liù

Lutèce (HM)
Madame Rochas
My Sin (HM)
Nahema
Nocturnes
Nude (HM)
Ombre Rose
Red
Rive Gauche
Salvador Dali
Scherrer 2 (HM)
Tamango (HM)
White Linen
Zibeline (HM)

FLORAL - AMBERY
Après L'Ondée
Balahé (HM)
Blue Grass
Caesars Woman
C'est la vie! *(HM)
Contradiction
DNA
Frangipane
Galanos de Serene
Grand Amour
Jaïpur Saphir
L'Heure Bleue
Moment Suprême
Oscar de la Renta
Panthère
Poison
Spellbound
Tiempe Passate
Tiffany

FLORAL - ORIENTAL
Aimez-Moi
Alchimie
Anné Pliska
Asja (HM)
Attar
Bijan
Burberry
Byzantine
Calla
Candie's
Charles of the Ritz (HM)
Chloé Narcisse
Coco
Cornubia
Di Borghese *(HM)
Diamonds and Rubies *(HM)
Dolce & Gabbana
Doulton
E.N.C.O.R.E. (HM)
Emporio Armani She
Escada
Fable
Fabulous
Fiamma *(HM)

Gai Mattiolo (HM)
Galanos (HM)
Galore (HM)
Gianfranco Ferré 20 (HM)
Glamour
Goddess
Good Life
Hanae Mori
Ici (HM)
Intoxication (HM)
Je T'Aime
Jil Sander No. 4
Joop!
La Coupe d'Or (HM)
Lelong
Les Copains (HM)
Longing (HM)
Mackie
Maroussia
Masquerade
Miracle (HM)
Moschino (HM)
Naomi Campbell
Narcisse Noir
Organza
Perhaps
Raffinée
Realities
Rose Cardin (HM)
Rush
Samsara
Secret of Venus *(HM)
Séxual
Sirène
St. John
Sui Dreams
Sunset Boulevard
Tocade
Très Chic
Trésor
Truly Lace (HM)
Truth Calvin Klein
Tuscany
Vacances
Van Cleef
Vanderbilt
Vendetta (HM)
Venezia
Venus de l'Amour (HM)
Verino (HM)
Volupté (HM)
Wings
With Love *(HM)
Zaharoff

FLORAL SEMI - ORIENTAL
5th Avenue
Boucheron
Byzance
Chamade
Désirade (HM)

Elizabeth Taylor's Passion
Hiris (♀♂)
Jivago 7 Notes

SEMI - ORIENTAL
Adrienne Vittadini (HM)
Alexandra
Allure
Ambrelle Canelle (♀♂)
Colors (HM)
Elige (HM)
Misuki
Parfum d'Hermès
Royal Delight
Tabarôme (♀♂)

ORIENTAL
Amber & Lavender
Angel
By Woman (HM)
Chaldée
CK Be (♀♂)
Coquette
Ellen Tracy
Émeraude (HM)
Fath de Fath
Fire & Ice (HM)
Guet-Apens *(HM)
Hot (HM)
Hypnotic Poison
Initial
Interlude (HM)
Maja (HM)
Nuit de Noël
Odalisque (HM)
Oh la la! (HM)
Ormolu
Realm
Royal Secret
Sacrebleu! (HM)
Santal Impérial (♀♂)
Shalimar
Shocking (HM)
Tabu (HM)
Tentations
Theorema
Ultraviolet
Vanilla Fields (HM)
Vanille
Vanisia
Zut (HM)

ORIENTAL - GREEN
Boudoir

ORIENTAL - FRESH
Nokomis (HM)

ORIENTAL - FRUITY
Angel Innocent
Casmir
Hugo Woman

Isadora (HM)
Jil
Lolita Lempicka
Magic
Stardust
Sun Moon Stars
Wish
Yohji

ORIENTAL - AMBERY
Anne Klein II *(HM)
Chantilly
Ciara
Dionne
Divine Folie
Guess? (HM)
Habanita
Le Feu d'Issey
Mania
Must de Cartier
Normandie
Obsession
Roma
Ungaro (HM)

ORIENTAL - SPICY
Cinnabar
Dioressence
KL (HM)
L'Heure Attendue
Ma Liberté
Nutmeg & Ginger
Opium
Parfum Sacré
Prélude (HM)
Teatro alla Scala (HM)
Tianne (HM)

ORIENTAL - AMBERY SPICY
Bal à Versailles
Magie Noire
Organza Indécence
Vol de Nuit
Youth Dew

CHYPRE
Bulgari Black (HM) (♀♂)
Cielo Napa Valley (HM)
Commes des
    Garçons (HM) (♀♂)
Enigma
Feminité du Bois (HM)
Fleurs de la Forêt
Guépard
Racquets Formula (♀♂)
Royal English Leather (♀♂)
Sandalwood &
    Cedarwood (♀♂)
Tabac Blond (HM)
Vetiver (♀♂)
Vetyver (♀♂)

CHYPRE - GREEN
Aliage
IO (HM)
Private Collection
Wrappings (HM)

CHYPRE - FRESH
4711
Création
Cristalle
Diorella
Eau de Rochas (♀♂)
Eau d'Hadrien (♀♂)

CHYPRE - FRUITY
Azzaro (HM)
Cocktail
Colony
Femme
Gem
Mitsouko
Que sais-je?
Talisman
Y

CHYPRE - FRUITY FLORAL
Cassini

CHYPRE - FLORAL
Animale (HM)
Aromatics Elixir
Chant d'Arômes
Coriandre
Diva
Eau du Soir
Fendi
Gucci No. 3 (HM)
Halston
Histoire D'Amour (HM)
Knowing
Ma Griffe
Montana Parfum de Peau (HM)
Niki de Saint Phalle
Paloma Picasso
Trussardi
V'E Versace

CHYPRE - FLORAL ANIMALIC
Azurée
Bandit
Cabochard
Cachet (HM)
Cuir de Russie
Empreinte (HM)
Givenchy III (HM)
Jolie Madame (HM)
Miss Balmain (HM)
Miss Dior
Moments (HM)

Mystère (HM)
Parure
Rumba (HM)
Ysatis

CITRUS
Acqua di Parma Colonia (♀♂)
Blenheim Bouquet (♀♂)
Carrière (HM)
CK One (♀♂)
Eau de Cologne du Coq (♀♂)
Eau de Cologne Impériale (♀♂)
Eau de Fleurs de
     Cédrat (HM) (♀♂)
Eau de Guerlain (♀♂)
Eau de Patou (♀♂)
Eau d'Orange Verte (♀♂)
Eau du Jour (♀♂)
Eau du Sud (♀♂)
Eau Fraîche by Caron (♀♂)
Eau Fraîche by
     Léonard (HM) (♀♂)
Etiquette Bleue (HM) (♀♂)
Grapefruit (♀♂)
Jean Nate (HM)
Le Temps d'une Fête (HM)
Lime, Basil & Mandarin (♀♂)
Ô de Lancôme
Paco (♀♂)
Pamplelune (♀♂)
Quercus (♀♂)
Route du Thé (HM)
Té (HM) (♀♂)
Verbenas de Provence (HM)
Zeste Mandarine (♀♂)

GREEN
Cerruti Image
Herba Fresca (♀♂)
Manifesto
Pheromone
Reverie

FOUGÈRE
English Fern (♀♂)
Epicéa (♀♂)
Jicky
Orange Spice (♀♂)
Royal Water (♀♂)

MARINE
Carita (HM)
Eau du Fier (HM)
Escape
Impérial Millèsime (♀♂)
Mare (HM) (♀♂)
Polo Sport Woman
Silver Mountain Water (♀♂)

MEN'S FRAGRANCES BY SCENT TYPE

FLORAL - ORIENTAL
Lalique

ORIENTAL
Bois du Portugal
Habit Rouge
Opium (HM)
Xeryus Rouge

ORIENTAL - GREEN
Envy (HM)

ORIENTAL - AMBERY
Obsession (HM)
Royal Copenhagen (HM)
Stetson (HM)
Tiffany (HM)

ORIENTAL - WOODY
Allure
Bijan
Contradiction (HM)
Escada
Hammam Bouquet
Héritage
Herrera (HM)
Jaïpur
Jordan
Le Mâle (HM)
Versace (HM)
Very Valentino

ORIENTAL - SPICY
Égoïste (HM)
Equipage (HM)
Jacomo de Jacomo (HM)
Lagerfeld
Santos (HM)

CHYPRE
Antaeus (HM)
Aramis
Déclaration
Emporio Armani He
English Leather (HM)
Green Valley
Oscar (HM)
Polo
Rocabar
Russian Leather
Salvatore Ferragamo
Vetiver (♀♂)

CHYPRE - GREEN
Fahrenheit (HM)
Grey Flannel (HM)

CHYPRE - FRESH
Coriolan (HM)
Pheromone (HM)
Voyageur (HM)

CHYPRE - SPICY
Bel Ami (HM)
Giorgio (HM)
Halston Z-14

CITRUS
Bois de Cédrat (♀♂)
Boucheron
Cerruti 1881
Cerruti Image (HM)
Chevalier d'Orsay (HM)
Eau Savage (HM)
Lord's

GREEN
212
Gendarme (HM)
Green Irish Tweed

FOUGÈRE
Avatar (HM)
British Sterling (HM)
Burberry (HM)
Candie's (HM)
Canoe (HM)
Cassini
Curve (HM)
Dolce & Gabbana (HM)
Drakkar Noir
Escape (HM)
Eternity (HM)
Façonnable (HM)
Hugo
Kouros
Lanvin
Michael Jordan
Pasha (HM)
Pleasures
Preferred Stock (HM)
Romance (HM)
Safari (HM)
Tommy (♀♂)
Van Cleef (HM)
XS (HM)
Yohji (HM)

FOUGÈRE - FRESH
Aspen (HM)
Cerruti Image (HM)
Cool Water (HM)
Kipling (HM)
Lauder (HM)
Navigator (HM)
Tsar (HM)

FOUGÈRE - AMBERY
Brut (HM)

FOUGÈRE - SPICY
Old Spice

MARINE
Erolfa
L'Eau d'Issey (HM)

HM: See Honorable Mentions
* Limited edition or discontinued. Some stock may remain available for a period of time.
♀♂: Unisex or shared fragrances.

COMMONLY USED INGREDIENTS IN PERFUMERY

For ingredients not listed, consult a dictionary or encyclopedia.

Aldehydes - Organic chemicals derived from natural or synthetic materials. Aldehydes add a vivid, quick quality to top notes. Variations can be powdery, fruity, green, citrusy, floral or woody.

Amber - A fossil resin from the fir tree. Prized for its tenacity, it also adds warm, leathery, powdery elements to a composition. The color amber refers to the color of the resin.

Ambergris - Secretion from the male sperm whale, often found floating in the ocean. The Chinese once used it as an aphrodisiac. Ambergris imparts a woody, balsamic odor. Substitutes are used more often today, because the natural substance is difficult to obtain.

Ambrette Seed - These plant seeds yield a musky floral, brandy-type aroma.

Anjelica - Oil from the root of the angelica tree, which is cultivated in France, Belgium, and Germany. It is musky and peppery, with a spicy green quality.

Balsam - Tree resins that exhibit a warm, sweet element. They are generally used as a base fixative.

Basil - A spicy herb with a green impression.

Bay Leaf - A tree leaf valued for its spicy, warm, almost bitter scent.

Bayberry - A shrub with berries, from which a waxy substance is taken. Bayberry adds a spicy, woody flair to fragrance.

Benzoin - Balsamic resin from the tropical styrax tree, used as a fixative, imparting a sweet, cocoa-like quality. Benzoin is found in Thailand, Vietnam, and Laos.

Bergamot - Oil produced from the peel of the bergamot fruit. The inedible fruit is of the citrus family and is about the size of an orange. The largest bergamot production comes from Calabria, Italy. The fresh, citrus essence is ideal in top notes and eau de cologne.

Black Currant Bud - (see Cassis)

Boronia - Essence taken from the flower of the boronia bush, which is mainly found in Australia. Often used in chypre blends, it leaves a spicy-rosy impression.

Broom - This produces a sweet, grassy odor. It is derived from the blossoms of the Mediterranean-area Spanish broom shrub.
Buchu - Substance from the leaves of the buchu herb. It yields a strong minty, camphor odor.

Bulgarian Rose - A highly valued flower in perfumery, grown Bulgaria's Valley of the Roses at the base of the Balkan mountain range, where a Turkish merchant began cultivation centuries ago.

Cardamom - Oil distilled from the cardamom plant, a member of the ginger family. It leaves a spicy floral impression. It is second only to saffron as the world's most expensive spice. In India, cardamom grains are chewed to freshen the breath.

Carnation - This flower gives off a spicy, sensual aroma.

Cassia Oil - Obtained from the leaves of an evergreen tree, valued for its spicy cinnamon-like quality. The oil is also used in cola drinks.

Cassie - Derived from the Acacia farnesiana bush, the cassie absolute produces a spicy floral flavor.

Cassis - Oil taken from the bud of the black currant fruit, which is also used in liqueur.

Castoreum - A secretion from the beaver that exudes a leathery quality and is used as a fixative.

Cedarwood - Oil obtained from the juniper cedar tree, which is native to Texas. An excellent fixative, it has a distinct wood tone.

Chamomile - A sweet, herbal odor with fruity notes, often used to balance floral compositions.

Cinnamon - Oil obtained from the bark and leaves of the cinnamomum tree, which is native to Southeast Asia and the East Indies. It imparts a familiar warm, sweet, spicy odor.

Civet - A glandular secretion from the civet cat, used as a fixative. Repugnant by itself, civet blends well and adds a warm, leathery, erotic tone to a composition.

Clary Sage - An herb valued for its sweet, subtle quality.

Clove - Obtained from the clove tree, clove buds are prized for their spicy sweetness. The tree is cultivated in Sri Lanka, Madagascar, and Indonesia.

Coriander - Oil from the coriander herb of the parsley family, valued for its spicy aromatic impression.

Costus - Essence from the root of the costus plant of the daisy family, lends warmth to Oriental blends. It has green, violet-like accents.

Coumarin - Obtained from the tonka bean and often created synthetically, produces a sweet, herbal, spicy, hay-like odor, similar to vanilla.

Cyclamen - Essence taken from the heart-shaped flowers of the primrose family.

Eucalyptus - Oil from the leaves of the eucalyptus tree, leaves a strong herbal, camphor impression. Discovered in Tasmania, it is widely cultivated in Spain, Portugal, and Australia and is well priced.

Frangipani - Oil from the sweet, jasmine-like flowers of the frangipani tree.

Frankincense (see Olibanum)

Galbanum - A gum resin valued for its leafy green, soft balsamic odor. Galbanum is used in many fragrances to provide a pleasing freshness, or green lift.

Gardenia - A heady white flower with a strong sweet scent.

Geranium - Oil made from the leaves and stems of the plant. Depending on the variety, it gives off a rosy, minty or fruity essence often used in rosy or spicy compositions.

Ginger - A woody, warm, spicy odor derived from the ginger plant.

Gums - Resins or balsams secreted from plants. Exhibiting a sweet tenacious odor, they are often used as fixatives.

Heliotropin - An aldehyde with a floral almond tone, found in pepper oil.

Honeysuckle - A highly fragrant vine flower but difficult to capture correctly. The essence of honeysuckle is usually re-created by blending a variety of florals.

Hyacinth - A sweet floral that imparts a green impression.

Incense - Made from gums and resins, produces a spicy aroma when burned.

Jasmine - Called the king of flowers, a sweet tiny white flower with a vibrant, smooth aroma. Jasmine is one of the most prized essences in the perfumer's palette. It is grown in France, Morocco, India, Egypt, and Spain and must be harvested before sunrise to retain the full amount of its delicate fragrance.

Jonquil - Highly fragrant essence derived from a flower of the narcissus family, rare because it is difficult to distill.

Labdanum - A dark resin obtained from the rockrose herb, valued for its leathery odor.

Lavender - From the flowering tops of lavender plants in France, Spain, Morocco, and old Yugoslavia, a sweet, light essence with woody floral accents. The oil is used in lavender waters, chypres, fougères, and florals. Lavender water is said to have been a favorite of Madame de Pompadour, mistress of Louis XV.

Leather - A smoky, sweet, animal odor crafted from the perfumer's palette. It is warm and persistent.

Lemon - Oil from the lemon rind. It is a zesty, sharp, refreshing essence, and is added to brighten many compositions, particularly eau de cologne.

Lilac - Since the essence released by the lilac plant and flower does not accurately portray its aroma, the perfumer re-creates the essence by using jasmine, ylang-ylang, neroli, and vanilla.

Lily of the Valley - Also known as muguet, lily of the valley is invented by the perfumer, using jasmine, orange blossom, rose, ylang-ylang, and chemical additives. The sweet essence is difficult to obtain from the natural flower.

Magnolia - A sweet, highly fragrant flower, also stubborn in releasing its essence. The perfumer re-creates the essence by blending rose, jasmine, neroli, and ylang-ylang with aroma chemicals.

Mandarin - Oil from the peel of the mandarin orange fruit, a brisk, sweet essence often used in eau de cologne.

May Rose - Also called rose de mai. The May rose from Morocco produces a rich, long-lasting oil prized for its full-bodied, diffusive qualities.

Mimosa - A green floral essence obtained from mimosa tree flowers and stems. It imparts a smooth, sweet aroma.

Moss - Earthy essences are derived from a variety of mosses: oakmoss, treemoss, lichen, seaweed, and algae.

Muguet (see Lily of the Valley)

Musk - A glandular secretion from the male musk deer of Tibet, China, and Nepal, used as a fixative in fine perfumes. It is valued for its woody, animal, erotic impressions, though nowadays it is often created chemically by the perfumer. Soft, sensuous, pervasive.

Narcissus - A highly fragrant yellow and white flower that produces an intense spicy, earthy, and sweet straw-like odor. Small amounts are often used to round off floral compositions. Native to Persia, the narcissus flower was carried to China over the silk route in the eighth century.

Neroli - Made from the orange blossoms of the bitter orange tree grown in France, Egypt, Algeria, and Morocco. It is light, sweet, and spicy and is used in top notes and eau de cologne. It was named for the Duchess of Nerola and was often used to scent gloves.

Nutmeg - Spicy oil derived from the seeds of the South Asian nutmeg tree.

Oakmoss - A lichen grown on oak trees. Its odor is earthy, woody, and slightly leathery. It is used as a fixative in many blends, especially chypre.

Olibanum - Also called frankincense. Olibanum is a gum resin from a tree found in Africa and Saudia Arabia. An outstanding fixative, its odor is spicy and balsamic, similar to that of incense.

Opopanax - Derived from a gum resin and similar to myrrh. A woody, sweet fixative.

Orange Blossom - From the white blossoms of the bitter orange tree. It adds a warm, spicy flavor that is often used in floral compositions.

Orange Oil - Produced from the peel of the orange, and often used in eau de cologne and floral fragrances. Refreshing, sweet, fruity, and crisp.

Orris - One of the most expensive ingredients used in perfumery. It is obtained from the iris plant, which is commonly cultivated in Italy. Its odor is violet-like and can be warm, sweet, woody, fruity or floral, depending on the quality.

Osmanthus - Produced from the flowers of the osmanthus tree, which is found in Japan, China, and Southeast Asia. It has a floral odor, with a hint of plum and raisin.

Patchouli - Oil obtained from the leaves of the patchouli plant, a superb fixative. Discovered in India, it is also cultivated in Malaysia and Indonesia. Its odor is earthy, dry, woody, and spicy. Patchouli is often used in Oriental and chypre blends.

Petitgrain - Essence derived from the leaves and stems of the bitter orange tree. It has a subtle woody tone similar to neroli. Sweet and floral, petitgrain adds freshness to a fragrance, especially eau de cologne.

Resin - Gum secretions from trees and plants, often used as fixatives.

Rose - Rose oil is also referred to as "otto" or "attar" of rose; these terms refer to perfume oil produced through distillation. There is a wide variety of roses, and the rich oil they produce has the familiar rose aroma, though undertones vary from honey to fruity, spicy to musk, and violet to green. Called the queen of flowers, it is one of the most precious ingredients in perfumery. Roses bloom just thirty days of the year and must be picked quickly, for they lose half their essence by noon. Centifolia and Damascena are popularly cultivated roses. The floral essence is used in rose water, chypre, and Oriental compositions. Rose water was said to have been a favorite of Marie Antoinette.

Rose de Mai (see May Rose)

Rosemary - Flowers and leaves of the evergreen rosemary herb of the mint family, distilled for use in perfumery. The oil produces an herbal note that is woody and slightly lavender-like.

Rosewood Oil - Oil obtained from the wood of the rosewood tree, the aniba rosaeodora of the laurel family. It gives off a rosy odor, sweet and subtly spicy. Rosewood is often added to eau de cologne.

Sage - A fresh, spicy odor from the sage herb.

Sandalwood - Oil from the sandalwood tree, the evergreen santalum album grown in India, Australia, and Southeast Asia, though the Indian province of Mysore supplies 85% of all sandalwood. The wood is valued for its aroma and its imperviousness to termites. The trees must mature at least thirty years for the oil to fully develop. An expensive ingredient, sandalwood oil is prized for its fixative quality. Its odor is powdery, balsamic, woody, and rich. Sandalwood gives a smooth finish to Oriental, chypre, and floral perfumes.

Styrax - A sweet balsam found on the styrax tree, an excellent fixative.

Sweet Pea - A flower oil produced from the fragrant flowering vine, valued for it light, delicate nature.

Tagetes - Essence produced from the tagetes flower, which is grown in Spain, Italy, and South Africa. The strong essence has an herbal, aromatic personality with fruity undertones.

Thyme - Derived from the flowering herb. Thyme smells sweet and herbaceous—ideal for eau de cologne.

Tonka Bean - Fragrant seeds from native South American trees of the Dipteryx family.

Tuberose - One of the most expensive oils, from a flower known for its rich, sensual aroma. Its cost is due in part to a painstaking processing called enfleurage, an oil extraction method whereby the flowers are pressed into fat, then the oil is separated with alcohol. Tuberose is a perennial plant native to Mexico. The sweet, honey-like aroma adds fullness to many floral fragrances and blends well with gardenia, jonquil, and hyacinth.

Vanilla - Made from the fruit and seeds of a climbing orchid vine. It has pods, or capsules encasing the beans. Vanilla is an impressive sweet fixative, used in many Oriental, amber, and floral perfumes.

Vanillin - Can be produced naturally from the vanilla pod, as well as certain balsams and benzoins. It can also be made synthetically. Its sweet, strong odor is similar to vanilla, but lacks the depth of vanilla. Vanillin blends well with vanilla to produce a round, full-bodied vanilla aroma.

Vetiver - A grass grown in Haiti, Réunion Island, Brazil, China, and Southeast Asia. It has a woody, earthy quality, enhanced by a moist balsamic accent. A superb fixative, vetiver is an important component in chypre blends.

Violet - The violet flower yields such a minute amount of oil that it is cost prohibitive to extract. Instead, the violet aroma is created chemically for use in perfumery.

Violet Leaf - Oil from the leaves of the violet plant, valued for its cucumbery green and peppery herbal aroma, with touches of violet and iris. Parma, Italy, is known for its violet production.

Ylang-Ylang - From Tagalog for "flower of flowers." This oil comes from the flower of ylang-ylang trees grown in Madagascar, Indonesia, Comoros, and the Philippines. The rich oil has a jasmine-like aroma and sweet balsamic accents. Used in many floral and Oriental compositions, ylang-ylang smooths and rounds bitter notes, adding warmth and grace.

BUYER'S GUIDE

Let your fingers do the walking! Most fragrances in this book are sold by department stores, independent perfumeries, duty-free shops, and Internet retailers. We've listed contact information for some boutique fragrances. For more information, try searching the Internet for a retailer or for the company's own web site.

(Note: All North American telephone numbers.)

Anné Pliska - (714) 532-3361
Antonia's Flowers - (516) 324-7109 or (800) 332-5558
Bijan Beverly Hills - (800) 992-4526
Creed - Neiman Marcus, Daniel Foxx,
   www.ashford.com, (877) CREED-NY
Guerlain Boutique By Mail - (800) 882-8820
Holzman & Stephanie Perfumes - (847) 234-7667,
   www.holzmansteffi-perfumes.com
Jean Patou Classics - www.ashford.com
Jo Malone - Bergdorf Goodman
Marilyn Miglin - (312) 943-1120
Perfumes Isabell - (800) 472-2355
Penhaligon's - (877) 736-4254, Saks Fifth Avenue in
   New York
William Owen - (561) 833-4076,
   www.williamowenfragrances.com

INTERNET RETAILERS:

www.ashford.com (jasmin.com)
www.drugstore.com
www.eve.com
www.fabulousfragrances.com
www.fragrancenet.com
www.gloss.com
www.hsn.com
www.macys.com
www.neimanmarcus.com
www.nordstrom.com

www.perfumania.com
www.qvc.com
www.saksfifthavenue.com
www.sephora.com

SEARCH THE INTERNET:

There are many good search engines; we've listed a few below. Remember to enclose the fragrance name or the company name in quotation marks for a more efficient search.

www.altavista.com
www.google.com
www.goto.com
www.lycos.com
www.msn.com
www.yahoo.com

For fragrance education and industry information, visit the following sites:

www.ctfa.org	*Cosmetic, Toiletry, and Fragrance Association*
www.fitnyc.edu	*Fashion Institute of Technology*
www.fragrance.org	*The Fragrance Foundation*

For more books and information on fragrances, or to join our mailing list, visit our web site at:

www.fabulousfragrances.com

BIBLIOGRAPHY AND SOURCES

"The Effect of Fragrance on the Mood of a Woman at Midlife," "Mood Benefits of Fragrance." *Aroma-Chology Review*, Vol. II, No. 1.

Beauty Fashion. January 1991 through May 2000.

Booth, Nancy. *Perfumes, Splashes & Colognes*. Pownal, Vermont: Storey Communications, 1997.

Booth, Nancy. *Scentsations*. Buckingham Impressions, 1998.

Bork, Karl-Heinz; Elke Doerrier; Arturetto Landi; Egon Oelkers; Peter Woerner; Lothar Kuemper. *Fragrance Guide: Feminine Notes, Masculine Notes*. Hamburg, Germany: Glöss Verlag, 1991.

Science & Technology. "No One's Sniffing at Aroma Research Now." *Business Week*, December 23, 1991, 82.

Chanel, Inc. *Chanel Fragrances*. New York: Chanel, Inc., 1991.

"How to Buy a Fragrance." *Consumer Reports*, December 1993, 765-773.

"All Passion Scent." *Country Living*.

"The Raison d'être of the Fragrance Foundation: Past, Present and Future." *Dragoco Report*, January 1991, 3-9.

Edwards, Michael. *The Fragrance Adviser*. Sydney: Distributed in USA by Crescent House Publishing, 1999.

Edwards, Michael. *Fragrances of the World 2000*. Sydney: Distributed in USA by Crescent House Publishing, 2000.

Edwards, Michael. *Perfume Legends: Feminine French Fragrances*. Sydney: HM Éditions. Distributed in USA by Crescent House Publishing, 1996.

Etherington-Smith, Meredith. *Patou*. New York: St. Martin's, 1983.

Fischer-Rizzi, Susanne. *Complete Aromatherapy Handbook: Essential Oils for Radiant Health*. New York: Sterling Publishing, 1990.

The Fragrance Foundation. *The Facts and Fun of Fragrance*. New York: Fragrance Foundation, 1992.

The Fragrance Foundation. *The Fragrance Foundation Reference Guide 1999*. New York: Fragrance Foundation, 1999.

The Fragrance Foundation. *Fragrance and Olfactory Directory*. New York: Fragrance Foundation, 1981.

The Fragrance Foundation. *The History, the Mystery, the Enjoyment of Fragrance*. New York: Fragrance Foundation.

Gaborit, Jean-Yves. Perfumes: *The Essences and Their Bottles*. New York: Rizzoli, 1985.

Happi. June 1994 through May 2000.

Israel, Lee. *Estée Lauder: Beyond the Magic*. New York: MacMillan Publishing Co., 1985.

www.jasmin.com/www.ashford.com. Creed Galleries. 2000.

Kaufman, William. *Perfume*. New York: E.P. Dutton & Co., 1974.

"History of an Ancient Art," "Lalique Parfums," "Recipe for a Fragrance." *Lalique Magazine*, Winter 1993, 4-11.

Lauder, Estée. *Estée: A Success Story*. New York: Random House, 1985.

Lawless, Julia. *The Encyclopedia of Essential Oils*. New York: Barnes & Noble Books, 1995.

"Scientists Say Aromas Have Major Effect on Emotions." *Los Angeles Times*, May 31, 1991, B3.

Monroe, Valerie. "How to Smell Really Wonderful." *McCall's*, September 1993, 140, 182.

"Scent System." *Mirabella*, October 1991, 142-143.

Morris, Edwin T. *Fragrance: The Story of Perfume from Cleopatra to Chanel*. New York: Charles Scribner's Sons, 1984.

Müller, Julia. *The H&R Book of Perfume*. Hamburg, Germany: Glöss Verlag, 1992

"The Intimate Sense." *National Geographic*, September 1986, 324-360.

"Discovery May Unlock Secret of Smell." *New York Times*, April 5, 1991, A1.

Newman, Cathy. *Perfume: The Art and Science of Scent*. National Geographic Society, 1998.

Ohrbach, Barbara Milo. *A Bouquet of Flowers: Sweet Thoughts, Recipes, and Gifts from the Garden with "The Language of Flowers."* New York: Clarkson N. Potter, Inc., 1990.

Olfactory Research Fund Ltd. *Living Well With Your Sense of Smell*. New York: Olfactory Research Fund Ltd., 1992.

Pavia, Fabienne. *The World of Perfume*. New York: Knickerbocker Press, 1996.

"Dollars and Scents." *Philadelphia Inquirer*, September 29, 1991, section J.

Pickles, Sheila. *The Language of Flowers*. New York: Harmony Books, 1989.

Scents & Style. November 1995 through December 1998.

"The Coming Age of Aroma-Chology." *Soap/Cosmetics/Chemical Specialties*, April 1991, 30-32.

Von Furstenberg, Diane. *Diane von Fürstenberg's Book of Beauty*. New York: Simon & Schuster, 1976.

Lab Notes. "Sniffing Heliotrope Helps MRI Patients Sit Still." *Wall Street Journal*, August 8, 1991.

"What the Nose Knows." *Washington Post*, July 26, 1992.

Women's Wear Daily. January 1994 through May 2000.

Green, Annette; Fragrance Foundation. Interviewed by author. October 1993.

Hayman, Gale; Gale Hayman Beverly Hills. Interviewed by author. October 1993.

Mosbacher, Georgette, and Paulsin, Lyn; Exclusives. Interviewed by author. October 1993

Nance, Bunni; Neiman Marcus. Interviewed by author. August 1993, October 1995.

Completed questionnaires, interviews, information, permissions, media kits and photography were supplied, in part or in total, by the following companies:

Adipar, Antonia's Flowers, Laura Ashley, Barclay Perfumes, Brandselite, Benetton Cosmetics, Bijan, Boucheron, Bulgari, Cassini Parfums, Caesars World Merchandising, Chanel, Liz Claiborne, Compar, Cosmair, Dionne Inc., Christian Dior, Erox, Escada, EuroCos, Marilyn Evins, Exclusives, Alice Fixx, The Fragrance Foundation, French Fragrances, Givenchy, Annick Goutal, Guerlain, Fred Hayman, Gale Hayman, Hermès Parfums, Jivago, Donna Karan Beauty Company, Key West Aloe, La Merveille Cie, Lancaster Group, Ralph Lauren Fragrances, L'Oréal, Parfums Lucien Lelong, Marina Maher, Marilyn Miglin, Jessica McClintock, Madeleine Mono, Georgette Mosbacher, Neiman Marcus, Niro, Nordstrom's, Olfactory Research Fund, William Owen, Parfums International, Parlux, Jean Patou, Perfumania, Prescriptives, Revlon, Riviera Concepts, Rochas, Chen Sam, Paul Sebastian, Tiffany, Ungaro, Vepro, Diane Von Furstenberg, and XEL.

To order more copies of *Fabulous Fragrances II* or to be placed on our mailing list, send postcard, call, fax or email. CRESCENT HOUSE PUBLISHING P.O. Box 718, La Quinta, CA 92253 • Tel: (310) 364-0551 • Fax: (760) 775-0501 Email: sales@fabulousfragrances.com

Additional copies of *Fabulous Fragrances II* are $29.95($U.S.) per copy, plus $4.50 shipping and handling. California residents add 7.75% sales tax. Visit our website at www.fabulousfragrances.com for ordering, fragrance news, and book excerpts. Join our Reader's Club!

To order more copies of *Fabulous Fragrances II* or to be placed on our mailing list, send postcard, call, fax or email. Visit our website at www.fabulousfragrances.com for ordering, fragrance news, and book excerpts. Join our Reader's Club!

NAME

COMPANY

ADDRESS

CITY/STATE/ZIP/COUNTRY

PHONE *(For questions on your order)*   EMAIL

Please send_____ (mark quantity) copies of *Fabulous Fragrances II* at $29.95 ($U.S.) $_____

Please send_____ (mark quantity) Purse Spray Fabulous by Jan Moran Eau de Parfum (Refillable) at $25 ($U.S.) $_____

Please send_____ (mark quantity) Basic 2-ounce Fabulous by Jan Moran Eau de Parfum Spray at $49 ($U.S.) $_____

Please send_____ (mark quantity) Grand Glamour 3.4-ounce Fabulous by Jan Moran Eau de Parfum Spray/Splash with Pouch at $95 ($U.S.) $_____

Please send_____ (mark quantity) copies of *Fragrances of the World* by Michael Edwards at $54.50 ($U.S.) $_____

Please send_____ (mark quantity) copies of *Perfume Legends: Feminine French Fragrances* by Michael Edwards at $120 ($U.S.) (Add additional $4.50 shipping–oversized.) $_____

California Residents add 7.75% sales tax $_____

Please add $4.50 shipping and handling for each item (Outside of U.S. $15, + $5 each additional item) $_____

TOTAL $_____

☐ Check or money order enclosed. Make check payable to: Crescent House Publishing.
CRESCENT HOUSE PUBLISHING P.O. Box 718, La Quinta, CA 92253 • Tel: (310) 364-0551 • Fax: (760) 775-0501
Email: sales@fabulousfragrances.com

☐ Visa/MasterCard/Amex Account # ☐☐☐☐☐☐☐☐☐☐☐☐☐☐☐☐

Expiration Date:_____ Signature:_____

☐ I'm not ordering now, but please put me on your mailing list.

To order more copies of *Fabulous Fragrances II* or to be placed on our mailing list, send postcard, call, fax or email. Visit our website at www.fabulousfragrances.com for ordering, fragrance news, and book excerpts. Join our Reader's Club!

NAME

COMPANY

ADDRESS

CITY/STATE/ZIP/COUNTRY

PHONE *(For questions on your order)*   EMAIL

Please send_____ (mark quantity) copies of *Fabulous Fragrances II* at $29.95 ($U.S.) $_____

Please send_____ (mark quantity) Purse Spray Fabulous by Jan Moran Eau de Parfum (Refillable) at $25 ($U.S.) $_____

Please send_____ (mark quantity) Basic 2-ounce Fabulous by Jan Moran Eau de Parfum Spray at $49 ($U.S.) $_____

Please send_____ (mark quantity) Grand Glamour 3.4-ounce Fabulous by Jan Moran Eau de Parfum Spray/Splash with Pouch at $95 ($U.S.) $_____

Please send_____ (mark quantity) copies of *Fragrances of the World* by Michael Edwards at $54.50 ($U.S.) $_____

Please send_____ (mark quantity) copies of *Perfume Legends: Feminine French Fragrances* by Michael Edwards at $120 ($U.S.) (Add additional $4.50 shipping–oversized.) $_____

California Residents add 7.75% sales tax $_____

Please add $4.50 shipping and handling for each item (Outside of U.S. $15, + $5 each additional item) $_____

TOTAL $_____

☐ Check or money order enclosed. Make check payable to: Crescent House Publishing.
CRESCENT HOUSE PUBLISHING P.O. Box 718, La Quinta, CA 92253 • Tel: (310) 364-0551 • Fax: (760) 775-0501
Email: sales@fabulousfragrances.com

☐ Visa/MasterCard/Amex Account # ☐☐☐☐☐☐☐☐☐☐☐☐☐☐☐☐

Expiration Date:_____ Signature:_____

☐ I'm not ordering now, but please put me on your mailing list.

CRESCENT HOUSE PUBLISHING
P.O. Box 718
La Quinta, CA 92253
USA

CRESCENT HOUSE PUBLISHING
P.O. Box 718
La Quinta, CA 92253
USA